THEATRE, TEENS, SEX ED

THEATRE, TEENS, SEX ED

Are We There Yet?

JAN SELMAN AND JANE HEATHER

With contributions from:
Shaniff Esmail, Brenda Munro, Tracy L. Bear, James McKinnon, and the Are We There Yet? Community-University Research Alliance

The University of Alberta Press

Published by
The University of Alberta Press
Ring House 2
Edmonton, Alberta, Canada T6G 2E1

www.uap.ualberta.ca

LIBRARY AND ARCHIVES CANADA
CATALOGUING IN PUBLICATION

Selman, Jan, author
Theatre, teens, sex ed : Are we there yet? / Jan Selman and Jane Heather; with contributions from: Shaniff Esmail, Brenda Munro, Tracy L. Bear, James McKinnon, and the Are We There Yet? Community-University Research Alliance.

Accompanied by DVD.
Includes bibliographical references and index.
Issued in print and electronic formats.
ISBN 978-1-77212-006-6 (pbk.).—
ISBN 978-1-77212-034-9 (pdf)

1. Sex instruction for teenagers. 2. Teenagers—Sexual behavior. 3. Participatory theater. 4. Drama in education. 5. Heather, Jane. Are we there yet. I. Heather, Jane, author II. Heather, Jane. Are we there yet? III. Title.

HQ35.S44 2014 306.70835 C2014-907167-1
C2014-907168-X

Index available in print and PDF editions.
First edition, first printing, 2015.

Printed and bound in Canada by *[name of printer]*.
Copyediting and proofreading by Joanne Muzak.
Indexing by Judy Dunlop.

The University of Alberta Press is committed to protecting our natural environment. As part of our efforts, this book is printed on Enviro Paper: it contains 100% post-consumer recycled fibres and is acid- and chlorine-free.

The University of Alberta Press gratefully acknowledges the support received for its publishing program from The Canada Council for the Arts. The University of Alberta Press also gratefully acknowledges the financial support of the Government of Canada through the Canada Book Fund (CBF) and the Government of Alberta through the Alberta Media Fund (AMF) for its publishing activities.

This book has been published with the help of a grant from the Canadian Federation for the Humanities and Social Sciences, through the Awards to Scholarly Publications Program, using funds provided by the Social Sciences and Humanities Research Council of Canada.

Canada

Canada Council for the Arts Conseil des Arts du Canada

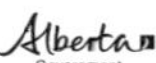

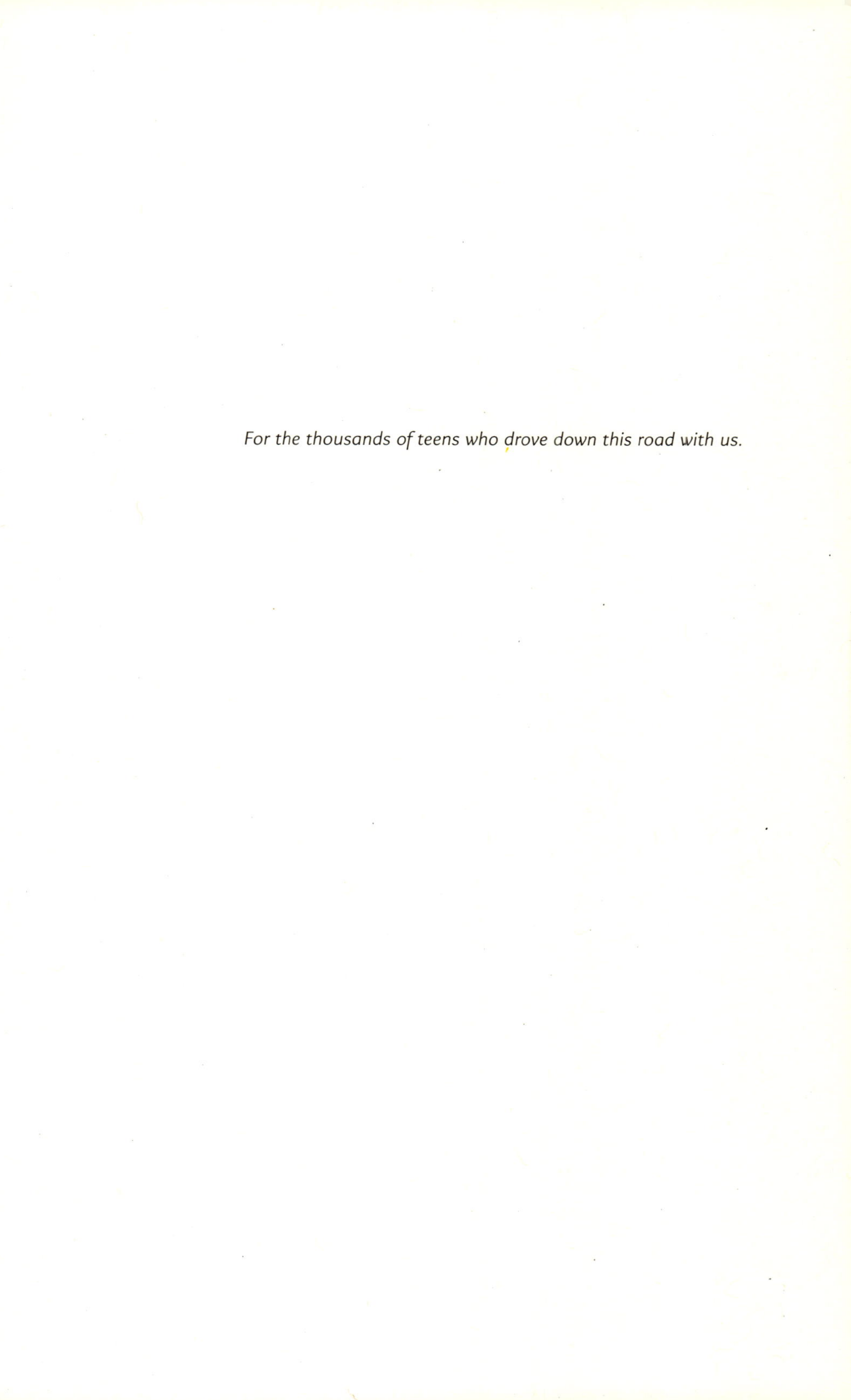

For the thousands of teens who drove down this road with us.

CONTENTS

PREFACE

CONTENTS

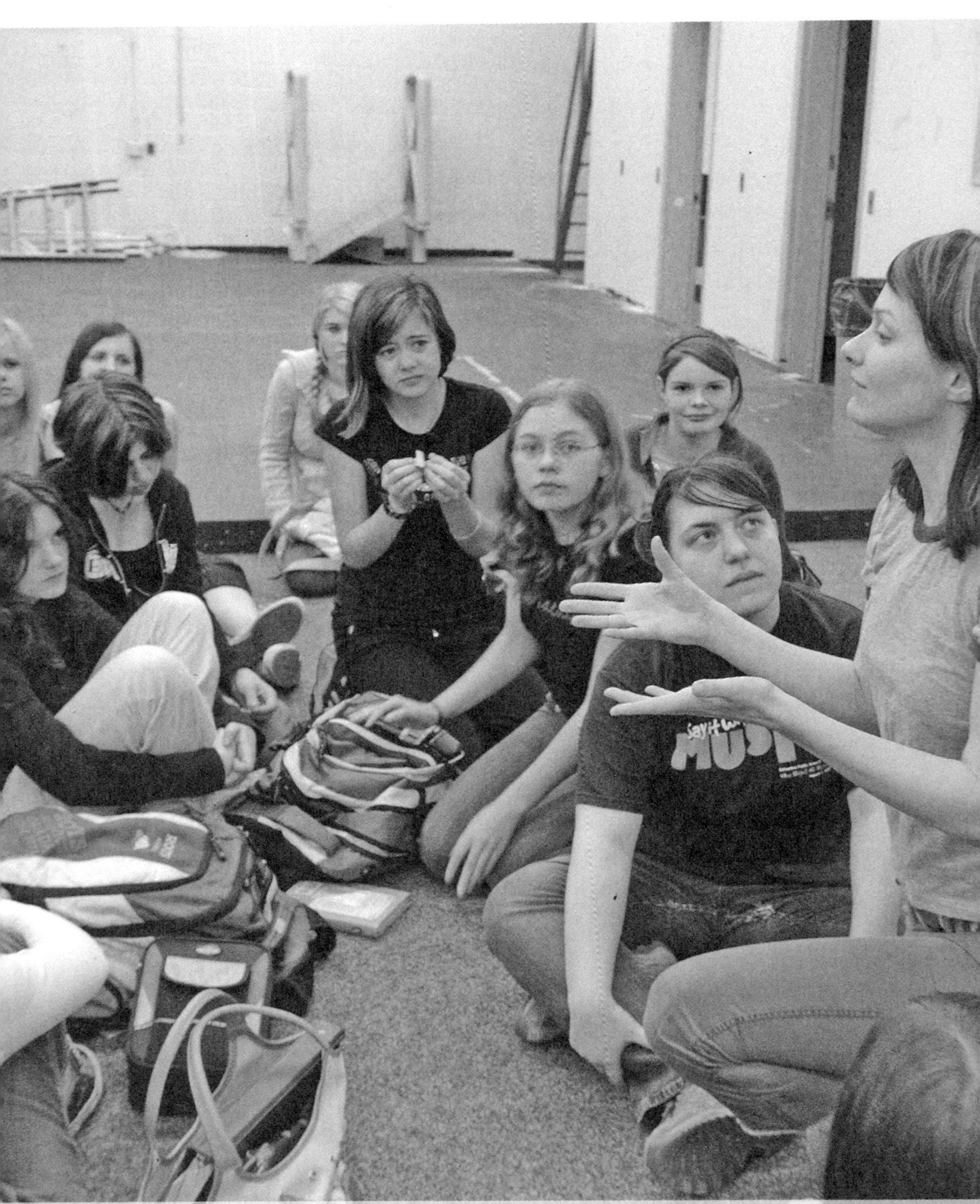

Kristi Hansen, Concrete Theatre. Photograph courtesy of Epic Photography.

ARE WE THERE YET? (AWTY) is an award-winning, participatory, sexuality education theatre program for teens. The interactive play and workshop are delivered to teens by a partnership of theatre artists and sexual health educators.

Two organizations in Edmonton, Canada—Concrete Theatre and Options Sexual Health Association (previously Planned Parenthood Association of Edmonton)—developed the project with playwright Jane Heather, and it has been offered annually to teens since 1998. In 2005, a national alliance of theatre artists, social science researchers, and sexual health educators received a major five-year research grant to assess the program and adapt it for other geographical and cultural settings. This opportunity led to extensions of the original project to new communities and new productions and adaptations of the play and workshop in disparate communities in Canada, including Aboriginal communities in Saskatoon and northern Saskatchewan, rural communities in Nova Scotia, many urban and rural areas in Alberta, and communities in Vancouver and Toronto. The Are We There Yet? Community-University Research Alliance (AWTY CURA) also developed assessment tools and conducted extensive qualitative and quantitative research, committed to determining and encouraging the most effective sex ed for teens.

Theatre of this kind (community-based, educative, social-change-focused) is a major global phenomenon. However, most of this work is short lived, and in-depth evaluation of its impact is rare. This book examines the field of transformative theatre, resting on the *AWTY* case study and the results of the associated and extensive interdisciplinary research project.

The need for effective sexuality education is extreme both in the Global North and the Global South. Educators, artists, and other adults seek effective, engaging programs that work. This book will be of value and interest to many kinds of readers including:

- Theatre practitioners
- Sexual health educators and organizations
- Teachers
- Professors of theatre, education, and social science
- Youth workers

- Peer educators
- Teens
- Other concerned adults and parents

How to Read this Book

Some readers will prefer to begin at the beginning and work their way through to the end. Some may start with the accompanying DVD, which focuses on participatory theatre techniques used in *Are We There Yet?* Others will prefer to read the section most applicable to their circumstances. Sexual health educators might, for example, turn to the chapters on the workshop or the theatre–sexual health partnership; theatre practitioners might first read the play; program assessors might first turn to the chapter on qualitative and quantitative research results. The book is a collection of many voices, and each contributes to different aspects of the project. Throughout, the book chapters are cross-referenced with others that expand on a particular point or provide additional information. We invite readers to dip into different parts of the book, led by their interest and curiosity.

The "Co-" in Co-Researcher, Co-Writer

Jan Selman and Jane Heather co-wrote this book, and some of our research partners contributed chapters. The research team influenced and informed each other all along the journey. Many other people's voices and experiences are represented here too (named or unnamed), including actors, directors, stage managers, teachers, sexual health educators, and thousands of teen audience members. All of these individuals were co-researchers on this project, but the words of the teen participants have been particularly important. Since the play was first produced in 1998, there have been approximately seven hundred performances in Alberta, Saskatchewan, Ontario, Nova Scotia, and British Columbia. We estimate that thirty-five thousand teens have participated in the play so far. What teen participants say, their insights, and how they describe their experiences, are front and centre in the book. Like most practitioners and researchers in this field, we endeavour to put the participants' experiences first. Quotes from teen audience members appear on almost every page and their candid, thoughtful, and often humorous remarks concretize everything else in the book. There are many kinds of research and researchers represented here, and each approach serves to illuminate the others. We hope that the interweaving of many voices, kinds of research, and perspectives captures the complexity, flexibility, and excitement of this kind of artistic and social intervention.

The *Are We There Yet?* DVD

A DVD accompanies this book. Using live performances of Concrete Theatre's 2010 production of *Are We There Yet?*, the DVD demonstrates participatory sequences and techniques for interacting with audiences. In addition, artists who have worked on Concrete Theatre's many productions, and Brian Parker from Options Sexual Health, who has an extensive history with the project, discuss values, methods, and approaches for this interactive play. The DVD is directed by Mieko Ouchi, who has also directed the play many times.

Acknowledgements

The authors acknowledge the contributions of all members of the Are We There Yet? Community-University Research Alliance. This includes research partners, artistic and administrative staff of theatre companies, and educators and other staff from health education organizations from across Canada. We also highlight some outstanding support by graduate students from several disciplines. Please see Appendix 5 for a list of the AWTY CURA partners and the AWTY website for a fuller list of participants: www.ualberta.ca/awty.

The AWTY CURA was funded by the Social Sciences and Humanities Research Council (SSHRC), as well as by contributions from each CURA member organization. The University of Alberta hosted the project, providing much support. Siân Williams's work was invaluable as the research project was developed, and three outstanding administrators of the CURA made it all possible: Kate Nunn, Anne Bailey, and Elizabeth Ludwig. The authors also thank Fern Swedlove and Joanne Muzak for their work copy editing various stages of this book.

The authors gratefully acknowledge the thousands of teens who participated in the play and workshops, met us in interviews and focus groups, filled in our questionnaires, and advised us as the project developed in each community.

All proceeds from this publication will go to Concrete Theatre Society, in recognition of the company's ongoing commitment to creating and producing meaningful theatre for youth.

part I

USING THEATRE TO MAKE CHANGE

Global Road Trip

THEATRE, COMMUNITY PARTICIPATION, CHANGE. Considerable activity around the world combines these three concepts. Theatre of this kind goes by many names: community theatre, community-based theatre, popular theatre, theatre for social change, theatre for development, applied theatre, drama-in-education, participatory theatre practice, theatre in health/education, transformative theatre, and more. From small street companies run on a shoestring to large well-established organizations with production budgets and payrolls, the variety and amount of this kind of theatre activity is extensive.

Views about potential values and roles of theatre are often polarized and, as Anthony Jackson (2007) points out, practitioners and critics tend to divide theatre broadly into two kinds: "first, high art that appeals to what is often described as our aesthetic sensibility, universal, timeless, free of that concern with current issues which usually renders the work before long hopelessly dated; and, secondly, the 'issue drama,' designed to raise questions, point a finger, change attitudes or even the world" (23). While we agree with Jackson that it is rare now for anyone to apply such a rigid binary to an analysis of kinds of theatre and that most would admit to some slippage between these categories, there continues to be a hierarchy of value applied to theatre based upon a division between art and instrument. This book focuses on useful theatre, theatre that is created to make a change in society. Further, it seeks to suggest ways that we can do so, ways that we can make the most of theatre's power. We argue that making the most of theatre involves first creating the best, most powerful theatre possible, and that pursuing this goal involves taking the performance and audience context into full account. Second, we suggest that artists and agents of change will have the most impact when they build strategic alliances with other agents of change. Finally, we report on and discuss a remarkable opportunity to test these assertions in-depth, while contributing to the problematic discussions about assessing and evaluating theatre's impact.

The postmodern project asks theatre artists and critics to challenge categories and dismantle hierarchies. Commentators such as Richard Schechner (2002), James Thompson (2006), and Anthony Jackson (2007) have begun to dismantle the either/or construct of "use or ornament"[1] and look at continuum, at blends and mash-ups of aesthetics and issues. We add our voices to this revisioning of theatre and its values. Schechner (2002, 23) identifies eight functions of performance: to entertain, make something beautiful, make or change identity, make or foster community, heal, teach, persuade or convince, and deal the with sacred and/or the demonic. While some think that theatre that foregrounds aesthetics accomplishes part of this list and that theatre for change fulfills another part, in fact theatre that seeks to be part of social transformation must be entertaining, beautiful, playful, and engaging—in addition to the other functions it plays—to be effective. Delight and education, art and instrument are entwined and dependent upon one another. Practitioners who use theatre for change understand this, and if they do not, their interventions will be largely ineffective.

Activist theatre work develops in a remarkably wide range of forms, styles, and processes. It is invented and reinvented everywhere. The following provides a small sample of some of the kinds of work being done in the world at the beginning of the twenty-first century.

> *Cardboard Citizens, London, England*

This company works with homeless adults and youth, using theatre to identify issues with homeless communities and educate people outside the community about homelessness. They also work in schools doing homelessness prevention. Much of their work is participatory and uses techniques developed by Augusto Boal. The company partners with many social service and education organizations and assists homeless people to access services. As they state on the "Who We Are" section of their website, "Cardboard Citizens change the lives of homeless and displaced people through theatre and performing arts" (2009).

> *Sistren Theatre Collective, Jamaica*

This company was established in 1977 to assist working-class and poor women in Jamaica to make social change using theatre. The company has performed a wide variety of work, from large musical spectacles that tour internationally, to community-based performances for and with youth, to short scenes that present women's points of view to governing bodies. Sistren is currently partnered with and funded by the United Nations Trust Fund in Support of Actions to Eliminate Violence against Women. The project is called *Tek It to Dem and Rise Up Wi Community 2008–2011*. On its website, the company states, "The central purpose and role of Sistren Theatre Collective is to provide consistent popular theatre that will reflect socio-economic issues as they relate to gender roles in an entertaining and educational atmosphere that influences society to change" (2013).

> *Women's Circus, Melbourne, Australia*

Created in 1991, Women's Circus teaches and performs circus-based pieces around women's lives and issues. Like Sistren, their work includes small intimate performances and large public spectacles. They introduce women of all ages and shapes to circus technique as a way to reclaim the body and create performances from their experiences. Women can take short courses or more intensive circus training. The company has a professional ensemble and several particularist groups, including youth, women suffering from eating disorders and personality disorders, and survivors of domestic and sexual abuse.[2] In the "About Us" section of their website, they state, "Women's Circus is a community arts company that presents innovative high quality circus performances and workshops to a diverse audience and participant base. The critical success of the Circus rests with our strong focus on creating a safe, supportive and stimulating environment in which participants can extend their skills, build confidence and have fun, and in presenting engaging, high quality public performances of social relevance" (2013).

> *Each One Reach One, San Mateo County, California*

This company works with incarcerated youth. The program includes one-on-one tutoring to assist the youth to complete a general education diploma and a one-on-one playwriting process. Professional playwrights are paired with youth and take them through a short, intense playwriting process. The plays are then given a staged reading by professional actors. The company uses a very specific playmaking process that focuses on metaphor. Youth write plays based upon their own lives and experience but are protected by metaphorical forms. This approach releases them from realism and allows them to come at stories and issues in a safe and theatrical way. The company also provides educational and employment opportunities and post-release links to community resources. "Each One Reach One diverts incarcerated youth from a life in prison to become productive community members through mentor-based performing arts and academic tutoring programs" (Each One Reach One 2013).

> *Roadside Theater, Kentucky, USA*

This is an Appalachian company located in rural Kentucky. Established in 1976, it works in its local community using storytelling, music, and theatre to celebrate the culture and history of the region and explore social and political issues raised by residents. They have long-term partnerships with several other ethno-drama companies, including Pergones Theater (a Puerto Rican company based in New York), an African American company, June Bug Productions, and Idiwanan An Chawe, a Zuni language theatre from the Pueblo of Zuni in New Mexico. Roadside Theater's process is based in story circles and incorporates the music, stories, and dance of the particular community they are collaborating with. The process is lengthy, and they commit to many years of development with each company or community group. They create and perform intercultural pieces, with both community and professional artists, and have many residencies with schools, universities, and communities. On their website, they describe themselves as "creating a body of drama based on the history and lives of Appalachian people and collaborating with others nationally who are dramatizing their local life. For Roadside, the purpose of theatre is to increase our understanding of ourselves and our empathy for others" (Roadside Theater 2013).

> *Budhan Theatre, India*

According to Safdar Hashmi, playwright, lyricist, actor, teacher, member of the Communist Party of India-Marxist, journalist, and founder of street theatre Jana Natya Manch, "if street theatre has any definite tradition in India, it is the anti-imperialist tradition of our people forged during the freedom movement. In other parts of the world it is the peoples' struggle for a just social and economic order" ("India Street Theatre" 2012).

Budhan Theatre is one such street theatre. The company was founded in 1998 and creates and performs street plays to examine issues faced by India's denotified tribes. These groups were declared "born criminal" by the British in 1911 and placed in forced labour camps. After independence, the Criminal Tribes Act was repealed and they were released. Poverty, discrimination, and high incarceration rates continue to oppress this community. Both adults and youth create and perform street plays about issues such as custodial death, abduction, beating, and torture of the Chhara and other tribal communities. The company states, "A population of some 60 million 'denotified tribes' can be found throughout India today. Since 1998, Budhan Theatre has performed street plays to raise awareness about the condition of such tribes. Their goal is to demonstrate that Chharas are not 'born criminals,' they are humans with real emotions, capacities, and aspirations" (Budhan Theatre 2013).

PEOPLE INVOLVED IN THIS WORK employ a very diverse range of creative processes, theatrical techniques, and approaches. However, a few central elements are generally held to be common to all: performance space, community participation, and the intention to make theatre that creates change.

The theatre work is often performed in unconventional or informal spaces. These companies' performance sites are often non-theatre venues such as schools, union halls, community centres, prisons, streets, public parks, hospitals, shelters, work places, or anywhere that has a particular connection or significance to a community.

The theatre performance and or the creation of the theatrical piece involves community members. This involvement might include participation during the creation process and/or during the performance itself. In the creation period, community members often contribute issues and stories. Sometimes this process is a theatrical investigation and sometimes it is based primarily in discussion, interview, or story sharing. In some cases, community members may act as consultants, collaborators, and/or writers in the creation of the script. Participating in the performance as an actor or shifting from spectator to active intervener—what Boal (1979) calls the "spect-actor"—during the performance is another way community members may be involved. Odd performance spaces and community involvement are usual for this branch of theatre, but it is the intention to make change that is the key defining element.[3]

NOTES

1. See Francois Matarasso's important study on the social impact of the arts, *Use or Ornament* (1997).
2. Schechner (1989, 4) uses the term *particularist*. He comments, "The second kind of casting and company making is particularist. Groups are formed according to gender or race or social class or disability or ideology or age."
3. See examples of such definitions in Burnham and Durland (1998), Kershaw (1992), Nelhaus and Haedicke (2001), Prendergast and Saxton (2009), Prentki and Selman (2000), and Thompson (2006).

1

GPS

Theatre to Make Change

CONTENTS

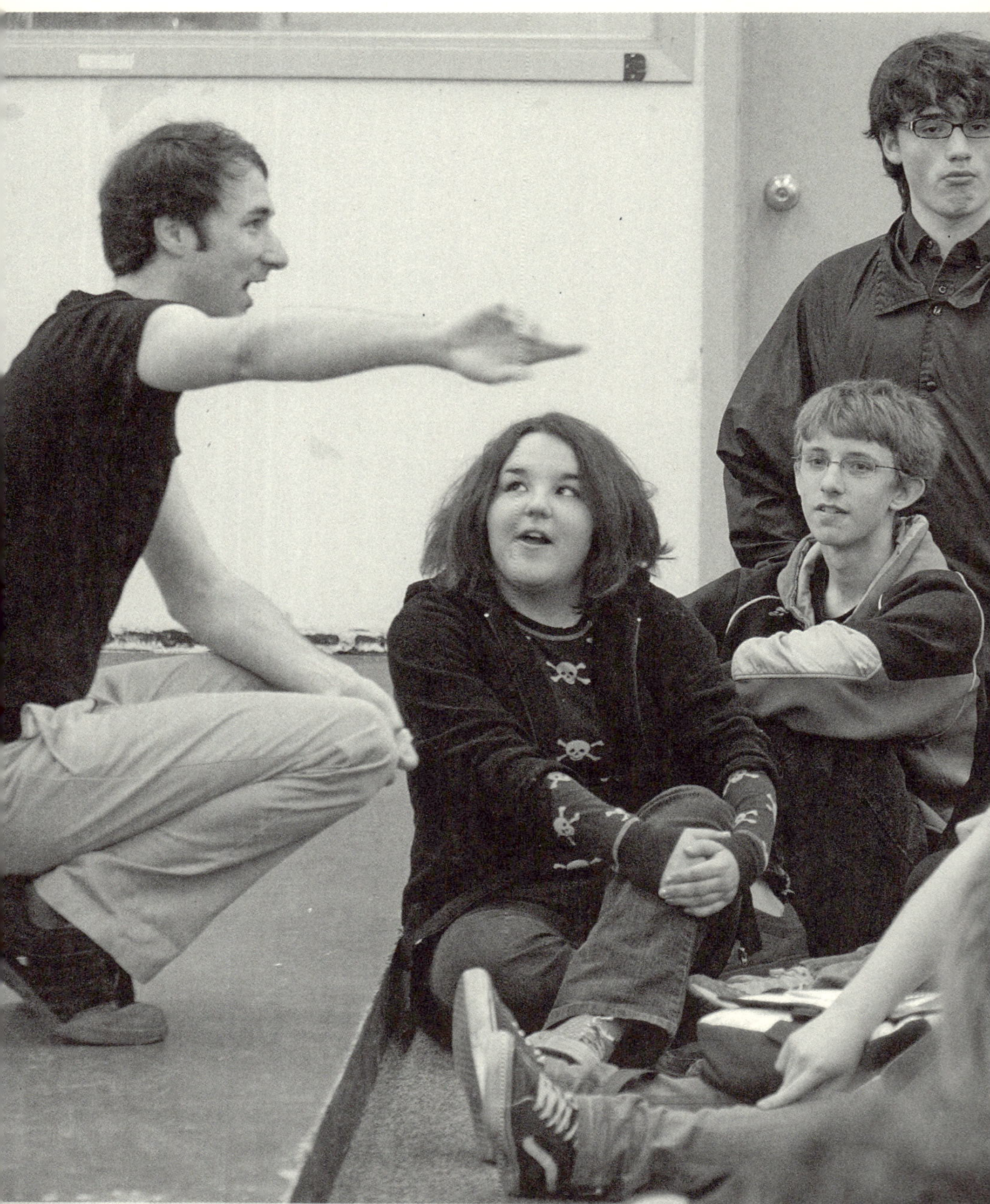

Jeremy Baumung and audience, Concrete Theatre. Photograph courtesy of Epic Photography.

Theatre for social change is created in response to a specific community context. The theatre is developed to reveal a community issue and contribute to change.

> *I like how they put it, how they made it, like, it was comfortable, they made a comparison with driving. We're comfortable with talking about driving so they tried to say, well think about it—talk about driving. So they made it [sex] comfortable to talk with before they even started talking about it.*
>
> —AUDIENCE MEMBER

THEATRE PRACTITIONERS who aim to make change via theatre maintain that engagement with the process and performance of theatre that is rooted in the issues, stories, and dreams of people who are underrepresented or underserved in mainstream theatre and society in general is part of a process of individual, social, and political change. Theatre, we assert, can be a means, mechanism, tool, and conduit for movement toward a more just world, but the degree of transformation is difficult to measure. Because theatre is performed live, it is never exactly the same from performance to performance, and it is ephemeral. Everyone who writes about the theatre struggles to convey what he or she saw to someone who did not. During a theatre event, spectators are bombarded with images, sounds, ideas, characters, and emotions. They are affected by everything on stage and everything going on in the audience and in themselves. Unless the theatre is truly awful, there can be no cool calibration of impact or change during the event. That an audience is engaged, that they "change" from bored to riveted or vocal, from skeptical to enthusiastic, from passive to active, can be seen and felt. After the event, describing and writing about what was seen and felt requires the deletion of all the languages and sensations that theatre uses to communicate. Only text is left—little soldiers marching across the page. The difference between how a human takes in theatre and the steady tread of printed text means the change that takes place for audience members is easier to see and sense than to write about. Nevertheless, these authors, and a number of others, try to do so.

Once change is on the table, there is a rash of questions. Change for whom? What kind of change? Why theatre? Why community-based theatre? How? How do you know it is working?

Change for Whom?

Widespread social and political analysis among community-based theatre practitioners suggests that those with the least power are in most need of a change toward justice. They argue that the change needed is not only internal but also external. Self-awareness, self-esteem, and healing are all possible personal and internal outcomes of a community-based theatre process and not to be sneered at. However, when a group moves beyond the personal to examine and challenge power structures and ideologies that negatively impact their lives and rights, the theatre they engage in tends to be oppositional. Although, as Prentki and Preston (2009, 13) point out, the tools and techniques of theatre for change can be used as well by the fascistically inclined, the work arises in most cases for, with, and by groups of people with little or less relative social and economic power. Indigenous populations, youth and children, the poor and working poor, women, the disabled, the elderly, immigrants, and cultural and racial minorities are all communities involved in theatre for change. Perhaps this is because these groups have a vested interest in change.

There is no doubt that the intentions and interests of a community in moving toward human development and change can be blocked or manipulated by granting bodies, sponsoring agencies, governments, and other power brokers. Further, well-intentioned theatre workers can make grave errors or misinterpretations of communities. There is no inherent, magical quality that provides immunity for theatre for change, and it is susceptible to all the same political machinations and power games as any other human endeavour. Taking action is always risky, as is stasis, and the values and politics of the choice to do something must always be weighed against the values and politics of doing nothing.

Why Theatre? Why Community-Based Theatre?

Some theatre artists (such as the authors of this book) seek (or stumble) upon a connection between what they know and understand about theatre and what they hope, long for, or discover about the world and its inequity. Artists who desire to expose the cost of war, the exploitation of humans by other humans, the vile ways that greed, mendacity, and solipsism devour the earth and the people on it, in short, the theatre artist who also considers him or herself an active citizen with agency, might write a play about the issue(s) that enrage or engage them most. Many fine and well-respected playwrights follow this path. They write often searing plays, performed in mainstream theatres, to mainstream theatregoers, but this experience can feel hollow. The artists have spoken their piece, presented their *cri de coeur* but it doesn't count for much. Theatre, in these circumstances, can seem like a good deal of effort for an insufficient change. Factors that can contribute to the sense of frustration include small audience numbers, many of whom agree with what's on stage, and no or little impact after the lights come up again.

Another kind of citizen might begin from an investment or membership in a particular community. Teachers, for example, human service workers, development workers, and others often begin with the same question: What can I do? A few proceed directly or indirectly to: What can theatre do? What is it about theatre that makes us think it has the capacity to effect positive social change? What kind of theatre is most likely to support and spark the change we want? And, who is the *we* in the previous sentence?

Books about theatre or drama normally devote some paragraphs to the pleasures of theatre, for audiences and participants. The immediacy, the ephemeral quality, the liveness, the courage of the performers, the ancient human ritual of being in a storytelling space together, are all part of the attraction of theatre. Anthropologist Victor Turner (1974) engaged with the concept of liminality and social drama to explore ritual and the process humans experience when they change from one state to another. Investigating the ritual structures and rules a culture employs to mark and shape significant changes, such as becoming an adult, he focused on the unstable state a person inhabits during the change—the threshold or liminal state. Turner argued that in the realm of liminality, "the possibility exists of standing aside not only from one's own social position but from all social positions and of formulating a potentially unlimited series of alternative social arrangements" (1974, 14). Schechner used these concepts to examine how theatre works and where we are when we watch or perform theatre:

> *A limen is a threshold or sill, a thin strip neither inside nor outside a building or room linking one space to another, a passageway between places rather than a place in itself. In ritual and aesthetic performances, the thin space of the limen is expanded into a wide space both actually and conceptually. What is usually just a "go between" becomes the site of the action. And yet this action remains, to use Turner's phrase, "betwixt and between." It is enlarged in time and space yet retains its peculiar quality*

> *of passageway or temporariness...An empty theatre space is liminal, open to all kinds of possibilities.* (2002, 58–61)

If all theatre is liminal, theatre for transformation, which often uses community stories, created in deep consultation with, and sometimes performed by community members, encourages and evokes some additional levels of liminality. Creators meld fiction and their sense of the truth, not to trick or create false authenticity, but for the possibilities that open up for audiences; fiction creates engagement and recognition but also the opportunity for anonymity.

Participation, which smudges or erases the border between stage and audience, also operates in a blended space, between observation and action. The disruption of the expected or normal makes the familiar strange—we look at it anew. This unbalancing, coupled with the betwixt and between nature of community-based theatre and participation, creates a little tear, a little shift, an opening where a new thought or question or a change might enter.

Community Participation in Process and Form

A commitment to using theatre to make change requires the invention and development of new forms of theatre and creation processes and the discarding and adaptation of old forms and processes. In this kind of work, the choice to use a particular process or form is driven by intention, an analysis of the issue(s) by the theatre practitioner and the groups and communities most impacted by the issue, as well as the artists' range of experience. Approaches are shared and traded and advanced, primarily through workshops and artistic collaborations. The literature is well behind the practice, but relevant publications are growing in number.

Ross Kidd, a Canadian adult educator and popular theatre organizer, contributed much to the field's conceptual understandings, critical capacities, and international cross-pollination through workshops, critical writing, and energetic dissemination. He promoted a basic analysis of action-based theatre work, suggesting that each project and planning process should examine the relative efficacy of creating theatre "for, with or by 'the people'" (Kidd 1979, 4). This formulation is useful in giving shape to the wide variety of theatrical forms and processes employed by people who seek to use theatre for change.

Theatre For

In the *for* category, the creation process will include community in some way, usually at the research and story gathering stage. Actors, directors, and playwrights engage community participants in determining the content of the play, and professional actors, students, or development workers perform the result. In some cases, Indigenous song, dance, or storytelling may be incorporated but the theatrical form often has much in common with more conventional theatre. Scotland's 7:84 Theatre Company and playwrights such as Sonja Linden of Iceandfire Theatre, a company that works with a variety of levels of participation, depending upon their project, approach the work in this way. Kidd (1979) critiques *theatre for* as not being sufficiently owned by the community, pointing out that this kind of work enables co-option and top-down decisions about what messages are good for people. *Theatre for* might be best if the intention is to bring the issues and concerns of a community to people outside that community.

Theatre With

Theatre *with* implies that community members create and perform with theatre practitioners or that audience members participate in the performance. The large number of theatre companies and groups around the world that use methods inspired by Boal's work fall into this category. Collaboration with a community (including participatory research and community members performing) might be used if uncovering issues and stories of that community is the focus. Participatory theatre is often chosen if an issue needs to be examined within a community. It is a strong choice of form when goals include working together on collective strategies and skill building to address an issue.

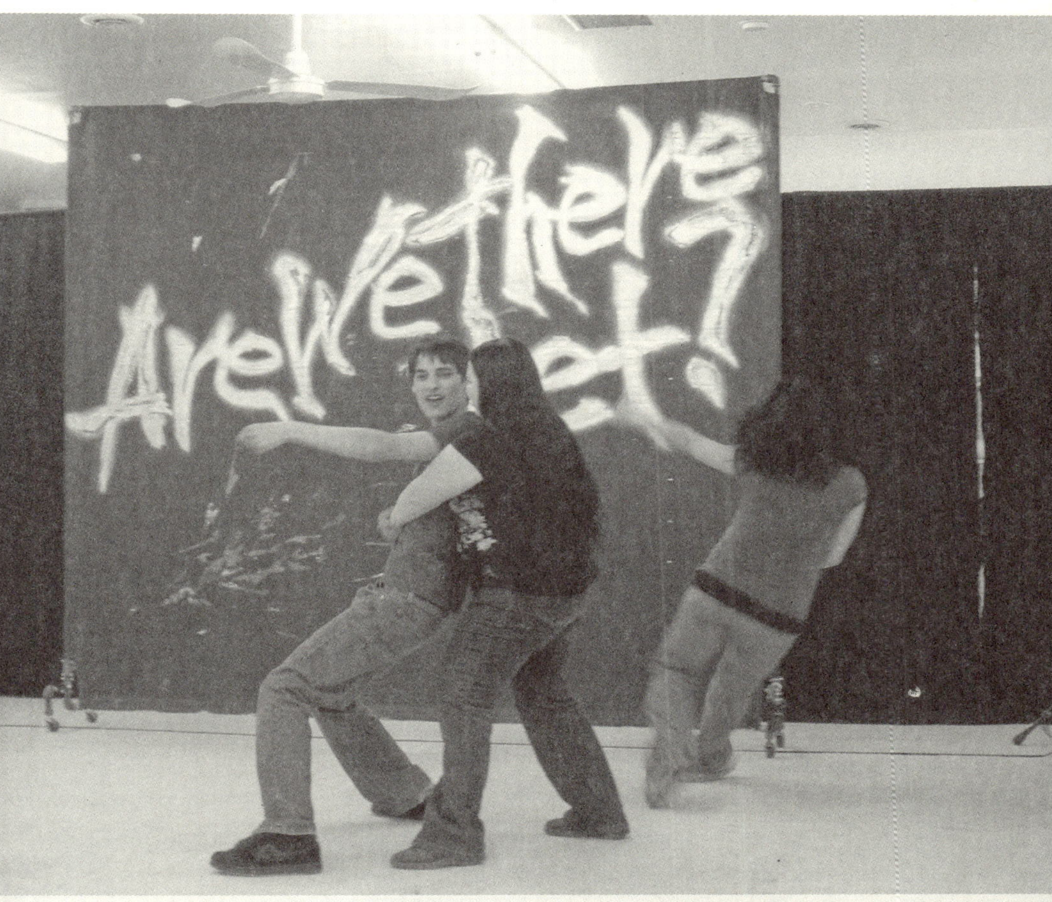

Clifford Cardinal, Jennifer Dawn Bishop, and Krystle Pederson, Saskatchewan Native Theatre Company. Photograph courtesy of Jane Heather.

Theatre By

In this case, community participants create and perform their own work about their own issues in a process usually facilitated by a theatre practitioner. Sometimes the work is issue-based, while at other times, a community seeks to celebrate its strengths and stories; of course, these functions overlap in most cases. This approach tends to be the most time-consuming and labour-intensive of the processes. Those who are directly involved in the creation and performance are the most impacted. Audiences are impacted as well but often to a lesser degree than the central participants. Examples of this approach include *My People's Blood*, a project about HIV prevention created with and by young adults in the northern Alberta Aboriginal community of Wabasca (Auger and Heather 2009); projects created by Marty Pottenger with Portland civic workers who performed their words in Art at Work (Korza, Shaffer-Bacon, and Assaf 2005); and the groundbreaking Kamiriithu Project in Kenya, led by Ngugi wa Mirii and Ngugi wa Thiong'o (Kidd 1983a; van Erven 2001).

The *Are We There Yet?* Example

Are We There Yet? is an example of *theatre with*. It is part of a global movement of theatre that is performed in non-formal theatre spaces using participatory theatre techniques "in the service of self development, well being and social change" (Prentki and Preston, 2009 14). In 1998, Concrete Theatre in Edmonton approached Jane Heather to write a play about sex for fifteen- to eighteen-year-olds. Concrete Theatre had recently completed a participatory theatre project (*Decisions, Decisions* by Mieko Ouchi) for twelve- to fifteen-year-olds, sponsored and supported by several human service agencies. One of those agencies, Planned Parenthood of Edmonton (now Options Sexual Health), was interested in continuing a partnership with a theatre company and developing a participatory theatre event for youth about sexual decision making and sexual health. *Are We There Yet?* is the result. It was performed annually in Alberta every year from 1998 to 2013, as well as across Canada, winning awards in Edmonton and Vancouver. The Are We There Yet? Program (AWTY Program), consisting of a participatory play (*AWTY*) and an interactive follow-up workshop, is delivered to teens in school settings by a partnership of theatre artists and sexual health educators. Its intention is to help young people make better, healthier decisions about sex.

In 2005, a national alliance of theatre artists, social science researchers, and sexual health educators, led by Jan Selman, received a major five-year research grant to assess the program and adapt it for other geographical and cultural settings. The research program, Are We There Yet? Using Theatre to

Address Teen Sexuality, was funded by the Community-University Research Alliance (CURA) program of Canada's Social Science and Humanities Research Council (SSHRC). The grant made possible new productions and adaptations of the play and workshop in four different communities in Canada, extensive qualitative and quantitative research, and the formation of a large national, interdisciplinary coalition committed to finding the best, most effective sex ed for teens.[1]

AWTY and the AWTY Program came about because many people over a long time worked to discover how theatre can be used to achieve a measurable social and educational end. *AWTY* also came about because many people worked to create a playful, surprising, serious, interactive, emotionally and intellectually engaging and entertaining piece of art. When best practice is sought, a careful balance between the aesthetic and the social is required.

Does It Work? How Can You Tell?

Despite the worldwide reach of this kind of theatre, it remains underreported, and assessment has been spotty. Anecdotal testimony from community participants, audiences, and theatre artists is quite common and often very moving. Some companies are able to assess and quantify ways in which the theatre has changed participants involved in their projects. Often, assessment has been linked to things that can easily be measured, such as numbers of participants. In some cases, theatre practitioners have returned to an area some years after the project or play to see what is remembered or if the work has had any long-term effect (Munier and Etherton 2006). There are a number of complex interrelated elements to consider when establishing proof that theatre works to make change. And there is pressure to do so. Funding for this kind of work and its integration into long-term education and development strategies are at stake. While the pressure to demonstrate efficacy is real, and such demonstrations are of value to artists, educators, and funders, the interplay of several kinds of change needs our attention.

The change may be an interior or personal one. We can only ask community participants what has happened to them and hear what they say. The experience of participating in a theatre event is often overwhelmingly positive. "It was fun, I liked it a lot, it was true, it was our story" are all common responses. Capturing a deeper response requires a lengthy interview and perhaps some reflection time for audiences, artists, and evaluators. These options may not be available to artists or assessors. Even with these conditions and tools, the experience and effect of creating, performing, or watching theatre are often subconscious or not readily articulated.

The theatre sits in a web of other social, economic, historical, and interpersonal influences and connections. Isolating the impact of a theatre component on a change is almost impossible. The change may have a long fuse—audience/participants may not see or feel the effects until long after they have dispersed and the project is complete. Longitudinal data is often particularly difficult to collect as audiences disperse. Keeping track of and re-interviewing audience members over a period of years could strengthen and deepen the evidence of lasting change; however, the logistics, infrastructure, and funding required for such a study are not readily available.

This book uses the AWTY Program and the research and evaluation project that surrounded it to examine questions about best practice in theatre that seeks to be transformative. It examines the use of theatre within education projects, focusing particularly on the pressing need for determining best practice in sexuality education for teens. The book reports on the team's pursuit of in-depth program evaluation and research. It also includes advice for others who might consider producing *AWTY* or a project like it. Just as no one play can cover all aspects of sex and sexuality for teens, no book could possibly cover all the ways theatre can be used to make change or all ways we might evaluate and assess theatre programs. It is our hope, however, that this book will encourage others to use theatre strategically and powerfully as they develop their thinking and practice of theatre and change.

It helped me put my thoughts and feelings to words—like they were always there but I never really thought of it.

—Audience member

NOTE

1. For a complete list of partner organizations, artists, and researchers, see Appendix 5.

2

INTERNAL COMBUSTION

Sexual Health Education: Urgency and Strategies for Change

Shaniff Esmail, James McKinnon, and Brenda Munro

CONTENTS

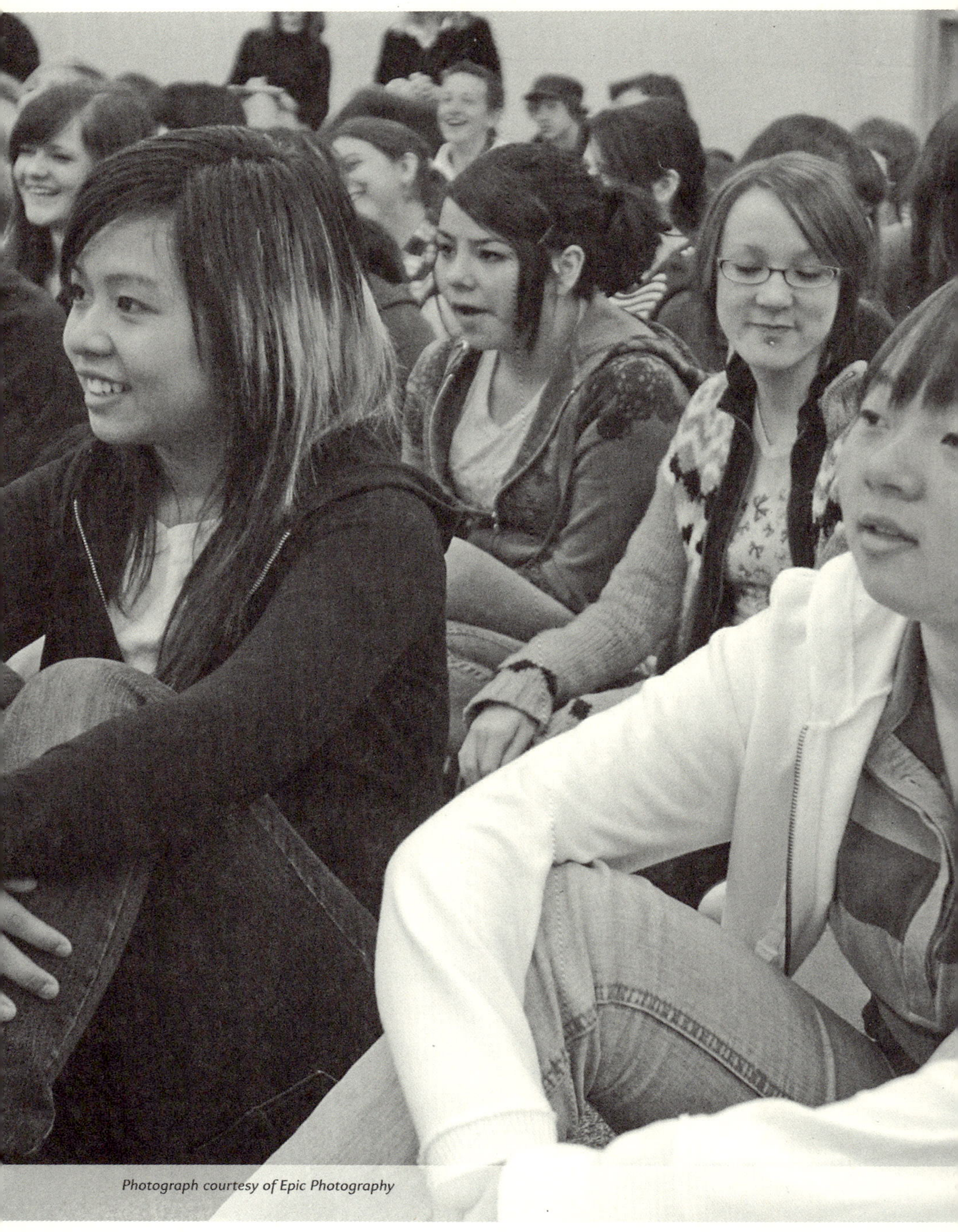

Photograph courtesy of Epic Photography

The AWTY project was created in response to ongoing pressing needs for effective sexuality education for teens. This chapter sets the context from which the work emerged—a context of urgency and an evolving understanding about sexuality education.

> *Well I didn't really pick anything out because I already knew a lot, but...I wasn't 100 per cent sure about when you're using birth control...I didn't know you actually had to use the condoms to stop like diseases, like a 100 per cent. I wasn't sure if you were taking birth control pills if that would be good enough.*
>
> —AUDIENCE MEMBER

ALTHOUGH SEXUALITY EDUCATION has been part of the public education mandate in Canada (and elsewhere) since the 1970s, educators have struggled with making it effective. Research shows that adolescents are having sex younger than ever and with more partners, aggravating the risks of negative outcomes such as sexually transmitted infection (STI), unwanted pregnancy, and negative or traumatic sexual misadventures, all of which can have painful, permanent, and even deadly consequences (Gavin et al. 2010).

With particular reference to *Are We There Yet?* this chapter builds a case for participatory theatre as an effective method for teaching sexuality education. The chapter outlines the problem of inadequate sex ed and its urgency, noting where past approaches have failed. We provide an overview of current theories on effective approaches to teaching human sexuality and demonstrate how participatory theatre techniques meet the criteria for an effective sexuality education program that does not merely transmit information but actually stimulates positive behavioural changes.[1]

A Global Concern

Since the 1980s, health and social issues related to sexual behaviour have become an important topic for professionals and academics in education, public health, and other fields (Gullotta et al. 1999). The sexual behaviour of young people is a particularly urgent matter in Canada and worldwide. In spite of the fact that sexual education has been widely taught in Canadian schools for many years now, the sexual behaviour of Canadian adolescents is as risky as ever (Gavin et al. 2010). Although the majority of teens in North America have knowledge and values consistent with responsible sexual conduct, many are unable to translate these values into positive behaviours (Zabin et al. 1984; Christopher and Cate 1984; McCabe and Killackey 2004). Research shows that adolescents are now far more likely to engage in sex before they finish high school than they were in the 1980s: approximately 25 per cent of Canadians will have had sexual intercourse by the age of sixteen (McKay 2000), with the majority of young Canadians initiating sexual intercourse between sixteen and nineteen years of age (Maticka-Tyndale 1997;

see Crockett, Raffaelli, and Moilanen 2003; Gavin et al. 2010; and Miller et al. 2003 for reviews).

In addition, teens are engaging in sexual activities with multiple partners and are not using condoms (Moore, Manlove, and Glei 1998; Wellings et al. 1998; Gavin et al. 2010). In 1996, the Canadian National Population Health Survey found that 29.4 per cent of males and 21 per cent of females aged fifteen to nineteen had had more than one sexual partner in the previous twelve months (Maticka-Tyndale 1997; Barrett and McKay 2000). According to the Canadian Association for Adolescent Health (2006), adolescents with multiple sexual partners appear to be compounding their risks, as they are more likely to: (1) have had sex for the first time before the age of thirteen, (2) not to have used a condom the last time, and (3) have consumed alcohol or drugs before having sex the last time (Kuortti and Kosunen 2009). As a result of such sexual behaviours, an increasing number of youth contract STIS and/or develop cancer, or experience early pregnancy and/or social and emotional problems (Gullotta and Adams 2006). Risky behaviours and practices are known to have long-term repercussions that affect both physical and mental health, and such practices and lifestyles have unknown effects on unfolding sexual identity and related self-regulations of impulses and desires. Thus, there is an urgent need for effective sexuality education, and the public health and education bodies, ranging from the World Health Organization (WHO) to the Population and Public Health Branch of the Canadian Government, recognize the importance of sexuality education as a preventative action (Health Canada 2003; WHO 2000).

In North America, there has been continuing debate about whether health initiatives should take place in the school system, a debate characterized by public clashes between parents, educators, politicians, and health care workers, which may itself constitute a barrier to effective sex education (Guttmacher Institute 2006). However, most educators, parents, students, and public health officials in North America are in general agreement that schools are an effective and appropriate location to provide youth with sexual health education. Schools already have a mandate to ensure that students gain the knowledge and skills needed to lead healthy, productive lives, and because sexuality is an important part of human identity and health, decisions relating to sex have lifelong consequences (Cairs, Collins, and Hiebert 1994; Health Canada 1994). In addition, both parents and adolescents overwhelmingly prefer sexual education to be taught in a formal setting: a study by Boyce et al. (2003), for example, found that 85 per cent of parents and 89 per cent of adolescents felt sexual health should be taught in schools. Therefore, several countries, including Canada and the United States, have adopted some form of formal sexuality education as part of their broader mandate, although parents are often allowed to choose whether to allow their children to participate in class discussions relating to sexuality and religion (Conn 2009).

So why has unsafe sexual behaviour in adolescents continued to climb, in spite of the widespread availability of sexual education and in spite of the fact that teens now report a generally high level of knowledge about the facts of human reproduction and the dangers of unsafe sex? How can we improve the strategies we use to teach sexual education in schools in order to achieve not only a high level of sexual health literacy, as it were, but also a reduction in dangerous sexual behaviour? To answer these urgent questions, we need to look more closely at the evolution of the goals and theories and methods of sexual education.

Evolution of Sexuality Education

Sexual education has gone through four generations of changes over the past two decades (Hubbard, Giese, and Rainey 1998), during which time both the objectives and the theories of educators have changed. Generally, sexual education has evolved from a relatively single-minded fixation on reducing teen pregnancy and sexually transmitted infections to a more comprehensive approach that seeks to promote positive outcomes as well as deter negative ones. Hubbard, Giese, and Rainey's (1998) survey sheds some light on how and why sexuality education has failed to achieve all the desired results.

The first generational approach emphasized knowledge about reproduction. The second, building on the first, added a values component with particular attention to decision-making and communication skills, based on the belief that if teens understood and implemented these skills, they would avoid risky behaviours. Although evaluations of these two approaches showed that student knowledge increased, the approaches did not appear to affect the behaviours that led to pregnancy and sexually transmitted diseases (Hubbard, Giese, and Rainey 1998); contemporary teenagers are well-aware of where babies come from and how to prevent the transmission of STIs, yet they still practice unsafe sex.

The third generation of sexual health programs was developed by opponents of the first two who "believed sexuality education should consist of a strong message that intercourse before marriage is dangerous and wrong" (Hubbard, Giese, and Rainey 1998). Hubbard, Giese, and Rainey's research indicates that this abstinence-only approach has had no demonstrated effect on the sexual behaviour of adolescents. As Mabray and Labauve (2002) point out, in their argument that an effective sexual education program facilitates teens' active involvement, the abstinence-only approach is ineffective because it does not allow teens to take ownership of their sexuality. Current literature indicates that, regardless of abstinence-only sex ed, many youth are sexually active in early adolescence, and while schools should not be expected to support these practices, they are responsible for protecting youth and minimizing the risks by providing proper education about safe sexual practices.

Finally, the fourth generation, theory-based approach that focused on prevention enhancement from a holistic and social perspective, known as Reducing the Risk, was developed by incorporating only those elements of previous approaches that demonstrated success. This approach, as elaborated by Hubbard, Giese, and Rainey (1998) includes six key elements: (1) a narrow focus on a small number of specific behavioural goals; (2) a foundation in social learning theory and social influence theories; (3) activities that personalize information on the risks of unprotected sex and how to avoid those risks; (4) training about social influences; (5) support for personal values and group norms against unprotected intercourse; and (6) exercises to develop skills. They also recommended training that emphasized these elements for persons delivering the program.

This approach proved more effective in reducing high-risk behaviours than the previous approaches. Results indicated that those who received the Reducing the Risk curriculum delayed initiating sexual intercourse, and that those who were already sexually active increased their use of contraceptives compared to the control group (Hubbard, Giese, and Rainey 1998, 243). Furthermore, in the Reducing the Risk group there was an increase in communication between students and their parents as compared to the control group. The fourth-generation approach to sexuality education, which stresses a comprehensive, multipronged approach to transmitting knowledge, skills, and behaviours, is the most promising method developed thus far.

A study by Langille et al. (2001) pursued similar questions from a different perspective by asking students themselves why they think sexual education isn't working. Their findings, like those cited above, demonstrate the importance of making the material personal and relevant to the students. The researchers interviewed young women in Nova Scotia about barriers to school-based sexual education and found evidence that collisions between pedagogical ideals and practical reality pose significant obstacles to effective sexuality education: sexual education fails either because of ineffective delivery methods or because the content remains too abstract and removed from actual lived experience. Langille et al. (2001, 253–55) identify four main concerns voiced by the participants: first, the lack of value placed upon sexual health education by schools; second, course material that is repetitive, uninspiring, and not personally relevant; third, a dissonance between what was taught in sexual health education and everyday experiences; and finally, concerns about confidentiality and loss of respect, as respondents expressed a need for a non-judgemental approach from the teacher. The participants also expressed concerns about a lack of depth exploring topics relating to sexual health, sexual practices, and sexual decision making. Langille et al. summarize the young women's views: "Methods of learning and testing were felt to be unrelated to the real world of sexual decision-making" (249). Student comments included, "some teachers will just skim through a part and not really go into what really [mattered]" and "a lot of things have been repeated. We don't really learn anything new" (249). Students also felt that topics were not covered or were purposefully avoided: "they never talked about sex itself [or] the consequences...They just kind of skipped over it" (249); "I was just worried that...if a teacher thinks I might be pregnant, does that mean they're going to change their opinion of me? Does that mean they're going to think less of me?" (253). The comments indicate that sexual education is teaching these students things they already know while some aspects of sexuality that are of most concern to teens are omitted. Thus, students who participated in the Langille et al. study are clear: they want a course that addresses real-life situations, not abstract theory. They wanted to know what effects the decisions they make will actually have.

To summarize, the aforementioned research all emphasizes that to be effective, sexual education courses must focus on teaching values, setting goals, and building interpersonal skills in an active and personalized way, and on empowering students and providing them with the necessary knowledge and confidence to make informed decisions. The question then becomes, how do we do this? How do we teach sexuality in ways that not only provide students with information, or even skills, but that actually induce safe, healthy, ethical sexual behaviour, since, as these studies indicate, simply admonishing unsafe and unethical behaviour does not work?

It should be noted—indeed emphasized—that content and attitudes are inseparable from methods of delivery. The earlier approaches to sexual health education failed not, or not only, because they focused on the wrong things but because they delivered their key messages in ways that were ineffective and often even incompatible with those messages; a program based on telling teenagers to sit passively and listen to lectures about how to be more assertive is inherently contradictory. Assertiveness entails skills and attitudes that require training and practice, so sexual health programs that encourage youth to take charge of their own sexual health will be more effective if they model the requisite skills. Students need hands-on opportunities to process what they learn and integrate it into their own behaviour. As such, sexual health programs need to consider alternative media and methods of delivery beyond the traditional rota of set lectures and educational films; they must become more interactive, both to be able to respond to the flexible needs of students and to provide examples of and opportunities to model the desired skills and behaviours.

The benefits of interactive and role-playing elements are confirmed in a study of the fourth-generation approach, conducted by Kvalem et al. (1996). Kvalem et al. based their program on cognitive and social learning theories and used the Solomon Four-Group Design.[2] They observed positive results, and stress that an effective program requires both repetitions of content and practical components such as role-playing.

Similarly, a study by Eisen, Zellman, and McAlister (1990) shows the positive effects of using social learning theory and the health belief model to influence the behaviour of teens. Social learning theory (SLT) predicts that individual behaviour is strongly shaped by observational learning: that is, when people see that others' behaviour achieves a desirable outcome, they are likely to mimic it. Thus, from the perspective of SLT, theatrical role-playing is an ideal medium for allowing participants to learn appropriate behaviours related to pregnancy prevention (Eisen, Zellman, and McAlister 1990, 263). The health belief model, briefly, postulates that people will take action to protect their health when they (1) perceive that they are vulnerable to a specific threat, and (2) believe that they can do so by taking a specific, reliable, action, the benefit of which will clearly exceed the cost. In order to take effective preventative action against pregnancy and STIS, then, teenagers need to perceive their vulnerability to those problems and feel that they can take preventative measures with relative ease and skill. Programs used as controls in Eisen's et al. study did not make use of observational learning strategies; while they covered topics such as biology, reproduction, STIS, dating, sexual values, norms and decision making, they did not focus on the teenagers' own perceptions of their susceptibility to and the seriousness of pregnancy, or contraception (264). Thus, Eisen et al. provide empirical evidence that programs based on social learning theory and a health belief model increase teenagers' base of sexual knowledge and improve their sexual decision making (269).

Ultimately, the results of these different studies by various researchers all point strongly to the same conclusion: the passive absorption of knowledge from lectures and videotapes does not work; for a sexual health education program to change participants' behaviours and have lasting effects, it must engage them on a personal level, and it must actively involve them.

Theory and Practice: When Sexual Education Works, What Is it That's Working?

The Critical Importance of a Comprehensive Approach

Research about sexual education consistently indicates that positive outcomes are most likely to occur when sexual health programs effectively integrate knowledge, motivation, and skill-building opportunities (Fisher and Fisher 1992), using a combination of educational media, in a carefully established, comfortable environment that encourages participation (Langille et al. 2001).

Research also indicates the importance of developing a comprehensive strategy, as opposed to a narrow approach that focuses on transmitting biological facts or obsessive reiteration of a single message (e.g., abstinence only, always use a condom, etc.), when planning and teaching curriculum (Kirby 2001). A wider range of sex-related information is needed to successfully change high-risk sexual behaviours (Christopher and Cate 1984; Greydanus. Pratt, and Dannison 1995; Kirby 1992; McKay 1993). In addition to age-appropriate or socially relevant information about both abstinence and contraception, sexuality education must comprehend a variety of topics and objectives, including information on relationships, decision making, assertiveness, and skill building to resist social and/or peer pressures (Government of Mexico 2008; Cohen 2005). Scientific evidence shows this type of comprehensive sexual education does not increase the number of sexual partners, accelerate sexual debut, or increase the frequency of sexual relations (Kirby, Laris, and Rolleri 2005). In fact, a review by Kirby (2001) concluded the opposite: comprehensive sexual health education programs resulted in delayed sexual activity, decreased frequency of sexual encounters, a fewer number of sexual partners among teens, and/or the increased use of contraception. Access to comprehensive sexuality education empowers students to make informed decisions about the initiation of sex and the use of protection (Government of Mexico 2008). Comprehensive programs work best because students themselves have comprehensive, eclectic needs (Greydanus, Pratt, and Dannison 1995). Sexuality is, after all, unique and individual (Hyde, DeLamater, and Byers 2009), and different students need access to different information. Abstinence-only approaches are of no use to a student who is already sexually active, and contraceptive-oriented curricula offer little to students whose main concern is how to negotiate differing sexual limits and boundaries with a partner. Only broad overview of a variety of sex-related topics can ensure that all students have access to comprehensive, accurate information, relevant to their paths and choices.

Theories of Successful Learning Activities: The IMB Model, Social Learning Theory, and Constructivist Learning Theory

As stated previously, traditional sexual education curricula have focused on transmitting information (about how to avoid pregnancy, how STIs are transmitted, how to use condoms, etc.), but research shows that a lack of information is not the problem. Adolescents are generally quite well-informed about sexual health, and yet many continue to practice unsafe sexual behaviour. What is required, then, are techniques that focus on modifying behaviour rather than just building knowledge. To this end, three key theoretical approaches can help guide teachers in developing effective sexuality education methods: the Information Motivation Behaviour (IMB) model, social learning theory, and constructivism. The IMB model, which is similar to Benjamin Bloom's (1956) taxonomy (information, motivation, and behavioural skills generally correlate with Bloom's familiar cognitive, affective, and psychomotor domains), proposes that learning activities need to be motivating to produce changes in behaviour (Fisher and Fisher 2000; Fisher and Fisher 1998). Accurate information about sexual health problems and practices is essential to dispel myths but will not, in and of itself, stimulate behavioural changes. In other words, an educational regime that seeks to effect behavioural change must activate emotional as well as cognitive interest. The best sexual education techniques, then, in terms of producing positive behavioural change, will be those that motivate such changes by engaging students at the emotional (i.e., motivational/affective) level.

Social learning theory follows closely upon the IMB model, particularly in its assessment of the importance of modelling and practicing skills. SLT suggests that observational learning and role-playing help students learn about skills and outcomes (Weiten 2001); that is, we learn about the world and how to negotiate it successfully by observing the actions of others and their consequences. In terms of developing effective sexuality education, this means that an effective sex education program will allow students opportunities to learn by observing others, and provide opportunities to practice modelling the behaviours and skills that are successful for others. Role-playing exercises, for example, create opportunities to experiment with modelling both successful and even unsuccessful behaviour and observing the results of both.

Finally, constructivist learning theory proposes that learning does not arise from passive absorption of information but from each learner's active construction of meaning from experiences. This approach allows students to interpret and discuss the meaning and implications of lessons (Pritchard 2007) because each individual learner has unique needs and approaches each experience from a unique perspective; thus, each can and should be allowed to learn what is important to him or her about any given experience. The more profoundly the learner is affected by the experience, and the more active the role they are allowed to play in shaping that experience, the greater the efficacy of the lesson. Therefore, the best practice for sexuality education, at least from the perspective of constructivist thinking, is to provide students with an engaging regime that makes them active participants in the learning experience and allows them opportunities to shape it for themselves and to take from it what is important to them as individuals. In addition, and to this end, a truly effective sexuality education program will simultaneously provide learning opportunities for the full spectrum of students, from those who are consciously abstaining from sexual experience to those who are actively pursuing it.

Educational Philosophy: Student-Centred Learning

Student-centred learning encourages student participation and ownership of learning. Student-centred teaching does not dictate what lessons are important to be learned; rather, lessons are guided by students' needs and wishes, not by teachers and administrators. Student-centred learning has several advantages. For one thing, it requires students to be active, responsible participants in their learning, which speaks to the principles of the IMB model discussed above. For another, it allows the students to identify and pursue objectives that are important to them. This is an important point in regard to sexual education because no educator can predict the entire range of his or her students' diverse needs in regard to sexuality, and as the aforementioned study by Langille et al. (2001) shows, many sex education programs simply repeat things that students already know while omitting topics that they consider critical. Knowledge of student abilities, interests, and learning styles helps teachers to choose the method used in the delivery of information and the range of information required.

Effective Delivery Methods: Participation, Humour, and Media

An effective sexuality education regime must be concerned not only with content and philosophy, but also the methods of delivery and the environment in which content is delivered. The aforementioned theories stress the importance of making the material personal and engaging the affective/motivational domain, which requires greater creativity in terms of delivery methods than the traditional (and demonstrably ineffective) regime based on the passive absorption of instructional videos and lectures. To this end, these theories stress the importance of participatory activities, which are more engaging, hold attention longer, and prove more effective at transforming knowledge into behavioural change, for all the reasons outlined above. But for participatory activities to work, students must feel safe, confident, and respected. Thus, an effective program must account for creating and maintaining a safe, positive environment. In this regard, humour and comedy are valuable tools. Although many teachers discourage humour in the classroom because of its tendency to undermine (their) authority, it is for that very reason a valuable tool for demystifying sex and empowering students with the confidence to deal with it on their own. Laughter dispels fear, tension, and anxiety and creates a positive environment that stimulates democratic participation, provided, of course, that the participants have no cause to fear that they will be its targets. In *AWTY* the targets of humour are never people, real or fictional, but ideas pertaining to sex. Young people themselves believe sexual education classes should provide opportunities for humour (Walker 2003), and studies have found that the judicious use of humour enhances participation, attention, and interest in what is being taught (Powell and Anderson 1985). Boys, in particular, often react negatively

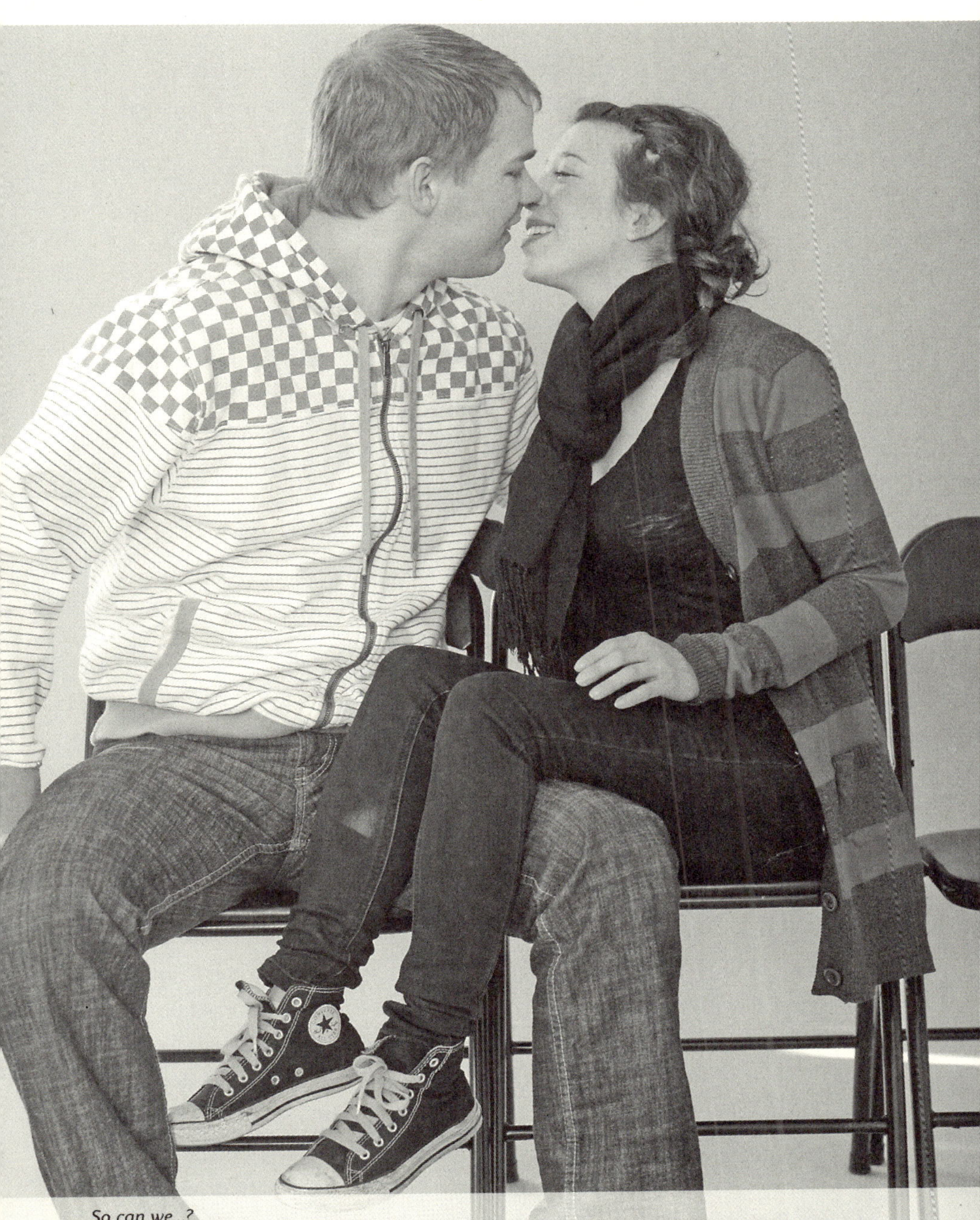

So can we...?
Cole Humeny and Ming Hudson, Concrete Theatre. *Photograph courtesy of Epic Photography.*

to sexual education classes, exhibiting poor behaviour and a lack of participation, but research has shown that boys respond favourably to humour (Cernerud and Olsson 2004), which enhances their participation in sexual education classes.

To summarize, adolescents are having sex younger and with more partners than in previous generations, and thus an effective sexual health education regime is needed more urgently than ever. It seems clear why previous programs have failed: because they provided information without motivating behavioural change; or because they presented the material in an abstract manner without connecting it to the material, lived experience of the students; or because they focused too narrowly on a single message without accounting for the diverse needs of the students; or some combination of these factors. It is also clear, therefore, that an effective sexual health education program that seeks to have long-term impact on sexual behaviour must accommodate a wide range of student needs and perspectives, address skills and motivation in addition to information, relate the material in a way that is engaging, personal, and relevant, provide opportunities to observe and model successful behaviour, and allow the students themselves to take charge of their learning experience through direct participation in a fun, safe environment.

The Advantages of Participatory Theatre-Based Sexual Education

Interactive theatre-based programs are uniquely able to incorporate the theoretical and practical concerns of sexuality education to enhance adolescents' ability to translate knowledge into productive, positive behavioural change. Participatory theatre shows great promise: it is effective at helping youth construct a healthy sexual identity, practice effective self-regulation, and develop skills to cope with difficult situations. Its open-ended, flexible format allows for comprehensive discussion of a wide variety of topics; it meets the theoretical goals of the IMB model, social learning theory, and constructivist learning theory; it is a student-centred approach driven by the interests and needs of the students; it combines several effective delivery methods, including active participation, role-playing, and humour; and its live immediacy, flexible content, and emotionally affective qualities make it a more suitable medium than lectures or films.

In addition, when performed by trained professionals from outside the school, like AWTY, participatory theatre-based sexual health education programs bring students into contact with reliable, trusted sources who have no inhibitions about discussing sex-related topics in public, are well-informed about such topics, and have no prior (or subsequent) social or institutional relationship with the students. These factors enhance the active discussion because the actors are not afraid of discussing the subject with the students (as some of their teachers are) and the students can ask them questions that they might not ask a teacher (who might judge them or betray their confidence to a parent, etc.).

Comprehensive Content

Participatory theatre is not ideal for transmitting facts and knowledge. Rather, its strength is in its flexibility and ability to respond to the unique needs of each audience and each spectator, providing students with the opportunities to explore a wide range of sexual health topics. Content in AWTY ranges from the exploration of personal opinions of participants to ways to identify and communicate personal boundaries and from strategies for safe and respectful sexual behaviour to discussing community resources and supports for both teens and adults. The play helps teens to sift through messages they receive from media, peers, and adults and to determine safe and respectful practices in their own worlds and relationships. Active discussion and audience participation helps to pitch the content of each performance to the specific developmental level and eclectic needs of the spectators because their needs and interests drive the discussion. Being able to select the content and control the field and level of discourse helps students integrate and synthesize knowledge into their current levels of experience.

Participatory theatre is well-suited to a program whose educational goals extend past the delivery of information. Traditional education methods teach youths the facts, statistics, and consequences of sex and unprotected sex but do not sufficiently address the skills, behaviours, and attitudes required to transform information into action. As a result, when students enter a difficult sex-related situation, behaviour can become reactive, guided by sensations, emotions, and a lack of relevant skills; they are unable to translate their classroom learning into practice. Teaching safer sex needs to integrate the roles of feelings and values, not merely provide step-by-step procedures. The teenage world is a complex integration of hormonal responses and social pressures, and there are too many variables for any one formula to apply to the many specific contexts in which students encounter sex and sex-related conflict.

AWTY addresses the need for skill development by focusing on problem-solving and communication behavioural skills rather than facts, figures, or proscriptions. Students are given the task of directing characters through challenging situations. Their suggestions are discussed, debated, and/or put into action, and the possible consequences of suggested actions are also enacted and discussed. This active discussion is fruitful and accessible to students with all kinds of different needs: those for whom the first sexual experience is still on the horizon may leave the session feeling more confident about their ability to deal with awkward situations when they arise, while those who are already sexually active may reconsider their behaviour or attitudes toward contraception, peer pressure, and so on in light of what they have discussed and observed.

Theoretical Basis

In addition to its facility for embracing a comprehensive range of topics and meeting the needs of the students, participatory theatre reflects the IMB model by providing accurate information in ways that motivate behavioural change. Adolescents are entering situations involving sex-related activities at a younger age than in the past (Moore, Manlove, and Glei 1998; Wellings et al. 1994; Wellings et al. 1998), and they need behavioural skills to feel comfortable negotiating boundaries without being overwhelmed by new experiences. Accurate information about sexual health problems and practices is essential to dispel myths but is not sufficient to transform behaviour. The motivation to translate knowledge into behaviours arises out of the development of conscious attitudes and values, which in turn depends on a sense of personal engagement and identification with the topic. Theatre, as a form, is totally oriented to creating personal engagement, empathy, and identification by performing situations and experiences relevant to the social contexts the students encounter. Participatory theatre, in particular, addresses behavioural skills through both role-modelling and role-playing. AWTY addresses skills such as open communication about sex and relationships, setting boundaries, respect for one's own and others' boundaries, being oneself, assertiveness, being ready for issues in the future and how to deal with them, and feeling more confident about the topic of sex and just being around someone you may be attracted to.

Theatre also coincides with the goals and techniques of social learning theory; indeed, the very practice of theatre is based on the theory that watching fictional representations of real situations has real effects on the behaviours and values of spectators.[3] Theatre, viewed from the perspective of social learning, is a form of modelling, which encourages vicarious learning through the observation of others. AWTY uses modelling when students watch actors represent other adolescents trying to negotiate relationship conflicts. Students observe others who are like them maintaining sexual boundaries, communicating with partners, and making sound decisions. Participatory theatre also incorporates the social learning theory by using role-playing to enhance self-efficacy. A student with high self-efficacy will believe that when he or she practices a skill like asserting boundaries that his or her partner will listen (Wieten 2001). Conversely, a student with low self-efficacy will feel that their skill level is not sufficient to produce a positive response. AWTY stimulates improved self-efficacy by giving the spectators opportunities to practice the target behaviours vicariously in a low-stakes, experimental environment (much like what video gamers and game developers call the sandbox mode): at various times in the play, the spectators are invited to stop the action and suggest alternative behaviours and strategies to help the characters negotiate their problems.

> *...it let you try out what you would have done and see how it panned out, and like...it felt good to know what other people were thinking and how like that matched almost what I was thinking, to know that I'm not alone where I'm standing on this issue.*
>
> *—Audience Member*

By allowing the spectators to direct the action in this way, participatory theatre also serves the objectives of constructivist learning theory. Constructivism is a hands-on approach that proposes that learning activities are most effective when they give students the opportunity to affect and change the world around them. Although the theory was developed in regard to acts of creating and manipulating tangible objects, it applies to acts of social creation as well: just as chemistry experiments are an important part of learning the natural world, social experiments are a critical aspect of any program that seeks to stimulate effective and positive behaviours in the social world. In participatory theatre, spectators are invited to stop, redirect, and contribute to the action at certain junctures, to give the characters advice or suggestions, and to help resolve conflicts. This kind of exercise raises the students' motivation through affective engagement, allows them to construct their own lesson from the experience, and enhances self-efficacy because a student who successfully intervenes in another relationship gains confidence in his or her decision-making and conflict-resolution skills—both of which are crucial for the construction of individual sexual identity. AWTY, for example, contains a segment in which two characters who are dating discover that they have different levels of comfort with sexual activity and learn how to negotiate their differences using suggestions from the spectators. The actors listen and react to the students' suggestions, allowing students to direct and explore the outcomes of situations in a safe and controlled environment. This type of learning allows each student to contemplate his or her own comfort levels and boundaries and construct a meaning from the experience. In the same session, students with different needs can construct their own meanings based on personal levels of comfort and familiarity: students who are sexually active may develop personal rules surrounding the use of contraception, while students with limited sexual experience may contemplate their boundaries and consider how they might negotiate differences with future or current romantic partners. Even if a student makes a bad suggestion (in jest or otherwise), the actors will attempt to put it into practice before moving on to solicit a more productive solution, and thus the student is rewarded with a sense of effectively exerting his or her agency to shape events. As a result, students become empowered and build self-efficacy

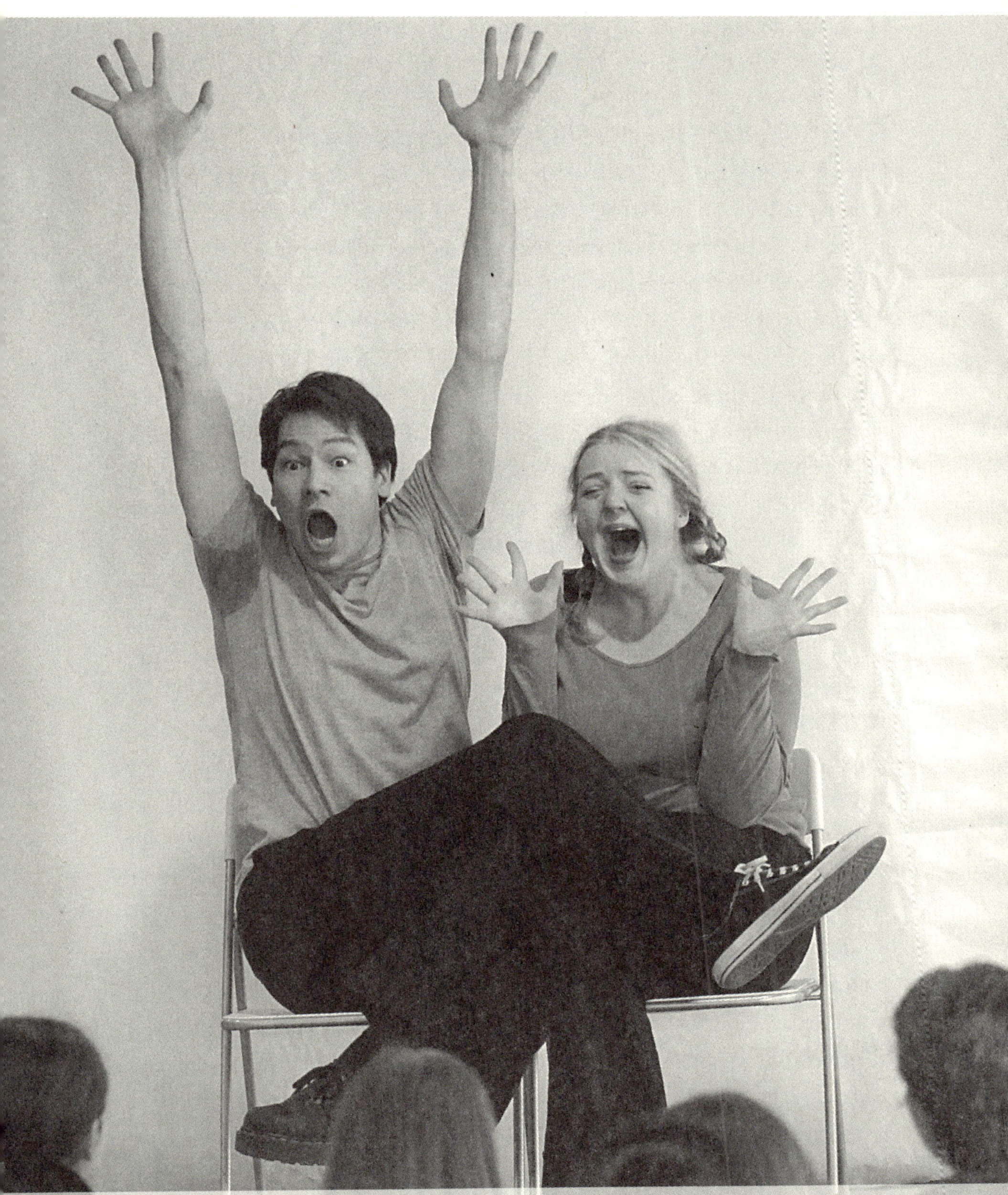

Ahhhhhh!
Jared Matsunaga-Turnbull and Jana O'Connor, Concrete Theatre. Photograph courtesy of Epic Photography.

because they learn ways to take charge of their lives and outcomes of their behaviour.

Educational Philosophy: Student-Centred Learning

Participatory theatre is an ideal medium for student-centred learning because it does not dictate what lessons are important to be learned but allows each student to take an active role in determining the content and direction of the performance. This style of theatre (more than traditional theatre in which the audience is discouraged from breaking the narrative frame or altering the plot) also accommodates opportunities for discussion in which the spectators share, listen, and discuss the consequences of characters' choices. Empathic involvement and "the opportunity to observe, analyse and form opinions regarding characters' actions creates a condition where audience members want to think" (Prentki and Selman 2000, 8). Furthermore through participation, students can claim responsibility for their own learning by directing the flow of conversation. The actors work as facilitators, allowing the students, within reason, to control their learning environment, to have a high level of choice, and to be actively involved in choosing activities (O'Neill and McMahon 2005).

Participatory theatre is an ideal medium for encouraging active, engaged learning about sexuality because it includes techniques for raising participation levels and attenuating or dissipating the fear and embarrassment that so frequently prevent frank, meaningful communication about sex. AWTY has two key strategies for creating a positive, productive, safe environment. First, the play and the actors employ humour and comedy to release tension, dispel anxiety, and signal their acceptance of the spectators. While the actors make it clear at the outset that overtly abusive, disrespectful, or offensive behaviour is unacceptable, they also undertake to honour any suggestion, however absurd or impractical. When students see their input will not be dismissed, trust and respect are built; and when impractical suggestions are played out, tension and anxiety are released through laughter. Humour also arouses affective interest, thus motivating participation. Furthermore, by treating the audience as a collective and encouraging the spectators to yell out suggestions as they please without asking permission or raising their hands, the actors enable situations and topics to be raised with relative anonymity,[4] as opposed to the traditional classroom situation, in which many students are afraid to signal publicly either their ignorance (by asking a question to which they fear everyone else already knows the answer) or their knowledge (by asking a question that would reveal an experience they don't want made public). The informal and even rowdy atmosphere of participatory theatre allows students innocuously to raise topics of grave personal import and see how certain choices might play out with no risk to themselves. Participatory theatre creates a safe and yet engaging atmosphere that encourages the spectators to talk about the situations on stage and, by proxy, in their lives.

Participatory theatre also provides a dynamic forum that integrates knowledge, motivation, skill-building opportunities, and environmental supports for sexual health. Students of traditional sex education classes have often complained that such classes do not provide enough access to information (Langille et al. 2001). In addition, research shows that knowledge acquisition alone does not change behaviours (Zabin et al. 1984; Christopher and Cate 1984; McCabe and Killackey 2004). While youth often have knowledge about sexual issues, they do not have the skills to deal with difficult situations (Gullotta, Adams, and Markstrom 2000). That is, they know how to get condoms and how to use them, for example, but they don't know how to broach the topic with a partner. To translate knowledge into action, students need practice negotiating "contraceptive use with sexual partners...[and]... how to access contraceptive services" (Health Canada 2003; Eisen, Zellman, and McAlister 1990, 263). Participatory theatre excels in this regard because it creates circumstances that are recognizable to teens and invites them to get involved in the fate of the characters and deal with the social and relational aspects of dilemmas and difficulties teens face. When they do so, they experience agency and success, and the self-efficacy and confidence noted as necessary for making healthy choices regarding sexuality (Health Canada 2003). Situations that are relevant to the social and physical pressures they face are explored in an emotive and engaged yet controlled and comfortable environment. The effectiveness of role-playing, a drama experience that is related to the experiential and participatory aspects of AWTY, has been proven empirically (Eisen, Zellman, and McAlister 1990) and is particularly helpful when encouraging the discussion of personal boundaries.

Conclusion

A review of the literature shows that traditional sexual health education is often ineffective for a variety of reasons: teachers do not feel prepared to teach sexual education and their students are not always comfortable talking with their teachers about sex; students do not relate to course material that either tells them facts they already know or tries to make them accommodate to a one-size-fits-all lifestyle; and above all, students are unable to translate facts from traditional sexual education courses into behaviour. New theories and methods of delivery are needed to enhance the effectiveness of sexual education.

Participatory theatre programs like AWTY addresses all the aforementioned shortcomings of traditional sexuality education practices and are examples of evidence-based sexual education (Fisher and Fisher 1992). The play is directly aligned with theories like the IMB, social and constructivist learning theories, and student-centred learning philosophy, all of which seek to engage and motivate students to take an active role in their learning. Participatory theatre is an innovative method of delivery for sexual health education insofar as it allows students to learn by observation and modelling, construct the experience into their own ideas about sexuality and sexual boundaries, and translate information into useful behaviour and skills that they can use to negotiate the unique and uniquely difficult social pressures they each face.

There is a global need for effective sexual education. Early successes suggest that innovative participatory theatre-based strategies and programs like *Are We There Yet?* are excellent, effective ways to engage and motivate students and catalyze their ability to transform knowledge into positive behaviour. We hope that such programs will expand nationally and internationally to decrease the worldwide incidence of negative consequences of sexual activity and make sexual health a way to increase quality of life.

NOTES

1. See Chapter 4 for a definition and more information on the structure and training involved in AWTY.
2. The Solomon Four-Group Design tests to see whether any part of the experiment—for example, the process used to recruit subjects before treatment—prejudices the subjects' response to the treatment. Social learning theory (SLT) is the theory that people learn better in a social context through interaction and observation; when we watch behaviours with positive outcomes, we are more likely to imitate them.
3. This theory, insofar as it pertains to theatre, is first laid out in Aristotle's *Poetics* in 4 BCE, and the idea that fictional representations influence real behaviour has remained a central tenet of theatre practice and criticism ever since. In fact, ever since Plato (writing even earlier than Aristotle) proposed banning poets from his utopic *Republic* because of their capacity to put dangerous ideas in the minds of their audiences, this has also been the central assumption of the enemies of theatre and other dangerous art forms throughout the last twenty-five centuries.
4. The context itself is quite public; but as opposed to the traditional classroom protocol in which a student must raise their hand and wait to be acknowledged, thus drawing the focus of the entire class upon him or herself, the AWTY protocol (specified by the actors at the outset) is to just shout out suggestions spontaneously and simultaneously. At a given moment, the actors may pick one option from among the general clamour and put it to use, and by belonging to the noisy collective, each participant is granted a modicum of anonymity.

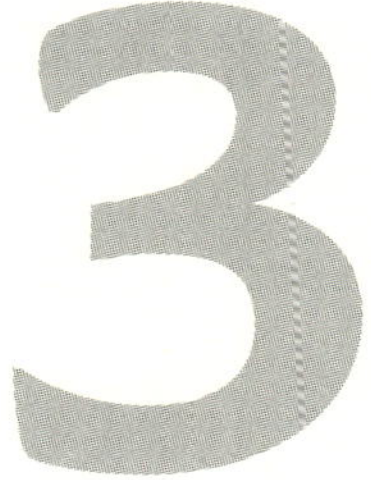

TEENS TAKE THE WHEEL

Are We There Yet? *The Play*

Jane Heather

CONTENTS

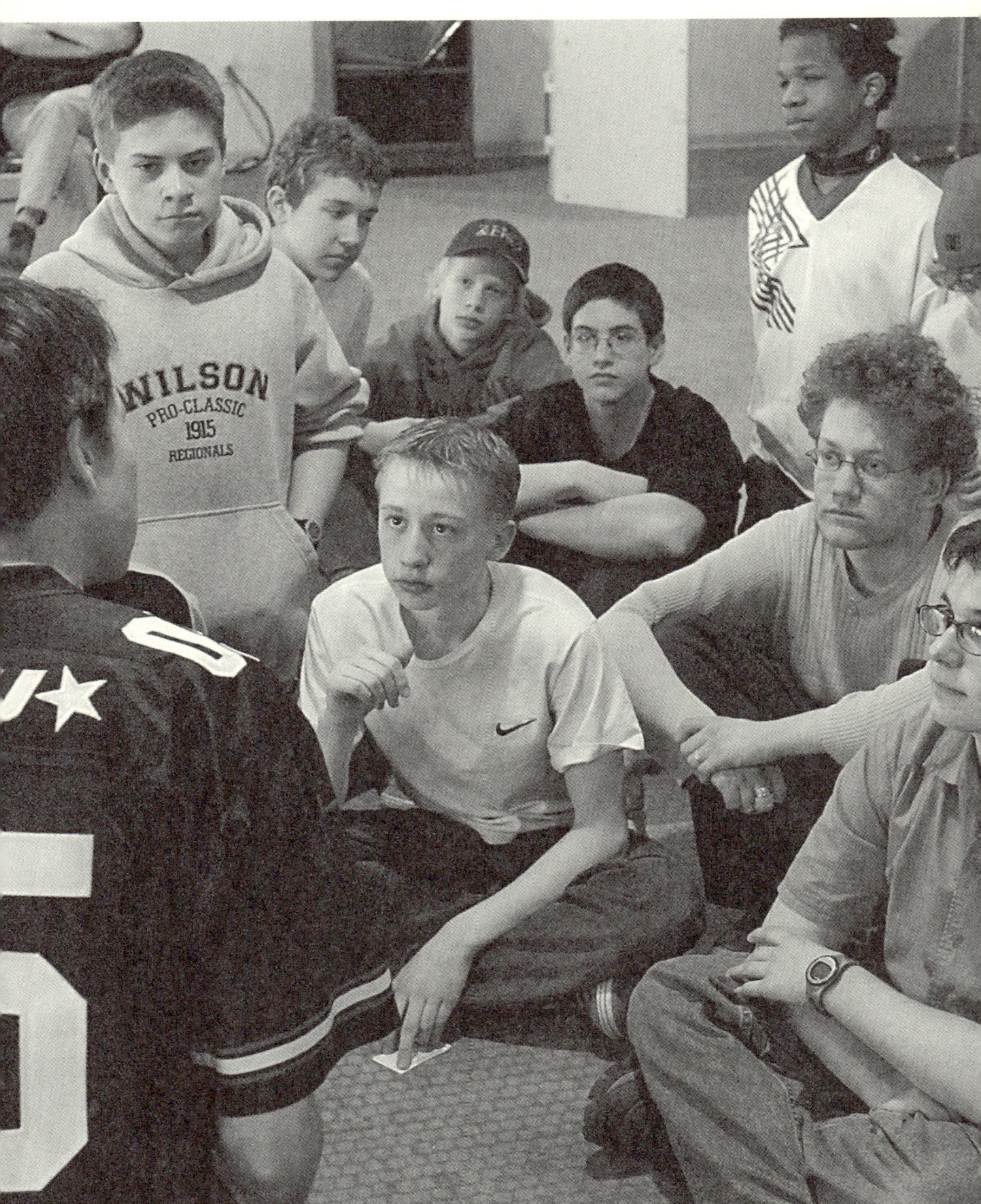

Jared Matsunaga-Turnbull and audience, Concrete Theatre. *Photograph courtesy of Epic Photography.*

Playwright Jane Heather discusses sources for *Are We There Yet?* and provides a scene-by-scene commentary. Also find the core script of the play, with notes about adapting it for particular communities.

> *I always knew you had to have boundaries but the play kind of put it realistically in my head that everybody needs to be strong about them and just, you need to take it at your own speed, and if you do decide to have sex, you need to be safe.*
>
> —AUDIENCE MEMBER

Introduction

THERE IS NO AVERAGE FOURTEEN-YEAR-OLD in Canada. Some are well into puberty, some are not, some are sexually active, most are not. It's a cusp time and the only thing we know for sure, is like it or not, they are becoming adults and sex is on their mind. It is the job of adults to ensure that children make the transition—safely, sanely, with love, support, and information. It is our responsibility to ensure their physical, emotional, mental, and spiritual survival. The development and refinement of this play and the companion workshop began with this foundational goal.

When this play became the subject of a research project and a social science-based assessment, I was asked by our research partners for something more concrete and measurable. To gather verifiable data that would determine whether a "treatment" was working, clear measurable goals were required. Artists are known to resist talking about the goals of their work. Some feel goals are for hockey players not artists, or that the work must speak for itself. In my world of popular theatre, the work does have goals that permeate all aspects, but even popular theatre workers are reluctant to try to fit everything into a linear equation.

Over time, I have returned again and again to the goals of the play. I began to realize that I had to overcome my reluctance to state what I wanted the play to do. I concurred that there needed to be clear goals in order to measure the impact of the play, and the ones I had written in response to our partner's request would be fine to design the evaluation measurement instrument, but there was more, a lot more.[1] I pondered the fact that one of the goals was a personal one: I want a better world.

I want to live in a world where every baby is loved, welcome, and wanted. In my world, little kids wallow around in the sensual joy of their own skin, and light, and air, and water, and other skin. In my world, every single adult celebrates his and her own body and the miraculous bodies of others. There is no shame attached to parts or functions. Kids know everybody masturbates but that it's a private thing. All kids from the time they are about five know how babies are born, know the fundamental things about their bodies and how they work. If a ten-year-old from here went to my world and said they didn't know about sex, birth control, and preventing infections, the kids in my world would think it was a joke. Then they would be shocked and outraged as only kids can be, then empathetic, then they would kindly and gently take this poor, ignorant alien through the whole thing, with pictures and demonstrations. If they got stuck, they'd ask an adult, any adult, because they would know that any questions they had would always be answered truthfully, patiently, and with tremendous love. Girls feel divine, in my world, just as they are, beautiful and powerful, and the boys feel the same. In my world, no kid turns on the TV and sees some poor miserable creature mutilated on camera to become beautiful. No girls give head to older boys to be popular or to feel wanted. Kids won't learn about sex from pop stars and the stone cold, dead, mercantile world of Internet porn. No unplanned, unwanted pregnancies, no date rape, no homophobia, no kids in the sex trade, no child porn, no unprotected sex. Condoms as a first resort. My prayers will have been answered about HIV.

In my world, when kids start to hit puberty they're so excited, so brave, so curious, so shy, so eager, so scared, so embarrassed, so exalted. Every adult cheers them on and congratulates them and tells funny stories about sex and growing up and growing old. When everybody gets together, the old women and men make the kids sit in their lap (even though they're too big for that) and they tickle them and whisper little joyful things. The old people tease each other and maybe cry a little, laugh a little.

The parents and aunts and uncles and friends of the parents take the kids aside for a solemn ceremony; some words of advice, some more jokes, some more crying. Then the best part begins (besides the dancing and eating and drinking but that happens later). The young adults, the twenty-somethings take over. They mostly don't have kids of their own, they may be single or coupled but what they all have is a healthy, positive attitude toward sex and a desire to welcome and help the newbies.

They are the people the kids want to become. They are confident, goofy, gorgeous, funny, and wise enough. They have already crossed the bridge that this next batch is about to attempt. It is perilous and high, narrow and oh so very swingy. Sure it's dangerous but it is so fun. Most importantly, they have no externally structured power in the lives of the kids. They aren't parents or any kind of family. They aren't teachers or people paid to teach you something. They're paid to play, to tell the truth in their mouth and their bodies, to tell the feelings, the costs, the rewards, and to listen to every syllable and every twitch. That's their job.

So they round up all the fourteen-year-olds (a few younger, a few older) and none of the fourteen-year-olds know exactly what will happen but the young adults are crazy excited and they drag them all off into a separate room and...together they engage in a fully funded, sustainable, community and government supported, participatory, best practice, live theatre event that is funny, engaging and proven to work.

No, we aren't there yet. I can't get the world I want, not all of it, but maybe I can get some of it. The goal of this project is to take a step toward creating the world I want.

Goals: Long-Term and Political

Are We There Yet? is based on politics. A complete understanding of the goals of the project requires, I believe, an unearthing of the politics embedded in the play. Adolescent sexuality has sides and we all have picked one.

AWTY has three controversial political principles related to ethics, decision making, and power. AWTY is:

- Sex positive
- Pro-liveness
- Pro-condom use

Perhaps the most unsettling thing for some adults and teens about AWTY is the goal of change—personal change, social change, political change, educational change, and policy change.

The desire for change comes from dissatisfaction with the status quo, a sense of urgency and a compelling question: Can't we do better than this? How teens learn about sex (usually) is disgraceful. The TV, the Internet, the movies, the pop stars, the advertising all inundate teens with sexual information and images. They are targeted as consumers and pressured to be experienced. We used to think it was about information. Adults (particularly parents) could see that shame and ignorance messed up many a life. But ignorance can be solved! No more girls who had never looked at their own genitals, who had no idea what intercourse was. No more boys who were just as clueless but were supposed to know everything. Education would break the death grip of monogamy and hetronormativity. As a culture we went from no information to all information, all the time. What a blow to discover that information doesn't necessarily change behaviour. Teens are still making poor decisions about their sexual behaviour and health—having sex without protection or birth control, early intercourse, unplanned and unwanted pregnancy. More information in a timely manner does help but not enough.

AWTY focuses on five things that help teens get beyond information and into the heart of the conundrum:

1. Permission and encouragement to talk about it all, to ask all the questions and to be heard in a respectful, safe, and positive atmosphere. To name and acknowledge all the things that go along with sex: embarrassment, fear, pleasure, anxiety, curiosity, exhilaration, and humour.
2. Active engagement with the real issues teens face, focusing less on mechanics and morals and more on personal relationships in all their complexity.
3. Collective, public problem solving where the audience is the expert.
4. Lots of ongoing support (during the play, workshop, and beyond) from trained sexuality educators.
5. A consistent genuine message from adults that we care about you, you are capable, you are worth listening to, you want to learn about sex, we want to help you do that, we can think of nothing we'd rather do than be in a room with you and sort out a bunch of stuff about sex. We don't want you to die, or get pregnant before you want to, or feel pressured into sex, or be shunned and bullied for who you are. You're becoming an adult and we welcome that, we're here to help you get there, safely, that's our job and we love it.

AWTY *is Sex Positive*

The power of life is everywhere, threatened by forces that work against it: toxic capitalism, greed, the wringing of the poor, nuclear arms, climate change, and war, war, war. The planet is soaked in death and still the kids are

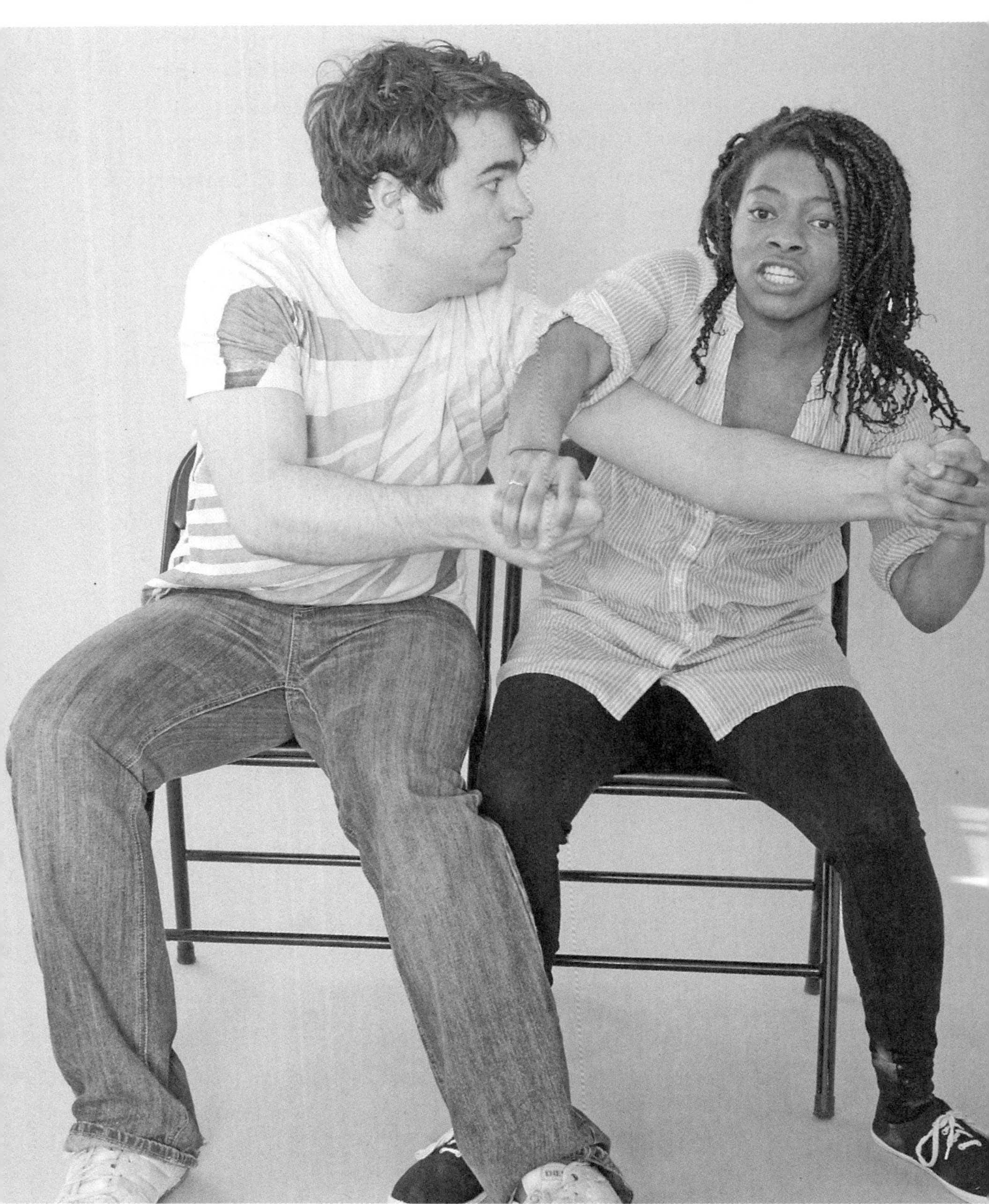

Put on the brake!
Garett Spelliscy and Monice Peter, Concrete Theatre. *Photograph courtesy of Epic Photography.*

screwing. Far too many of them experience sex as painful, degrading, brutal, and sometimes fatal. But sex can be so many positive things as well—a bit of solace, a moment of tenderness, a release of glory, intimacy, breath, sweat, skin, dreams. No human can live without it. A space and time to explore their exquisite, holy bodies. Feeling fresh and alive in the morning, feeling your sex tingle between your legs as you walk to school. Seeing the one, the heart leaping, breath-stopping moment of pure agonizing delight.

Although the play is very tightly focused on the giddy sexuality of teens (their lives, feelings, and dilemmas) and the delivery of the play is through the minds, bodies, and sprits of young adults (slightly less giddy but still juicy), the heart of the play is the voice and thinking of grandparents. I am particularly attentive to what grandparents have to say about the play. I listen hard to the youth audience but grandparents are very significant. In pre-contact Cree culture (I am told) grandparents taught youth about sex. This makes perfect sense to me. Parents are too messed up about their own sexuality and their kid's sexuality to dig deeply into the required conversations. Children are, after all, the living proof that parents had sex. Somehow talking to the person who is the result of you having sex is too messy and embarrassing. But grandparents, they aren't connected to the teen by sexuality at all.

Not very many grandparents have seen the show, but the two I know who have seen it said things of great value. An elder at Beardy's (a reserve in northern Saskatchewan) said, "This is good, we should do this," and a grandmother in Saskatoon said, "it took me to the place I was. I shared that story about date rape in my community." Both of these elders are watching and not watching a play. They are watching fourteen-year-olds (the audience) watch twenty-five-year-olds (the performers), both of whom are grandchildren. Neither said a lot of words but they said a lot.

They endorsed the play, they understood the play, and we understood each other. Contact with grandparents was brief, but it revealed to me things in the play that I had not seen or heard before. By unpacking their comments, I constructed this grandparents' list of true things about sex that is the subtext of the play:

- You are becoming a sexual being
- Sex is great
- Sex is long

- Sex gets better over time, particularly for women, but for men too
- Nobody should ever be forced to have sex
- You have a right to the pleasures of sex
- You have the right to say yes
- You have the right to say no
- You have the right to say maybe, later, I changed my mind, my orientation, my gender, my life, my body, myself
- You have to right to some ease about sex
- You have the right to choose

AWTY *is Pro-Liveness*

Sex happens between people who are in the same space. One can have cyber sex but nobody ever got pregnant or an STI from a computer. To achieve really good sex ed—sex ed that helps prevent sexual disasters and promotes positive sexual experiences—you need to actually be in the same room. Sex is between humans; education about sex has to be between humans. A DVD isn't going to do it. Why would you even try to talk about sex on a screen?[2] On screens everybody hides. Performers hide. They can't see you and they are only allowed to show, say, or do what the director and editor allow. Audiences also hide. The performers can't see you—even if the little ball of fur or whatever looks directly into the camera and talks as if they can see you, they can't. Hiding, I believe, is what has what has got us into this mess. Hiding behind embarrassment, behind shame, behind fear, behind ignorance. Hiding because it's easier. Who do we imagine we're fooling? Not adolescents. Actors can hide in conventional shows but not in participatory theatre. When an actor tries to hide in participation, they are never completely successful. Ready or not, you will be seen. What happens in the room between teens and actors in a participatory play, the way the audience and the actors "see" one another, is the opposite of hiding. Everyone is in liminal space, what Victor Turner (1967, 97) describes as "a realm of pure possibility whence novel configurations of ideas and relations may arise." People move and are moved together toward a common goal in a playful and unfettered way; they create a moment of *communitas*, another Turner concept.

When I was in Northern Saskatchewan in spring 2008 I saw this happen. Four actors came into the school, four Aboriginal actors. Each one totally beautiful, totally themselves, totally talented, flawed, vulnerable, courageous. Gods.

What happens when the Gods come to your school and talk to you? When you laugh with them, talk about sex and relationships and how to talk to the girl or the guy? What happens when they demonstrate how to show yourself, your heart, your fears, your desires? The actors are Gods but also confused, yearning, funny, awkward youth, just like you. And just like you, they are often in a lot of pain. The way the actor and the character flickered in and out of focus, first one then the other then both together, was electric. Was it good sex ed? Yes, but it was something else too, something impossible to quantify. Something that can only happen face-to-face.

I just don't think you can get to the good stuff: respect, love, wait, listen, respect, build a relationship, wait, love, unless you do that in the event's form as well as content.

Sexuality education should be as close to good sex as possible:

- In close proximity
- With people you trust and respect
- Lots of laughing and honest communication
- Lots of chances to talk, listen, try, fail, change your mind, risk
- Between people whose power relationship is not coercive, institutional, or family-based

Neil Postman (1969, 19), respected critic, theorist, and educator, says, "the critical content of any learning experience is the method or process through which the learning occurs."

Participatory theatre is the method.

AWTY *is Pro-Condom Use*

Condoms have to be normal. Totally normal, ubiquitously available. Everybody should know what they are, how they work, what they do, where you can get them, and how to talk to a partner about using them. The more normal condoms are, the safer kids can be. How can condoms be normalized? By talking about them, in public, in the gym, frankly, and without embarrassment or lying. Most of the audience knows the mechanics but the real barriers to condom use are generally not discussed. Those barriers need to be identified and dismantled.

The character of Mac reveals his (and others') most intimate fears of not being big enough and losing his erection. Would a real teenage boy talk about these things to his peers or his partner? Probably not, but theatre can make that happen, and both boys and girls can hear, from their peers, very good advice about how to overcome internal and external resistance. Everything about condoms is vulgar, hilarious, or both—let us not try to pretend otherwise. Making them normal could increase teen use.

It is noteworthy that, although unplanned pregnancy rates in adolescent populations are dropping (in the Global North), STIS and HIV are on the rise. Globally, HIV and STIS are still rising, particularly among the poor. In Canada, infection rates are rising in Aboriginal communities, the urban and rural poor of all colours, women, intravenous drug users, and once again among gay men. Can normalizing condoms and increased condom use solve that? No. Condoms aren't a panacea, but they are one crucial prevention strategy. And until a cure is found we need to promote that strategy enthusiastically.

Are We There Yet? is also pro-choice. Although no character is pregnant and abortion is never mentioned, the other pros embedded in the play signal this position subtextually.

I have continued to write and refine the goals of the play in response to the wide variety of comments and criticisms the play provokes. Every adult who sees the play has an opinion, and they usually don't hesitate to tell me. I listen hard to those who have a complaint or problem. The variety of comments and the contradictions they reveal mirror the culture's conflicted feelings about teens, gender, and sex. No ninety-minute play can do everything every adult wants, but, that so many adults are eager to be engaged in thinking, talking, and arguing about how theatre can help create change for teens is tremendously positive and hopeful. AWTY will continue to evolve, but perhaps it will also launch new plays that further serve the needs of youth and of the adults that care about them.

> *Like it made it a bit less alien, kind of, like yeah. Just to hear adults talking about it and talking about it so openly. It's like oh, ok, this is alright.*
>
> *—Audience member*

Are We There Yet?

A Participatory Play for Teens

Jane Heather

Commissioned by Concrete Theatre

In Conjunction With

Planned Parenthood Edmonton

A PDF of the playscript is available from the University of Alberta Press.

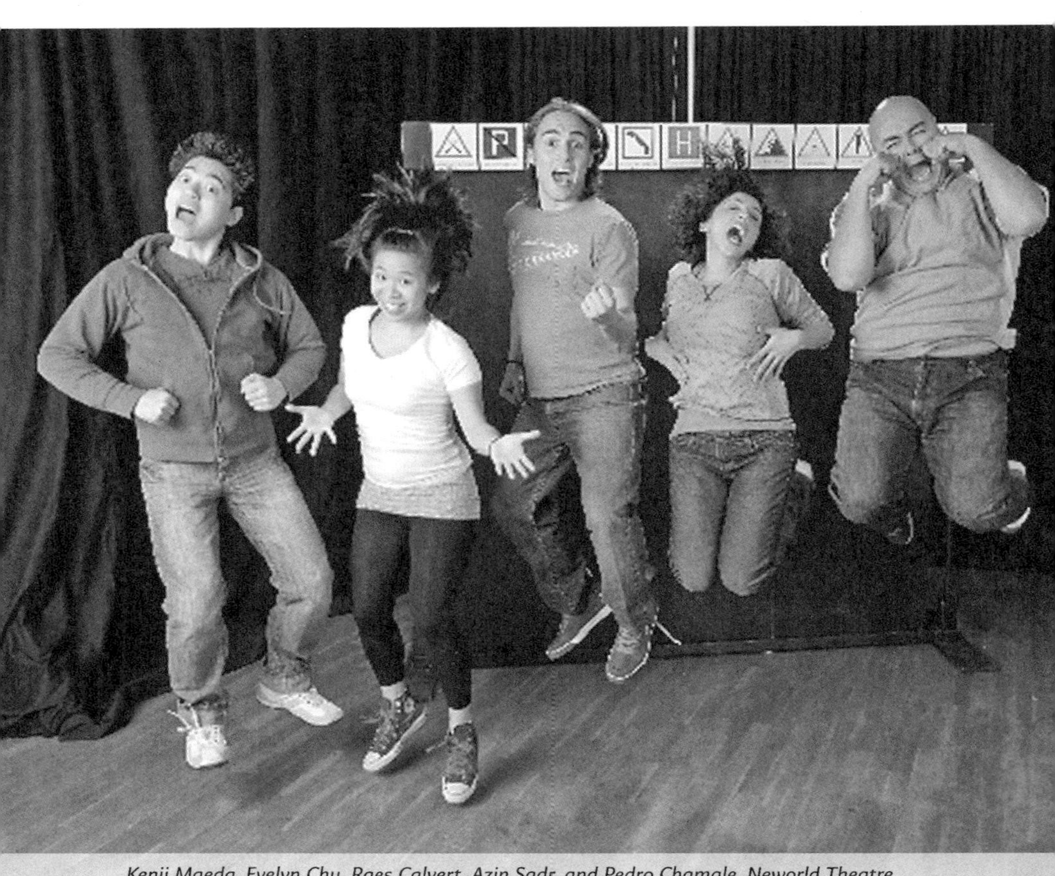

Kenji Maeda, Evelyn Chu, Raes Calvert, Azin Sadr, and Pedro Chamale, Neworld Theatre.
Photograph courtesy of Tim Matheson.

Are We There Yet? was commissioned and produced by Concrete Theatre in 1999 in partnership with Planned Parenthood Edmonton. The original production toured junior high schools in Edmonton, Alberta.

Cast

Adam Blocka
Jared Matsunaga-Turnbull
Daniela Vlaskalic
Uma Viswanathan

Thanks also to Beth Graham who assisted in workshopping the original script.

Director
Elyne Quan
Stage Manager
Jessica Rose
Planned Parenthood Heath Educator
Tracy Duncan

Acknowledgements

This play is the work of many hands. Every theatre artist and every sexual health educator who has ever worked on a production of the show (and there have been many) has put their heart and brain into developing the script. Over time there have been many additions, cuts, rewrites, and tweaks. Some artists and educators have had a long commitment to the show and therefore have had more opportunity and desire to influence the script. The work, thoughtful comments, suggestions, and insights of artists and educators have shaped and sharpened the play and my thinking about participation, teens, sex, and theatre's capacity to make positive change.

So when I say I wrote the play I mean I wrote it in a participatory process with many others. For their love and their courage I am indebted to:

- Elyne Quan, who worked on the script, wrote the Josie monologue, and directed the first two productions of the show;
- Jared Matsunaga-Turnbull, who worked on the script, acted in, and directed several productions;
- Mieko Ouchi, who worked on the script and directed many, many productions;
- Caroline Howarth, who worked on the script and directed several productions;
- Jan Selman, who worked on the script and co-directed the participation for most of the productions;
- Tracey Byrne and Gina Puntil, who stage-managed the show many times, watched over actors and audiences with intelligence and love, and created a great stage management report template that stage managers across the country used;
- Brian Parker, who developed and refined the role of the sexual health educator;
- Concrete Theatre and Options Sexual Health Association.

How to Read this Play

Like any play script, the best way to "read" this play is to see it. Watching the play with its intended audience (teens) would provide the clearest and most complete picture of how the play works. However, as that is probably not possible, the next best way is to read the script while watching samples of the participatory sequences on the accompanying DVD. This combination can begin to give a sense of what cannot be scripted: the participation. Finally, it is important to remember you are not the intended audience for the play (unless you are a thirteen-, fourteen-, or fifteen-year-old, in which case, I hope you get to see it sometime). Given all that, it might be helpful to take yourself back in time to when you were in grade nine. Try to remember the itchy, bubbling, breathless, anxiety-provoking response to the word *sex*. Imagine yourself jostling and sliding down to the gym or library to see a play (or presentation as it is often called) about sex. Now stay in that frame of mind to read the play.

The script is a map (like any script) and a good deal of work has been done to make the map as useful and consistent as possible. The scenes can be read just as any scripted scene can be read but the participations must, to a certain extent, be imagined. Each participation has a particular intention, and a number of tools and techniques are outlined at the beginning of each scene. Each participation is shaped by its intention and by the incremental deepening that develops over the course of the play. The tools and techniques are markers, written primarily for directors and actors to help them make their way through what is unknown territory for most.

Let your teenage mind come up with the most profound, outrageous, obscene, witty, naïve responses to questions characters and actors ask the audience. Be assured that every one of them and more has come out of the mouth of a teen audience member. Now imagine yourself as the actor and consider how you might respond, stay in character, honour the contribution, and keep steering toward the intention. The DVD focuses on the participations and will give you a clearer picture of what happens in the room between the actor and the audience.

The play has no story, per se, no character arc, no unity of time or locale. It does, however, have a structure, and the characters and scenes, though skeletal, are not without substance, complexity, and a solid core. Upon first reading, they appear insubstantial, even negligible; this is intentional. There needs to be a lot of room for the actors, in concert with audiences, to make flesh. In each participation, audiences are engaged in building characters and/or giving advice about the action characters should take. Characters absorb audience's words, attitudes, and stories and take them back into the scene with them. Actors can change characters' class, degree of sophistication, maturity, boldness, or shyness, depending on who is in the audience. Characters should represent the specific performance's audience. Actors play what they see.

> *Because it is a participatory show, there's an absolutely different feel with every single audience and there's an absolutely different feel with every single combination of group, the dynamic is always different. So there are times when I feel like I need to sort*

of dial it down and, and meet the kids where they are. The way that the students are talking, the way that the students are approaching the subject, informs your body, informs your voice. I have an Annabel dial where when I feel the kids are on one level, she's at it too. I approach her with my edges slightly rounder. And then if there's a group of kids that are a lot more urban and are dealing with a lot more things, I'll dial her up, my edges get a lot more sharp.

—*Nadien Chu,* AWTY *actor,*
Concrete Theatre

Reading this play is much like reading any play except the reader (like the audience) is a co-creator in a very concrete and immediate way.

Script Options

There are three key elements in the play that should be adapted to particular community circumstances.

Cultural References and Teen Argot

There are a few places in the script where the generic can be made specific. For example, Carol Ann says, "We both love science fiction and graphic novels" (page 80). In the Vancouver production of 2008, "science fiction" was replaced with "*Battle Star Galactica*." Now that this program is no longer on TV, directors and/or actors might find another specific cultural reference that resonates with the immediate audience. In the "Practice Your Skills" section at the end of the play (page 93), the Clay characters phone, Skype, email, and text when one is trying to reach the other. In some communities, these technologies may not be as ubiquitous as they are in others. Research with local teens will determine which references are appropriate for them. Expressions and cultural references have a short shelf life; the script published here is a guide, and each company will choose the expressions and details that best reflect their audience. Given that, it is important to remember that teen style and slang changes very quickly and is not universal, even in the same geographic region. Something that is cool and popular in one school is unknown in another. A balance between specificity and inclusivity is encouraged.

The Monologues

There are four monologues published here, but in a ninety-minute performance only three can be performed. Usually companies cast four actors and if that is the case, it is important that one actor be outside the monologue section, to act as a host and guide for the audience. Therefore, only three of the four can be performed in any one show. There are a number of factors to consider when choosing the monologues. When time is a factor, as it often is in schools, companies have chosen to perform only two of the monologues in each performance. Some companies alternate between Josie and Mateo, always performing Hal and Annabelle and one of the other two. In communities without LGBTQ[3] services for youth, companies could consider using the Mateo monologue if online services are available, but would need to modify the monologue. Without the Mateo monologue, there is very little LGBTQ content in the script, and that is a significant weakness. However, if services mentioned in the monologue are not available, as is the case in many rural areas, it may be unethical to suggest that help is available when it is not. This is a difficult contradiction to resolve and each producing partnership of theatre and health organizations need to make a choice that works best for their community and youth audiences.

Health Partner Role in the Script and Definition of Abstinence

The definition of abstinence in the script was developed by Options for the original production. In each region, the health partner worked with the theatre company to write a definition that worked for their agency and community. For example, in Nova Scotia, when Instructor Two did the Drawing the Line exercise (page 75), the actor did not include the scripted line, "giving or receiving oral sex." In this case, the health partner's definition of abstinence did not include oral sex. For each production, the sexual health agency or health practitioner will need to write a definition of abstinence, which may be different from the one in the script (page 75).

Other Possible Adaptations

The script was adapted to three different communities and regions between 2005 and 2010. In each case, specific references and theatrical images were created to fit the particulars of that teen audience. Please see Chapter 7, "Customized: Adapting *Are We There Yet?* for Community Specificity" for some examples of the Aboriginal, rural, and urban adaptations.

Are We There Yet?

As students enter, ACTORS *mingle, welcoming and chatting with them. They give out cards with names and numbers of helpful resources for teens and make contact with as many of the audience as possible. When everyone is in,* ACTORS *gather on stage, signal they are changing into character and that the show is starting. This may include a choral gesture, donning a costume piece, a sound effect, and/or announcing the title of the play. One possible signal is actors quickly assemble a "car" using chairs, getting into the car and assuming "character" poses: the anxious mum, the bored teen with iPod, the annoying little sister, the map-reading dad. As one, they say: (Some companies may discover this first image/intro is not necessary. In that case actors begin with Welcome...).*

Actors: Are We There Yet?

Actor A: Welcome and hello to you all (ACTORS *adjust what they say to what's comfortable, cheery, and not too dippy.*) I'm [Actor's Name],

Actor B: I'm [Actor's Name],

Actor C: I'm [Actor's Name],

Actor D: I'm [Actor's Name],

Stage Manager: I'm [Stage Manager's Name], the Stage Manager,

Actor D: And we're from [Theatre Company].

Sexuality Educator: And I'm [Educator's Name] from [Name of Health Organization].

Actor A: And together we're presenting *Are We There Yet?*, a show about sex.

Actor B: Sexual decision making.

Actor C: Sexual health.

Actor D: Sexual choices.

Actor A: It's a funny thing about the word "sex,"

All four ACTORS *say the word with a different emotional value, e.g., sexy, frightened, confused, embarrassed.*

...all you have to do is say it and all kinds of questions, feelings, and thoughts start rolling around inside us. That can make it hard to talk about. (*To* AUDIENCE) So what are some of the feelings people get when they hear the word "sex"?

> *Just a Minute (Participation One)*

Intention: *This participation is to develop the audience's comfort with participation, to demonstrate that actors will use audience members' specific suggestions, and to give the audience a good laugh in order to break the tension.*

Method: *"Just a Minute" is a fun game. For the audience, it is a low-risk, no fail way to give input and see their ideas used by the actors.*

Techniques: GATHER *lots of ideas from as many audience members as possible; use their suggestions for the game.*

ACTOR A GATHERS *lots of ideas from the* AUDIENCE.

Actor A: We're going to play a game called "Just a Minute." This is how it works. We're going to take those words you just gave us and do something with them. (ACTOR A *assigns a feeling to each of the other actors.*) They now have one minute to say everything they can about this word and how it relates to sex. The rules are: they can't repeat, they must maintain eye contact with the audience, and they can't stop or pause. So is everyone ready? In three, two, one...

ACTOR A *blows a referee's whistle. The three* ACTORS *begin to speak directly to the* AUDIENCE, *simultaneously improvising on their "feeling" assignment.* ACTOR A *monitors and prompts them, looking for infractions, reminding the actors of rules, and building the competition and suspense. She or he leads a countdown of the last five seconds then blows the whistle to stop the game.*

Actor B: Fear, excitement, confusion, embarrassment, lust (*list begins with the feelings the Audience has suggested and adds some or all of these*) are all feelings we have when we think or talk about sex.

Actor C: Today you're going to see some situations and hear some stories about people your age. Sometimes the characters won't know what to do or what to say and then we will ask for your help.

Actor D: Lots of help. Your ideas and input are really important.

Actor B: The rules for participating are very simple.

Actor A: Everybody has a right to express their opinion, so respect the ideas and suggestions of others.

Actor B: Watch your language and no put-downs.

Actor C: Don't be shy. We want to hear from everyone.

Actor D: You may see something during the show that brings up a memory or a feeling that is upsetting or a question that needs an answer.

Actor A: During and after the show, [Educator's Name] from [Name of Health Organization] will be here to answer any questions you have that we might not be able to answer.

Actor B: I have a question. What is [Name of Health Organization] exactly?

Actor A: [Educator's Name]? (*e.g., Steven?*)

Sexuality Educator: (*Provides a brief description of what the organization does.*)

Actor A: Thanks, [Educator's Name]. (*Turns to* AUDIENCE) You know, if you think about it, learning about sex is a bit like learning to drive.

Actor D: Everybody thinks about it, everybody expects to drive some day but there's so much to learn!

Actor A: All the mechanics, steps for starting it up, safety procedures and equipment, how to signal, passing, rules of the road, figuring out the intention of the other drivers, dangerous driving and how to avoid accidents.

Actor B: When you're learning to drive you take lessons and Driver's Ed, you write a test, get your learners, and finally, you take your road test. Even with a licence you might not drive for years. With sex, most people don't get a lot of training, they have to figure it out on their own.

Actor C: And, everybody talks about driving: how to drive, when to drive, what driving is like, drinking and driving, accidents, good drivers, stupid drivers...but sex? Well that's a different story.

Actor D: But what if learning about sex was like learning to drive?

ALEX enters. Alex "ages" through the show, from fourteen to about seventeen years, as lessons become more complex and topics more serious.

Alex: Mum, when can I learn to drive?

Parent: You're only fourteen, you're too young to drive.

Alex: Some kids in my class already drive.

Parent: What? Who?

Alex: I don't know. I just heard about it. They snuck out and took the car for a spin around the block.

Parent: My gosh, it's so dangerous. They could have been hurt or killed. Driving is difficult and potentially fatal. So many things can go wrong.

Alex: That's all anybody ever says to us. It's dangerous; wait until you're older. They make it sound like we can't do anything right. I just want to try it.

Parent: I guess it's time for your first driving lesson.

Alex: Yeah? Who's the instructor?

Parent: Well, for your first lesson, me.

ALEX *reacts.*
PARENT *puts on Instructor costume.*

> *Know Your Vehicle (Lesson One)*

Parent/Instructor One: Lesson One: know your vehicle. What you need to know before you start the car.

Mechanics and Equipment

PARENT/INSTRUCTOR *uses two cartoon (not anatomical) diagrams of the human body, one male and one female, and points to different body parts through the demonstration.*

Parent/Instructor One: The engine (*points to heads*): the control centre, everything is routed through here, including the gas pedal and the brake pedal. Signal lights (*mouth*): to signal to others when you want to slow down, stop, or change direction. The windows and mirrors (*ears and eyes*): must be kept clear to hear and see incoming messages and signals. Other standard equipment includes: gps (*heart*), headlights (*breasts: boys and girls*), stick shift (*boy parts*), glove compartment (*girl parts*), trunk (*indicate back of drawing*), and various other knobs, buttons, dials, gauges, etc., scattered through the vehicle (*whole body sweep*). Drivers should be thoroughly familiar with their own equipment before starting the car. Drivers should also become familiar with the equipment of other models. Let's watch the film.

Puberty and You

Cheesy Film Host: (*Music*) As you approach puberty you will notice that your body and the bodies of your friends are changing (*MALE and FEMALE enter*). Girls are becoming women, boys are becoming men. Girls begin to menstruate and now it is possible for them to become pregnant (*FEMALE gets an attack of cramps*). Boys' voices begin to change (*demo from MALE*). Both boys and girls will notice many other physical changes. Girls will begin to develop breasts (*FEMALE picks at shirt, crosses arms uncomfortably*). Boys' testicles will descend and his penis will become larger (*MALE is a little uncomfortable around the crotch, picks at his pants*). Both will notice hair (*both look down pants, out to AUDIENCE, over to each other, out to AUDIENCE*) where there was no hair before. Both boys and girls will notice their perspiration has a more pungent odour (*both sniff their armpits*). And they begin to notice each other (*they look at each other in a starry-eyed way*).

Parent/Instructor One: So Alex, any questions?

MALE and ALEX fire out questions, as if talking to themselves.

Alex: What is oral sex exactly?

Male: Can you masturbate too much?

Alex: Can you damage your body if you have sex too early?

Male: When is too early?

Alex: What does an orgasm feel like?

Male: How will I know if the other person is having an orgasm?

Alex: Why are my breasts two different sizes?

Male: Is pornography real?

Alex: How do lesbians do it?

Male: Am I gay?

Alex: Why do boys only want one thing?

Male: How do you know if someone likes you?

Both: Am I normal?

Parent/Instructor One: Alex? Alex?

Alex: (*turning back to PARENT*) What?

Parent/Instructor One: Any questions?

Alex: No.

Parent/Instructor One: Well, if you think of any, let me know.

Alex: Sure Mom. So is that it...with the parts and everything? Now can I drive?

Parent/Instructor One: After one lesson? I don't think so.

Alex: Well, what else?

Parent/Instructor One: Reading and interpreting signs and signals. And a new instructor.

PARENT/INSTRUCTOR ONE hands over Instructor costume to INSTRUCTOR TWO.

> *Signs and Signals (Lesson Two)*

Instructor Two: Lesson Two: Signs and Signals. Once you are familiar with the vehicle, knowing how to read and interpret the signs can be the single most important way to prevent accidents. Sending and receiving clear signals will help you stay in control of the situation. Stop, yield, proceed with caution are all signs you need to be able to recognize in yourself and others. Sometimes, however, the signals aren't clearly sent so they can't be clearly received.

This is Delphi and Marcel. They're in grade ten and have been dating for a month. They like each other but the road they're on has a few potholes.

MARCEL'S house. He is watching TV on the couch. DELPHI knocks, MARCEL opens the door. The last time they were together things went badly.

Marcel: Delphi!

Delphi: Hi.

Marcel: Hi.

Delphi: Can I come in?

Marcel: Sure, sure.

Pause.

Delphi: What are you doing?

Marcel: Just...watching TV.

Delphi: Is this that show you were telling me about?

Marcel: Yeah.

DELPHI moves to watch TV.

Delphi: Marcel, are you mad at me?

Marcel: No. Are you mad at me?

Delphi: No. (*Pause*) Well...I guess I better go.

Marcel: No. No, don't go. I want you to see this. Sit down.

Delphi: Okay.

She chooses to sit near him on the couch. Awkward silence. He "fakes" a big yawn and stretch and eases his arm around her.

Delphi: I'm kinda hot.

Marcel: Oh sorry (*moves away*).

Delphi: No, I mean...I'll take my sweater off.

Marcel: Okay.

She does. They sit. DELPHI leans over and kisses MARCEL on the neck.

Marcel: Delphi!

Delphi: (*very fast, prepared*) Marcel, I want you to know I wasn't comfortable before but now it's okay.

Marcel: So, can we...?

Delphi: Yes. (*They kiss. MARCEL wants to go further, DELPHI pushes him away. This action happens two or three times.*) That's enough.

Marcel: What? What did I do?

Delphi: You don't get it, do you?

Marcel: No, I don't.

> *Setting Boundaries (Participation Two)*

Intention: *To encourage clear communication (verbal and non-verbal) about sexual boundaries.*

Method: *Ask the audience to identify the problem, explore possible consequences, and then suggest ways to solve the problem.*

Techniques: *GATHER to get lots of ideas, then PROBE to explore some of the ideas more deeply.*

Instructor Two: Okay, these two seem to be having trouble. What do you think is happening?

GATHERS from the AUDIENCE; they will likely identify communication issues, among other things.

PROBES. E.g. What do they mean when they say [communication]?

Okay, great. Let's check in with them.

GATHERS from the CHARACTERS.

Instructor Two: Marcel? What's going on with you?

Marcel: Okay, yesterday I went over to her place and we were kinda makin' out and stuff and then she pushes me away and we got in a fight. So now she comes over here and she tells me we can make out, so I go to make out and then she's like, "no we can't."

Instructor Two: So how does that make you feel?

Marcel: It's pissing me off.

Instructor Two: And Delphi, what's happening with you?

Delphi: I just feel like he doesn't understand what I want.

Marcel: I don't know what you want.

Delphi: Well, that's obvious—

Instructor Two: (*Interrupts them*) Okay. So you feel like he doesn't understand what you want, and you don't know what she wants...(*turns to AUDIENCE*) So what does this mean for these two?

WAITS for the AUDIENCE to process the scene, then GATHERS ideas, and PROBES to deepen discussion.

Does this mean they may have to break up?

GATHERS and PROBES.

Let's ask them. Do you two want to break up?

They look at each other. They have never considered this.

Marcel and Delphi: (*Slowly, checking out each other's reaction.*) No. No, I don't want to break up either.

Instructor Two: So you do want to stay together. But you seem to be having some trouble with the physical side of your relationship...Can you talk about that?

Delphi: Yeah, well I like the stuff we're doing now. I wouldn't mind doing more stuff. But I don't necessarily want to go all the way.

Marcel: I like the stuff we're doing too. I'd like to go further, but we don't have to go all the way.

Instructor Two: When you talk about not going all the way are you talking about abstinence? Does anybody know what abstinence means?

GATHERS a very few definitions from AUDIENCE then turns to SEXUALITY EDUCATOR for clarification.

[Educator's Name] is there anything you'd like to add?

Sexuality Educator: I really like what everyone said. You're right, abstinence means not having intercourse, but there are lots of ways to be physical and intimate that aren't intercourse. It all depends on your personal boundaries.

Instructor Two: Okay, personal boundaries. What does "personal boundary" mean to you guys?

Briefly GATHERS AUDIENCE'S ideas.

Thanks. (*Turning to MARCEL and DELPHI*) Can I do an exercise with you two?

Marcel and Delphi: Okay.

Instructor Two: (*To CHARACTERS*) Okay, now the exercise I'm going to be doing with you deals with your personal boundaries. I'm going to get you two to close your eyes. (*To AUDIENCE*) Now this exercise is for these two but you can do it as well. (*To CHARACTERS*) Imagine you have a felt pen. Now I'm going to list off a bunch of intimate activities. When I get to the point where I reach your personal boundary, the point that you're not comfortable with, I want you to draw that line in your mind. Does everyone understand? Good. (*The CHARACTERS listen without revealing their personal boundaries.*) Okay, holding hands. Is that your personal boundary? Hugging. Kissing. Kissing with tongue. Rubbing genitals while dressed. Getting naked together. Touching each other's genitals when you're naked. Bringing your partner to orgasm with your hand. Giving or receiving oral sex. Okay, open your eyes. Wherever you drew the line is a personal boundary for you.

Marcel: (*To DELPHI*) Where did you draw your line?

Delphi: You first.

MARCEL whispers into DELPHI'S ear.

Delphi: My line's in a different place. (*Both look at INSTRUCTOR TWO.*)

Instructor Two: So their lines are in different places. What does this mean for them?

GATHERS *from* AUDIENCE.

PROCESSES AUDIENCE *ideas, challenging them to explore the consequences of their suggestions for each person. (Often "compromise" is suggested, but discarded once the implications of this solution are explored. See Appendix 1.5.) The processing leads the* AUDIENCE *to recommend that the person whose boundary allows more sexual contact needs to slow down, for now.*

SUMMARIZES *the advice from the* AUDIENCE.

So you two heard all that? Seems like you're going to have to talk about this. And Marcel? You're going to have to respect Delphi's boundary. Are you ready to try that?

MARCEL *and* DELPHI *check in with each other, they want to follow this advice.*

Marcel and/or Delphi: Sure, we'll try.

MARCEL *and* DELPHI *acknowledge the* AUDIENCE *and exit.*

Instructor Two: Those two have got a lot of talking to do. Thanks for your help in getting them started.

ALEX *enters.*

Alex: Okay, being really clear, getting your signals straight. But what if you get into it and you find out you put your boundary in the wrong place?

Instructor Two: Well, you and your partner will have to talk.

Alex: What if you want to change your mind?

Instructor Two: That would be...more talking.

Alex: But if you're in love, I mean really in love, don't you just know what the other person is thinking?

Instructor Two: Sometimes, but most people can't read your mind, they're guessing. So unless you're telepathic you have to use the old-fashioned method: (*together with* ALEX) talking.

Alex: Okay! But I can drive now, right? I mean if I want to and my partner wants to. If we've talked. Are we there yet?

Instructor Two: You're getting closer. You can practice sending and receiving signals accurately to help protect yourself from common driving mistakes. But some hazards are more difficult to handle. And for those you move to lesson three.

INSTRUCTOR THREE enters, INSTRUCTOR TWO exits.

> *Safety Equipment and Procedures (Lesson Three)*

Instructor Three: Lesson Three: safety equipment and procedures. They can save your life. When we watch people driving in films or on television, sometimes it looks like this:

Studley Muffin and Creamy Delight Go for a Spin

Music, something steamy, glossy, and Manhattan or California. Black leather and white chocolate. STUDLEY MUFFIN and CREAMY DELIGHT perform pre-driving ritual: very stylized, sexy, slightly campy. As they move toward the car, SMARMY ANNOUNCER speaks.

Smarmy Announcer: It's just a natural human experience. Everyone just instinctively knows how to do it. Your first experience will be spontaneous and wonderful. When the time is right you'll just know. Just one look! (*They give each other a long look.*) So jump in and you're off! Zero to sixty in three seconds! Feel the excitement, feel the thrill.

Once they are in the car:

Studley: Oh Creamy Delight, with you I'm in paradise!

Creamy: Oh Studley Muffin, your technique is magnifique!

Studley: So smooth! So controlled!

Creamy: So powerful, so...je ne c'est quoi.

Instructor Three: Well, sometimes driving can be like that...let's rewind (*ACTORS rewind the action until they are out of sight again*)...but often, it's more like this:

ACTORS re-enter as more ordinary teens. They enact a driving ritual, getting into a car, awkwardly, the opposite of Creamy and Studley. During the course of the scene both actors take the wheel.

Creamy: Oh man, I'm driving.

Studley: Am I doing it right?

Creamy: This is fun!

Studley: This is fast!

Creamy: This is...

Studley: Holy hacky sack, what was that?

Creamy: A sign, we were going too fast to read it.

Studley: It's a cliff!

Creamy: Put on the brake!

Studley: I don't know where it is!

STUDLEY *leans over to look at his feet.* CREAMY *grabs the wheel.*

Creamy: Seat belt! I forgot my seat belt!

STUDLEY *grabs the wheel again.*

Studley: Oh man! I thought you'd have an air bag!

Creamy: Me! I thought you'd have one! Pull over! I thought you said you would pull over!

Both: AHHHHHHHHHHHHH!!!!! (*They go over the cliff and are thrown from the car. They crawl from the wreckage.*)

Creamy: I thought you knew how to do this. Didn't you take Driver's Ed?

Studley: Yeah but...well, I skipped a lot.

Creamy: Me too...it was so boring.

Studley: Were you wearing a seat belt?

Creamy: No. I hope I'm not...

Studley: You don't have any diseases...do you?

Creamy: Do you?

Instructor Three: Studies show and when we talk to you we find out that young drivers know quite a bit about safety equipment and procedures. You know what to use to prevent unwanted pregnancies, sexually transmitted infections, and HIV but you have a lot of questions.

Instructor Four: Which of these questions do you think is the most asked by young people about condom use?
Number 1. What size should I buy?
Number 2. What brand is the most effective?
Number 3. How do I bring it up with my partner?

INSTRUCTOR *gives a beat in case* AUDIENCE *wants to respond, then continues...*

And the answer is...How do I talk about condom use with my partner? Let's look at different ways to raise this touchy topic.

When is the Right Time to Talk about Condoms?

JERI (female) and SAL (male) are at a locker talking, CHRIS (male) enters.

Jeri: Hi Chris.

Chris: Hi Jeri.

Jeri: This is my friend, Sal. Sal, meet Chris.

Chris: Hi Sal. How do you...feel about using condoms?

Instructor Four: Too soon.

BEN and FERN in stand-up bed (a sheet), fully clothed. They are asleep and in each other's arms. Simultaneously they: (1) Wake up with a start, (2) Look at each other, (3) Lift sheet to look at their naked selves, (4) Look out to AUDIENCE. FERN exits, taking the sheet; BEN exits covering his parts.

Instructor Three: Too late.

MAC and CAROL ANN under a blanket, lots of heavy breathing, moans, etc.

Carol Ann: Mac wait! Wait a minute.

Mac: Wha...?

Carol Ann: I have to go, I left the stove on.

Mac: What? The stove?

Carol Ann: (*Babbling, emerging, adjusting clothes*) Nobody's home, there's curtains right by the...(*exiting*) Sorry.

Mac: (*groans*) Carol Ann.

Instructor Three: Too indirect.

> *Talking Protection (Participation Three)*

Female Participation

Intentions: *To identify appropriate places, times, and methods (with emphasis on actual words to say) for raising condom use with a partner; to address some of the barriers to condom use, including reasons for hesitancy to talk about it.*

Method: *Ask the audience to identify the problem, explore possible consequences, and suggest ways for the characters to talk about their concerns.* PLAY OUT *and* TEST *these suggestions.*

Techniques:
DEFINE *Carol Ann's problem*
BLOCK *for depth*
PLAY OUT *(improvise) suggestions with* COACHING *from audience.*

CAROL ANN *comes back out. It is the next day and she has been worrying and sleepless since the previous night.*

Carol Ann: (*To* AUDIENCE) Man, last night was close. Too close. Me and Mac... we're great together. We're both weird in the same way. We both love science fiction and graphic novels. He always makes me laugh. And I know we both think we'll have sex someday. But then...last night, I was really shocked. You know how some girls say they got pregnant 'cause they got swept away? Like they didn't know what they were doing? I always thought that was a bunch of crap, an excuse. A smart girl like me with a great boyfriend like Mac, well that was never going to happen to us. Suddenly, it's happening and I'm thinking...we need a condom. I was so scared I just...ran out of there. (*She sets up the question for the* AUDIENCE.) Now I don't know what to do. I'm meeting Mac in a few minutes at the mall. What should I tell him?

CAROL ANN *pauses,* WAITS *to see if* AUDIENCE *responds, if necessary asks a* SECOND QUESTION (*What shall I say to him?*). *She* GATHERS *suggestions from* AUDIENCE *about her embarrassment and fears.*

Carol Ann: Okay, I'll try.

CAROL ANN *goes into the scene.* MAC *is waiting for her at the mall. He's mad.*

Carol Ann: Hi Mac.

Mac: Hi. You want to talk.

Carol Ann: Yeah...about last night.

Mac: How's the stove? No fire?

Carol Ann: It's fine.

Mac: I waited all night for you to call me and when you didn't I expected your dad to show up and kick my ass or something.

Because MAC is so angry, CAROL ANN is unable to PLAY OUT much of the advice she got from the AUDIENCE. She comes back out for more advice.

She PLAYS OUT their suggestions and returns to the AUDIENCE when she needs more help. She PROBES and DEEPENS the discussion by revealing her embarrassment and fear. With COACHING from the AUDIENCE, she finally manages to get it out.

Mac: (*Relieved*) Great. Wow. Okay. That's it? I thought it was going to be something bigger. Like you wanted to break up with me...

MAC and CAROL ANN assure each other that they still care about each other, they don't want to break up. MAC is incredibly relieved and goes out to the AUDIENCE.

Mac: (*Whoops*) Yeah! All we have to do is use condoms. Oh yeah...condoms.

Male Participation

Intentions: *To DEEPEN the discussion about the importance of wearing condoms and explore male perspectives about barriers to condom use.*

Method: *Mac and the audience have a confidential conversation about his private fears and hesitations about using condoms.*

Techniques:
BLOCK a decision to get and wear condoms by NAMING fears and deterrents
'YES BUT...' YES he loves any ideas about how to get out of condom use, BUT what could the consequences be?
BLOCK and PROBE, so audience works to convince Mac that nevertheless condom use is vital

Mac: We could use condoms, I guess but...well, everybody knows it's just not as good for the guy. Like, it reduces the sensation, that's what my brother says. And we don't have infections so maybe we don't need them...

MAC GATHERS and PROBES AUDIENCE ideas about why wearing condoms is important. He loves alternatives to condoms, but then BLOCKS with questions, doubts, and fears about effectiveness, comfort, availability, and CAROL ANN'S response. In this way, the AUDIENCE works harder and develops strong arguments for condom use. MAC is talked out of his initial position and agrees with the AUDIENCE that condoms are important, but he has other concerns...

Mac: Okay, okay, but...well, I've been thinking about it. Like how to get them. So I went to look, just check it out, a few weeks ago. I was just casually going up and down the aisles. I started to sweat, my mouth was all dry, and it was really embarrassing. I passed the condom rack three times and I couldn't do it. The pharmacist was staring at me, the other customers, the lady at the till. I can't buy them, I'm too nervous.

GATHERS *from* AUDIENCE.

Where else can I get protection?

GATHERS *ideas then* BLOCKS, *taking into account specific audience circumstances, such as cost, distance, quality, etc. Once these barriers are overcome,* MAC *is now completely ready to go buy or get condoms.*

Mac: Great! I'll [*or* Me and Carol Ann we'll] just go get some and—(*he turns to talk to her but has a sudden thought. He turns back to* AUDIENCE). So like...we get them and then...me and her are getting it on, all smooth and shivery and warm and...you know...and suddenly...Time to get your condom.

So first you have to turn on the light. Then you find it and open it and put it on and squeeze the air out and meanwhile what's she doing? Waiting for you, watching you...you feel like an idiot and...What if she sees you and you aren't...what she expected? What if everything just...fades away? What if she laughs? I don't know. I don't think I can do it.

MAC *gets advice about how to talk to* CAROL ANN *about his fears. He deliberately gets advice from both boys and girls in the* AUDIENCE. *He goes back to* CAROL ANN.

Mac: Carol Ann I think we should go get condoms and use them but...(MAC *references the* AUDIENCE *and uses their language and some of their suggestions. He concludes with...*) Don't laugh, okay?

Carol Ann: Ever?

Mac: No I mean, if it's...weird, or...something happens or...

Carol Ann: Okay, I won't laugh.

Mac: Promise?

Carol Ann: Mac, I'll have to laugh if it's funny and well...condoms are funny and we're both weird. It'll be okay. Come on, let's go buy them.

Mac: Okay, okay, I think I'm ready.

They acknowledge the AUDIENCE *and begin to exit.*

Carol Ann: Can I laugh if I'm surprised?

Mac: No.

Carol Ann: How about if I'm pleased?

Mac: Maybe. I know, you can laugh if I'm laughing.

Instructor Three: So Mac and Carol Ann have decided to go and get/buy condoms. Thank you very much for all your advice. I think you really helped them out.

If any misinformation was provided during the participation, INSTRUCTOR THREE *asks the* SEX EDUCATOR *for clarification. Thanks them for their help.*

Alex: (*entering*) I can do it, I know I can. I'm totally revved. I can corner, I can signal, I can brake and accelerate, I have all this safety information. So that's it, right?

Instructor Three: Whoa, whoa, yes you have a lot of information, but there are a few other things to keep in mind.

Alex: Like what?

Instructor Three: Sometimes things don't go as you expect.

> *Dealing with Obstacles (Lesson Four)*

ANNABELLE, HAL, JOSIE *and/or* MATEO *enter.*

Annabelle: I'm Annabelle. I'm twenty-one and in my second year of college. I went to a party last Christmas with my friend Mina. What happened there changed my life. I was raped. When I first got there, I was having a great time, drinking, partying, and then I met this guy, got talking to him and then kissing him, after that...big blank. I woke up on the floor between the bed and the wall in the room where everybody had put their coats. I had vomit all down my sweater, my skirt was up to my waist, my shoes and socks and underwear had disappeared. I felt like dying. I tried to find my friend but she was gone. I had to walk out through the living room. Trevor, this guy I liked, wouldn't even look at me. Nobody helped me; they wouldn't even make eye contact. Some of the guys were laughing and making comments.

When I got home my family went berserk. My brother wanted to kill the guy. My mum called the Sexual Assault Centre. I didn't want her to.

I figured I got drunk, it's my fault. And that's what some of you are thinking. I know that. Every time I tell this story, I see it in people's eyes. "She got what she deserved." But I see other things as well. Sometimes I see eyes that say, "That happened to me too." And so, I tell my story to let them know you're not alone, and you can survive. I'm learning to sort out what happened to me. Slowly, I'm beginning to understand that yes, I can take responsibility for my own behaviour, what I can't take responsibility for is what he did to me. Being drunk doesn't excuse what he did. They taught me that at the Sexual Assault Centre. They were great. They believed me. They said it was normal to feel angry, ugly, suicidal...all the things I was feeling. They gave me support and counselling. One of the women went with me to the hospital and the cops. I didn't press charges because I couldn't be sure who it was. It's been over a year now and I survived. My life was broken but I'm starting to put it back together.

Hal: I'm Hal, nineteen. First off, I'm not a pervert or anything. I'm not some big rapist or stalker, okay? I'm just a normal guy. Well, you just do what everybody does. In grade seven all the guys snap the girls' bras. You stand around outside the school and yell stuff at them as they walk by. "Hey, bet you can't touch your elbows behind your back..." "You've got the biggest... eyes I ever saw on a girl." You get the picture. It was like a competition, who could get a good one off, make everybody laugh. I knew it didn't make the girls feel very good, most of them, well I guess all of them but... they never said. In high school all the guys ever talked about was scoring. Scoring, scoring, nailing her tonight. Man, if those guys scored as much as they said they did...I knew they were lying but I didn't know how much. I was sixteen, still a virgin and really horny all the time. So I started seeing this girl that everybody said was easy. She wasn't but I tried everything, bought her stuff, told her I loved her, told her I was going to die if I didn't get laid. And one night we did it. I forced her. I didn't like, use violence or threats, I just pressured her until she gave up. She didn't want to, but she didn't want to break up either. So I won. But it didn't feel like I won, and we broke up anyway.

My sister is a school counsellor and I looked at this pamphlet she had about date rape. I guess I knew before but I didn't really put it all together. Finally I did. I sexually assaulted my girlfriend in grade eleven. I wish I hadn't. I wish I could go back and tell her. I'd tell her that I'm sorry. I hope she'd forgive me but I don't know if she would. This last winter I helped coach the junior high wrestling team at my old school. And I tell the guys, "think about how you'd like to be treated and treat girls like that. Why not try to find a way to behave around them so they feel good about themselves and their bodies, instead of like it's open season and any jerk can make a comment about them or hit on them any time?" And you know what? I think they're getting it.

Josie: My name is Josie. I'm eighteen. When I first started junior high I wasn't very popular. I had a few friends but wasn't part of the in crowd. Actually I wasn't part of any crowd. I felt like I didn't fit in and most of the time I felt invisible. And then...I think I just decided that I was going to change things. I used my allowance and babysitting money that I had saved and I bought a new me, new clothes, new hairstyle, everything. I made friends with some of the popular guys...I mean I flirted with them. A lot. And they started to notice me. And I loved it. I felt...finally worth something because I was getting noticed. And then it started getting crazy. I was going out all the time, hanging out at parties and stuff. There would always be lots of drinking. And one night in grade eight I was at this party and this guy who had been talking and laughing and hanging around me all night said we should go upstairs to the bedroom to talk where it was quieter. And I went with him. And we talked for a while. And then we started making out. Like really making out. And the next thing I know we're naked and having sex and I'm not thinking of the consequences or anything and he's not wearing a condom and it's awful. But at the time I thought it was great. I felt grown up because I had just done something most of the other girls at the party had never done. So I kept having sex, at first just with this one guy every once in a while and then more with other guys. Most of the time I would be going out with the guy but sometimes it was just sex at a party. And the whole time I thought I was so...cool. And then one day I was on Facebook and saw a post between two girls from school about how I was easy and a slut and would screw anything in pants. I couldn't believe it. My first reaction was that they were jealous but then I realized they weren't too far off. And I went home and cried. Who was I? Just something the guys could screw? What went wrong? Things changed after that. I stopped going to those parties and hanging out with that crowd. I cleaned up my act. I stopped drinking and didn't have sex in high school at all. I have a boyfriend now and things are really good with him but I'm always afraid that he'll hear about some of the stuff I used to do. I told him some of it but not all. And it's hard, you know. I mean I've changed but...it's hard enough living down reputations that aren't true...Imagine how hard it is to get over the ones that are.

Mateo: I'm Mateo, twenty-two. It started when I came out to Cherish in grade ten. No. Wait. It started way before that, like in grade one. I knew I was gay but I didn't know I knew, or I didn't know how to know. Gay! I couldn't be that. It was a swear word or weird or gross. I just knew I wasn't like other people so I figured I must be an alien in a human body. Me and Cherish were this unit in high school. She was fearless and funny; we were perfect together except...for the sex bit. That was really confusing. I'd be kissing her and suddenly I'd get this...like, she'd morph into this guy at school, Sunil. Whenever I saw Sunil my whole body turned to grape Jello. One morning I looked in the mirror and thought, well...just say it. So I did. "I am gay." I realized I wasn't an alien disguised as a human, I was a human.

I had to tell Cherish but I didn't want to hurt her or...or lose her. We got a little drunk at a dance and I spilled. There was yelling, stomping around, crying but finally we had a big hug and we were okay.

I didn't make her promise to keep it secret. She told one other person and by Monday morning it was all over school. It was pretty ugly, some of it, whispers, rumours, people hissing "faggot" at me as I walked down the hall. You know that naked at school dream? I was living it.

I started ditching a bunch. I would have been happy to never go back, just become a game tester that never graduated. But no, I had to finish. So I go and I'm at my locker, trying to chill and this guy comes up to me. I didn't know him, just some guy and he says, "Mateo, right?" I flinched 'cause, you never know. And he says, "Call the Pride Line, they're cool." And he hands me this card. That was a huge moment for me. I didn't know it at the time.

I did check it out, after a few weeks. I went to the youth drop-in and met some kids and adults who...it was like they knew me, inside and out.

They helped me get through those last two years of high school. Cherish too, she was great.

I've been living with Paul for two years now. His family is kind of old-school, sort of conservative, he's out to some of them, some know and pretend not to. Some will just never accept it. There's nothing you can do. You can only accept yourself, like, know yourself, be yourself.

Instructor Two: The experiences you've shared with the students are really hard to talk about. Thank you. I have a question to ask each of you. Why is it important for you to tell us your stories? Annabelle?

Annabelle: After I got raped, I started to cut myself and I wanted to die. My mum made me get help. If she hadn't I don't think I'd be here so...the important thing is to talk to someone, get some help and support, and not to blame yourself. Don't go through this alone.

Instructor Two: Hal?

Hal: Guys don't want to know. Most guys. I didn't. I had to step up...take a look at myself, say..."yeah that was me, I did that." It sucks. But, I want to respect myself and so...I have to respect other people. I hope my story helps others make better decisions.

Instructor Two: Josie?

Josie: Well, like Hal said about respecting yourself, but also about keeping yourself safe. And not just safe from infections or pregnancy but emotionally safe, you know? Feeling good about who you are and what you do. And if you have made a choice that doesn't feel right anymore, you can always change.

Instructor Two: Mateo?

Mateo: I just want...Maybe some guy or girl sitting out there is me, me when I was younger—confused, hurting, scared maybe. A guy I didn't know helped me out, and I can do that too. So, younger me, check out Youth Understanding Youth or call the Pride Centre.

Instructor Two: Thank you for sharing your stories Annabelle, Hal, Josie, Mateo.

ANNABELLE, HAL, MATEO, and JOSIE exit.

Young drivers make many choices when they get behind the wheel. Sometimes things go wrong. Recovering from a crash is hard, but with help, it can be done.

ALEX enters.

Alex: Man, I thought this was going to be easier. So how long does it take to get it all together?

Instructor Two: Well, the fact is...your whole life. Learning about sex is like learning to drive but it's not exactly the same. Sex is way more complex and difficult and it's also way more enjoyable and fun. Human beings aren't machines, and sex isn't just mechanics, signalling and safety equipment. But knowing about those things can help you prepare to make choices about abstinence, becoming sexually active, birth control and ways to prevent the transmission of infections, and what to do if something goes wrong. You never get to be an expert; you just learn more skills over time. Practice helps and Lesson Five is your chance to practice your skills.

> *Practice Your Skills (Lesson Five)*

Coach A (female): This next section is called "Practice Your Skills." It's a chance for you to take the wheel so let's review the rules of the road. Everyone has the right to express their opinion so respect the ideas and suggestions of others.

Coach B (male): Watch your language and no put-downs.

Coach A: And don't be shy. We want to hear from everyone.

Coach B: As we go along we'll add a few more rules. First we're going to bring out these "two lumps of Clay"...

CLAY CHARACTERS enter.

Coach A: ...and mould them into your ideal fantasy guy and girl.

> *Negotiating Complex Issues (Participation Four)*

Intention: *To build skills in negotiating complex issues.*

Method: *Audience groups (formed by gender) create characters and advise them through difficult moments in their relationship.*

Techniques: *Audience MOULDS living Clay and COACHES their Clay characters through complex situations.*

Step One: Stereotypes

Coach A: Now we need to split you into two groups. Guys on this side and girls on the other.

COACHES split group into two, by gender. FEMALE COACH teams with FEMALE CLAY; MALE COACH teams with MALE CLAY.

Coach B (male): I'm going to take this lump of Clay (*male*) over to the girls.

Coach A (female): And I'll take this lump of Clay (*female*) over to the guys.

COACHES take their lumps of CLAY over to their respective groups. AUDIENCE MOULDS the CLAY by answering the COACH'S questions:

- *What does he/she look like?*
- *What is his/her personality like?*
- *What is she/he into? Likes?*
- *What is his/her name?*
- *What is a saying they use?*

CLAY exits to get ready.

Coach A: Okay, our Clay [Name given by Audience]...

Coach B: ...and our Clay [Name given by Audience]...

Coach A: ...are going to get ready. While they're getting ready we can go over a couple of rules.

Coach B: Number One: Foul. No inappropriate suggestions or comments. You know what they are.

Coach A: Number Two: When we blow these whistles it means the scene has come to an end or that we need to move on.

Coach B: Or it's getting a little too loud and we need to quiet down. Okay, can we get a place these two can meet? Where would be a good place for our ideal guy and girl to meet for the first time?

COACHES GATHER suggestions and pick one.

Coach B: Okay, they are going to meet at the [location]. (*Calls to CLAY*) [Name given by Audience] How are you doing back there?

CLAY CHARACTER responds, using his saying.

And [Name given by Audience] how are you doing?

CLAY CHARACTER responds, using her saying.

Coach A and B: Okay! In three, two, one...(*Blow whistles to begin scene*).

CLAY CHARACTERS emerge in outrageous stereotyped form. One at a time, they establish their location, two or three of their traits and then they notice each other. There is an instant attraction, played big. They meet and get close very fast, usually with the help of a few cheesy pickup lines or moves.

COACHES whistle down the action before it goes too far.

Coach A: Well, what do you think of these two? Girls, what do you think of [Female Clay Name]?

Quick GATHER from the girls.

Coach B: And guys, what do you think of [Male Clay Name]?

Quick GATHER from the boys.

Coach A: How realistic are these characters? (*Brief AUDIENCE response*) So these two need some adjustments. I'm going to take [Name] over to the girls for a tune-up...

Coach B: ...and I'll take [Name] over to the guys for some realignment.

Step Two: Real People

COACHES take CLAY over to their new team (girls with girls and boys with boys). Each team creates a new, more realistic character, someone who would go to their school, is their age, etc.

CLAY sheds the stereotype costume pieces. COACHES and CLAY (out of role) work with their group to develop new answers to the previous questions and make some new decisions. Questions include:

- *What do you think about his/her name? Do we need to change it?*
- *What about her/his personality? What is he/her like?*
- *What is his/her favourite subject?*
- *What does he/she like to do? Hobbies? Sports?*
- *What's a saying he/she says all the time?*
- *What about a pet peeve? Something that really bugs him/her.*

After all the information is offered, CLAY repeats all the changes back to his/her team, gradually taking on the characteristics. The COACHES prompt for a final detail:

Coach A and B (in their groups): Now she/he is sounding pretty perfect so far. Can we get a personality flaw to make her/him more realistic?

CLAY takes in the suggestions, selects one and EXITS to get ready.

Step Three: Meeting Someone

Coach A: While these two are getting ready we're going to go over two more rules. Number Three: no interference. That means no cross coaching. Girls, you can't tell the guy what to do and guys, you can't tell the girl what to do. You are responsible for your character only.

Coach B: Number Four: Time Out. The characters can call a Time Out if they need help from you and you can call Time Out if you see some place to offer a suggestion.

Coach A: The goal of this section is to help your Clay out and to give them advice to get through their lives. We're going to be dealing with how to negotiate through a relationship. Today, we will be focusing on a heterosexual, girl-guy relationship. The same issues can apply to same-sex relationships.

Coach B: Absolutely! Now we'll get them to meet in (*GATHERS a different more realistic place or sticks to the same location if it is appropriate.*) (*Calls*) [Clay Characters' Names], how are you two doing back there?

CLAY CHARACTERS answer with the saying given by their team.

Coach A: So we'll start the scene...

Coach A and B: ...in three, two, one...(*whistle*)

CLAY CHARACTERS come out, see each other, have an instant attraction and call TIME OUT.

They rush to their team to ask advice on how to approach the other. They GATHER suggestions, then go back into the scene.

Using the suggestions, and with SIDE COACHING from their team, they PLAY OUT a brief scene until they have established some kind of communication and have introduced themselves to each other.

One of the COACHES blows the whistle and the CLAY CHARACTERS freeze.

Step Four: Asking Someone on a Date

Coach A: Okay, it looks like they're talking and getting along. We're going to jump ahead in time two weeks. They've both run into each other a few times, but neither one's had the courage to ask the other one out.

Coach B: The goal of this section is to have one of them take the plunge. It doesn't matter which one asks. So at [location]...

Coaches A and B: ...in three, two, one...(*whistles*)

CLAY CHARACTERS improvise meeting. Both want to ask the other on a date, but they are hesitant. There are OBSTACLES. They need advice and GATHER ideas from their team. CLAY and COACH can ask their team: how should I ask, what should I say, what will she or he think of me, what if she or he says no, etc. The COACH returns the team and the CLAY back to reality when necessary.

When a date is agreed on, COACHES blow their whistles and the CLAY CHARACTERS freeze.

Coach B: Okay. Good work everyone.

CLAY thanks their team and exits.

Step Five: Dealing with a Relationship Crisis

Coach B: Now let's say they went out on their date and everything went great. They like each other and decided to keep seeing each other. They have now been dating for three months but a conflict has arisen. It's time for them to have a serious private conversation. Where could they have this talk?

COACHES GATHER from AUDIENCE and select a location.

Coach A: Okay, great, but before they have their talk, let's have them out here to find out what's been going on in their relationship. [Clay Name] and [Clay Name] can you come out here?

CLAY CHARACTERS rush out to their teams to give them a short update on the relationship and the issue he/she is struggling with. In this section there is a sense of sharing something very serious among friends.

They have been going out for three months. Five days ago they had consensual sex. They had safe, protected sex and both agreed to do it willingly. Afterwards though, one character decided that they aren't ready for sex and would like to take a step back in their relationship. The other character felt comfortable with sex and would like to continue having it. But they haven't talked about any of this. The character who was comfortable has been trying to get in touch for five days but the other has not returned the calls, texts, emails, etc. They are about to meet. Both are worried about what is going to happen next. They need advice on how best to proceed.

They GATHER *advice from their teams.* CLAY *thanks team and enters scene.*

Coach B: So at [location]...

Coaches A and B: ...in three, two, one...(*whistles*)

This is the most complex and difficult negotiation in the play. CLAY CHARACTERS *attempt to bring up issues discussed with their teams. Throughout this scene* CLAY *asks for and applies their team's advice. There are many* OBSTACLES. *With the* AUDIENCE'S SIDE COACHING, CLAY CHARACTERS *attempt to renegotiate their relationship. They work through these stages:*

1. *Emotional fallout and obstacles*
2. *The news from one character that he or she wants to stop having sex for now*
3. *Renegotiation of personal sexual boundaries*

When the CHARACTERS *have made substantial progress* COACHES *stop scene at a natural end.*

Coach B: So how are these two doing?

GATHERS *a few insights from* AUDIENCE.

Coach A: (*To* CLAY CHARACTERS) Did you feel like all your issues were addressed?

CLAY CHARACTERS *answer.*

> *Wrap Up*

Coach B: Okay, so these two are off to a good start. Who knows what the future may hold for them. They may stay together...they may break up. Only time will tell.

Coach A: Can we get one last piece of advice for these two before we send them off to the rest of their lives? (GATHERS *from* AUDIENCE) Thanks.

CLAY CHARACTERS *thank their teams.* CLAY *and* COACHES *shed their personas.*

Actor A: You guys gave great advice. [Educator's Name] will be coming back to do a workshop with you on (*Checks with* EDUCATOR *who provides the day*).

Actor B: We're going to be setting up for the next show/packing our stuff away so if any of you have any questions you would like to ask one of us one-on-one, feel free to just come up and say hi.

Actor C: Nobody has all the answers and what may be okay for one person may not be okay for you. So check in, ask questions, and use the resources on those cards we gave you to help you out when you need it.

Actor D: And we appreciate your questions, comments, and your participation. Thanks guys...

All: Bye!

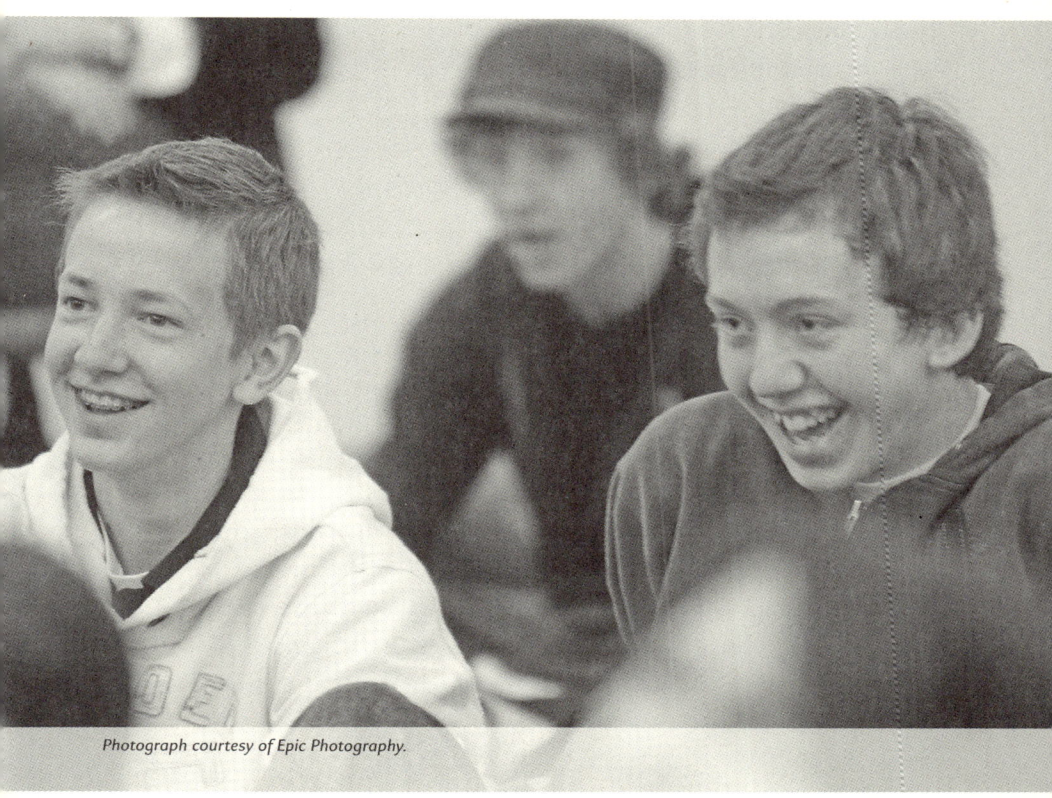
Photograph courtesy of Epic Photography.

UNPACKING THE PLAY

> *Everyone has the same questions and stuff, you're normal. You might not feel it like yet...you might think you're alone, like you don't know what everything's about, but then other people are acting like they know what everything is but they don't really know either so...You kinda, like, think you're alone, but you're not.*
>
> —*Audience Member*[4]

Are We There Yet? is a series of short scenes and progressively longer and more complex participations. If the audience is not engaged with the characters and the situations, if they don't see themselves on stage, then they won't help. There is no show if the audience doesn't advise the characters, so in a pretty graphic and visceral way we know the characters and situations represent what this audience faces because they always talk—a lot.

> *It was like…a teenager's perspective on the issue and like how the adults would… help us get through this, and we all talked about that and how cool we thought it was…at first we thought…maybe it was adults…trying to look into us, but it ended…that it was our way of figuring stuff out. It was…almost the entire play was based around what we were thinking.*

Participation

The participation in AWTY is the result of many years of experimenting and testing. The participation begins when the actors, stage manager, and sex educator enter the school. No matter how they're feeling, they are always thrilled to be there. Any student, teacher, or staff member that sees them sees the people who are here to do the sex show. How they walk and carry the set, how they talk to each other and welcome the audience keeps saying the same thing: yes. Yes, we're here to talk about sex; yes, it's funny; yes, it's hard to talk about; yes, it's human; yes, it's how you got here; yes, it can kill; yes, it's on your mind; and yes, it's normal.

> *It's really interactive so you find it more interesting. It's not like some of those plays where it's just…they're doing their thing but it's like we're not even here.*

Students tend to have a finely tuned detector for the false *yes*. The early participations are designed to allow them to test the trustworthiness of the show and the actors. The degree to which they trust the show not to preach, talk at them, retreat into embarrassment, avoid the tough questions, or otherwise betray them, determines the degree and depth of the participation.

Intentions Scene by Scene

"Just a Minute" (page 68)

This participation sets the tone for the show and takes the first formal step toward establishing trust.

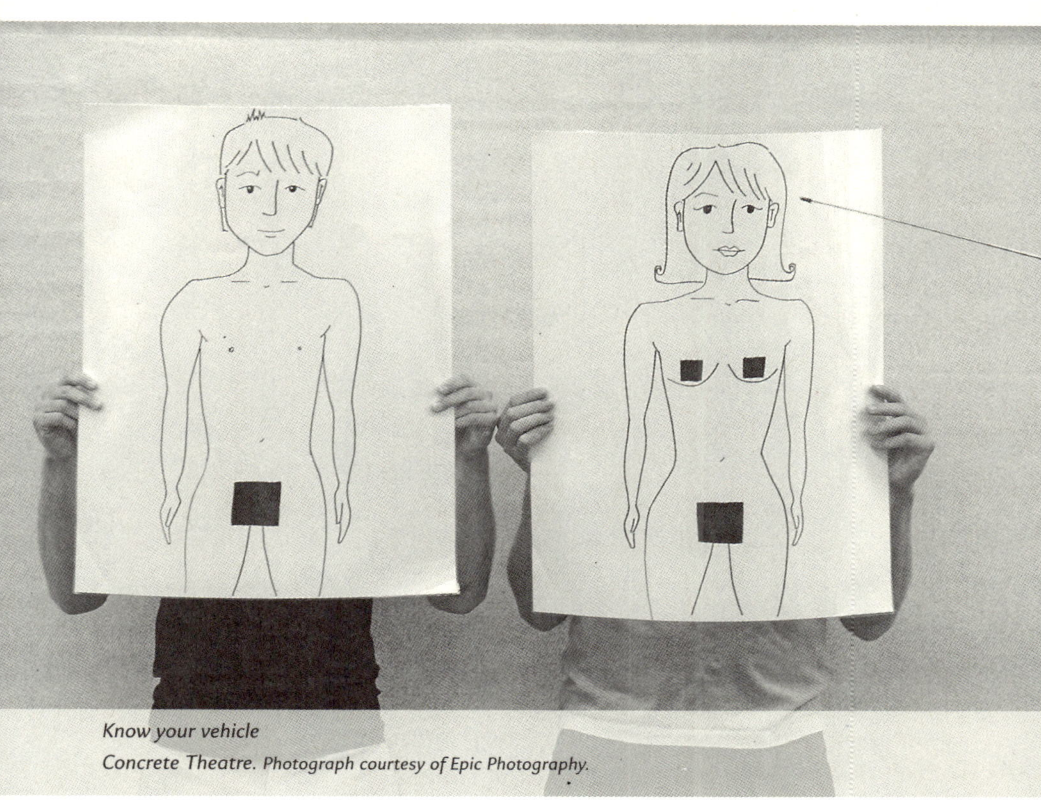

Know your vehicle
Concrete Theatre. Photograph courtesy of Epic Photography.

Tone

Tone is signalled from the first and most important question: How do you feel? Not: what do you do? Not: what do you know? Not: how does reproduction or a condom work? But *how do you feel?* Immediately, those feelings are fed back, heightened, and theatricalized. Actors take the feelings the audience names and make them into stories. Those first brave students to talk to the actors get a reward. A sex educator might do the same thing: ask for feelings, collect them, and then say, "that is normal." But what the actors do is make it normal. The actors have pretty much free rein to tell whatever story they want about sex, in a minute, without pause, while making eye contact with audience members. Usually students will name embarrassment, horny, and shy. The stories the actors tell are often funny and always true.

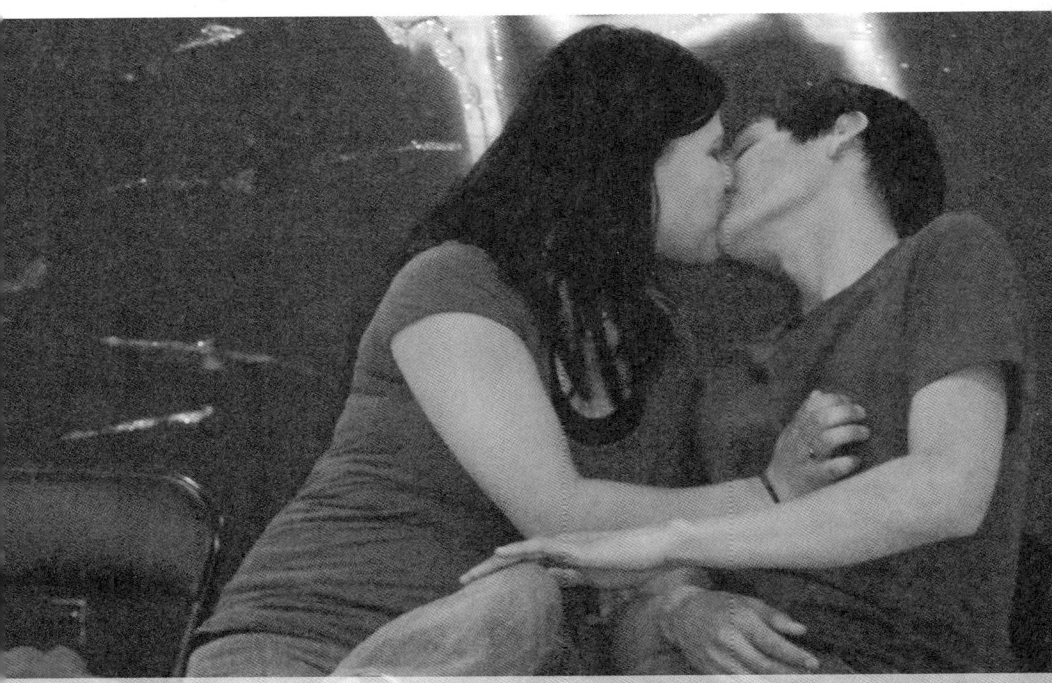

Signs and signals
Clifford Cardinal and Krystle Pederson, Saskatchewan Native Theatre Company. *Photograph courtesy of Jane Heather.*

> *They (actors) weren't shy because some of the guys they came down and they talked to us. They sat down on the floor and we talked. It was good, I liked it...They were all really happy to be there. You could tell.*

Trust

Is it real participation or is it phony? Do you really hear what we say or only what you want to hear? Will you really talk about sex or only about mechanics and morals? Can I trust you? This participation is low-risk for audience and high-risk for actors.

[I liked] the part that you weren't scared to make a suggestion and they would go through with your suggestion. You get to say whatever you want even if it's...like, funny or doesn't make sense.

"Know Your Vehicle" (page 70)

After this participation the driving metaphor is introduced and the student driver gets her first lesson.

There is no participation in this section as its intention is to provide information and build common language. It is impossible to determine where students are at in terms of sexual knowledge so "Know Your Vehicle" (with cheesy drawings) and "Puberty and You" (the 1950s puberty film) aim to name the parts and allow for both real and feigned sophistication. Even if every single student is totally knowledgeable about puberty and their bodies, they are engaged and entertained by how the driving/car metaphor is extended, and they recognize the puberty film in tone if not in fact.

The last piece of this section is a long list of all the questions that teens (or at least these character teens) have but can't ask. By the magic of theatre, they all get spilled out but the adult/parent instructor can't hear them, only the audience. This models that characters will want to ask the audience things they may not feel able to ask their parents or other adults.

When the girl's trying to talk to her mom it seemed as though the mom was trying to just get her off the entire idea of it; parents aren't necessarily comfortable discussing sex and relationships and so they are not always helpful if we have questions or concerns.

"Signs and Signals": Marcel and Delphi (page 72)

The scene where the male and female are both saying they are ready, neither knows what the other is talking about—just assumed that the other knew but it is important to talk about it to make sure both people understand what is going on.

Setting Boundaries: Part One (page 72)

The intention of this participation is to have the audience consider and discuss delaying sexual intercourse. The audience helps the characters move from inarticulate longing and miscommunication to being able to identify personal boundaries and communicate them to a sexual partner. Unlike life, however, there is an instructor who can intervene and a group of peers who can help. As is usual, the characters are much less articulate and much more embarrassment bound than most of the audience. The audience knows what the problem is, the characters do not. The audience is the expert on feelings and expressing them.

> *You didn't have to participate if you didn't want to, but...it's really easy for us to tune out and, like, just not pay attention. But the participation thing made you pay attention...our input really had a big impact on them.*

Part Two (page 75)

The other intention is to clearly articulate sexual activities that are not intercourse and to define abstinence. In this case, the audience is not the expert. They may all know it, but they are not asked to generate the list. That is the job for Instructor Two and Sexuality Educator, the adults in the room. This is for safety and to keep building trust. There is a right answer to *what is abstinence?*[5] and there is a list of sexual activities. The actors don't go on a fishing expedition to get the correct answer. Kids have to put up with the humiliation of fishing all the time in school. This guess-what-I'm-thinking method is insulting and an anathema to participation.

> *The boundary thing was pretty cool, made me think about other people's boundaries not just, like mine.*

Part Three (page 76)

Once the characters and the audience have drawn the line for their personal boundary and the characters have communicated that to each other, the power goes back to the audience. With information and language to express that information, the characters need to negotiate. Again, the audience is the expert on feelings and expressing them.

Well...[I learned] ways to say no, and there are like ways to talk with your boyfriend or girlfriend kind of thing. The way of, like, communicating with a partner.

"Safety Equipment and Procedures" (page 77)

This participation has quite a long set up. Similar to the 1950s sex ed film at the beginning of the show, pop culture tropes and the driving metaphor are employed.

"Studley Muffin and Creamy Delight Go for a Spin" (page 77)

The puberty film communicates that we know and acknowledge the pitiful sex ed most students receive in school, and the first part of the Creamy Delight/Studley Muffin scene acknowledges the aberrant sex education kids get from pop culture and the media. Although these sections are not participatory, they are central to establishing communication between student and actor. If nothing else, it communicates that we (adults) are ashamed of the pathetic and appalling way in which we have neglected you in terms of sex. First we put a medical drawing of fallopian tubes on the overhead and call it sex ed. Then we saturate the very air with porn and tell you to practice abstinence. Sorry, we'd like to make it up to you a bit.

Like a really good way to relate with teens and cuz...teens we don't want to sit in the class and have someone just talk about "Oh, here's a condom" and you know, they actually made it funny so we can relate to it.

Studley Muffin and Creamy Delight enact two metaphorical driving scenes. In the first, they are sophisticated, sexy, powerful "drivers." In the second, they are more like real teen "drivers," awkward, embarrassed, eager. The thrill of driving gets away on them, and they get in an "accident." In the scene that leads to participation, the couple (Mac and Carol Ann) is in a similar situation.

"When is the Right Time to Talk about Condoms?" (page 79)

After the teen driving accident, the instructor takes the stage again to introduce condom use and the issues teens will explore in the next section of the play. The instructor asks the audience to identify which question teens

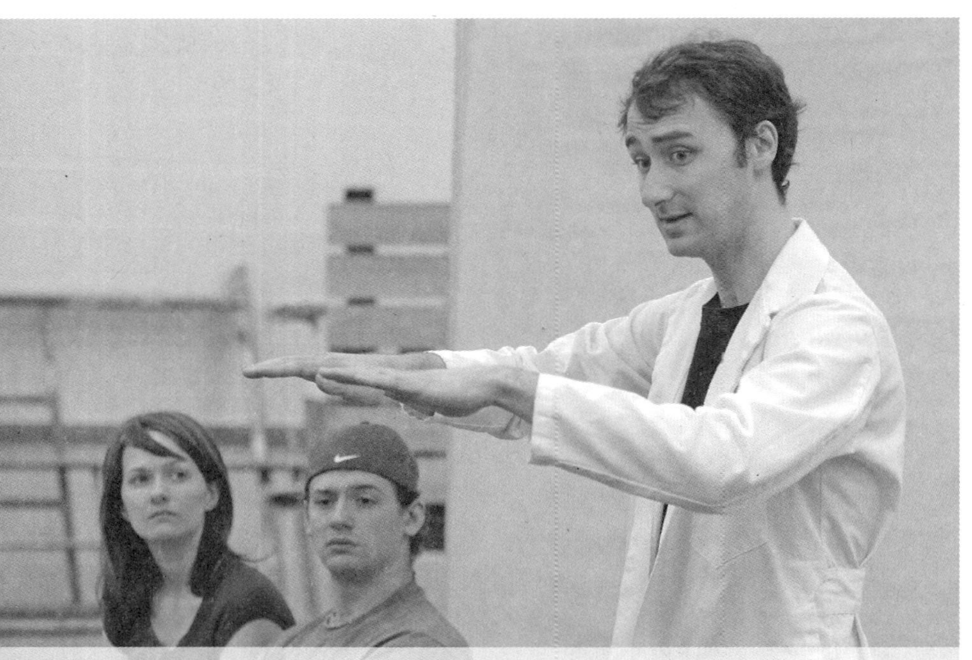

Personal boundaries
Kristi Hansen, Ryland Alexander, and Jeremy Baumung, Concrete Theatre. Photograph courtesy of Epic Photography.

ask most often about condom use and offers three possibilities: (1) What size should I buy? (2) Which brand is most effective? And (3) how do I raise condom use with my partner? Teen audiences are offered a chance to participate here and offer their opinion about the most commonly asked question. With or without audience input, the instructor informs them that questions teens ask most often about condoms use is number three, how do I bring up condom use with my partner?

> *Like everyone's always telling us to take precautions like birth control and condoms or whatever, but they never tell us like how to talk about it with anyone. It was a more realistic way to talk about it.*

The audience then sees three short scenes where this "touchy topic" is handled poorly. The intention of these non-participatory short scenes is

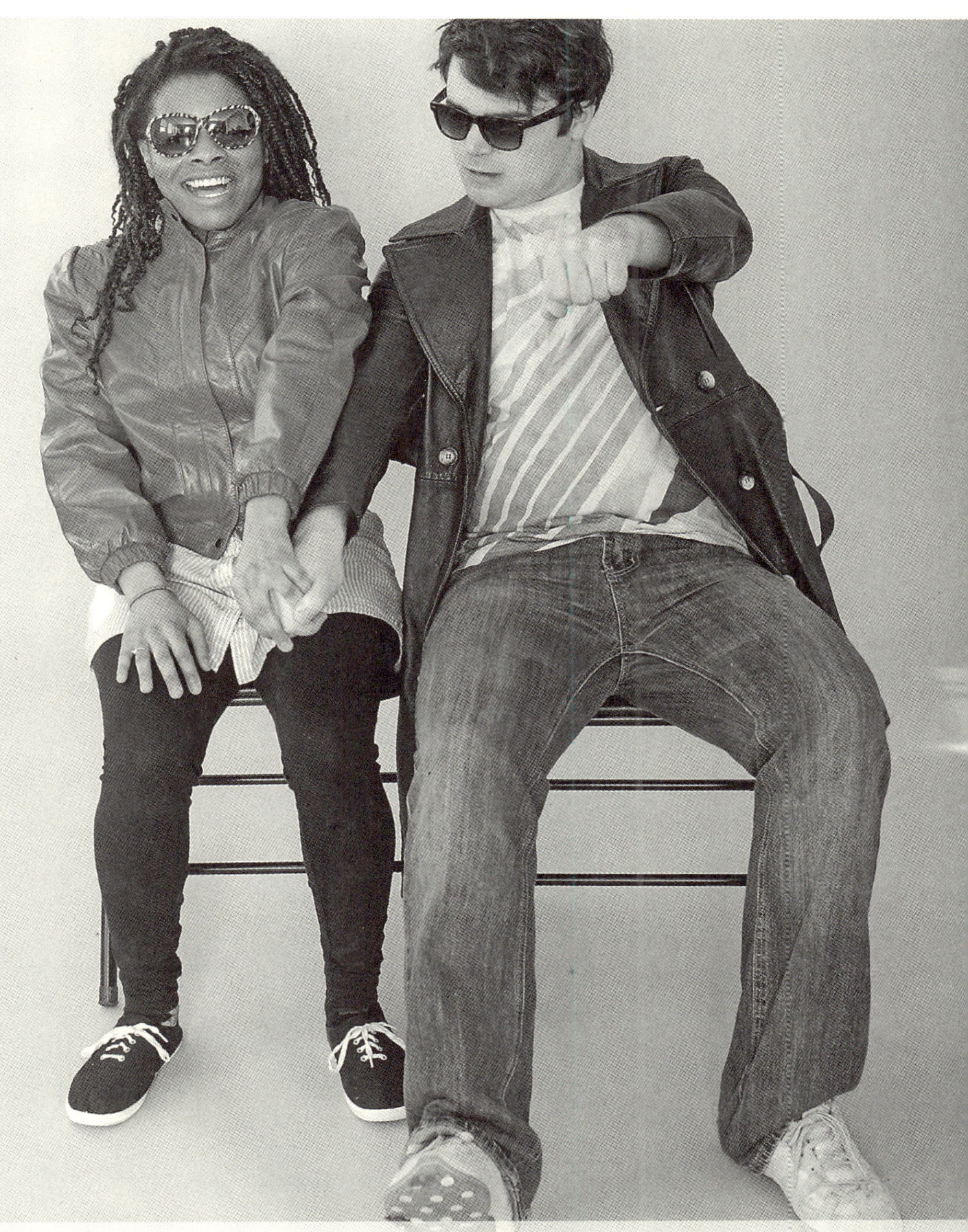

Your technique is magnifique
Monice Peter and Garett Spelliscy, Concrete Theatre. Photograph courtesy of Epic Photography.

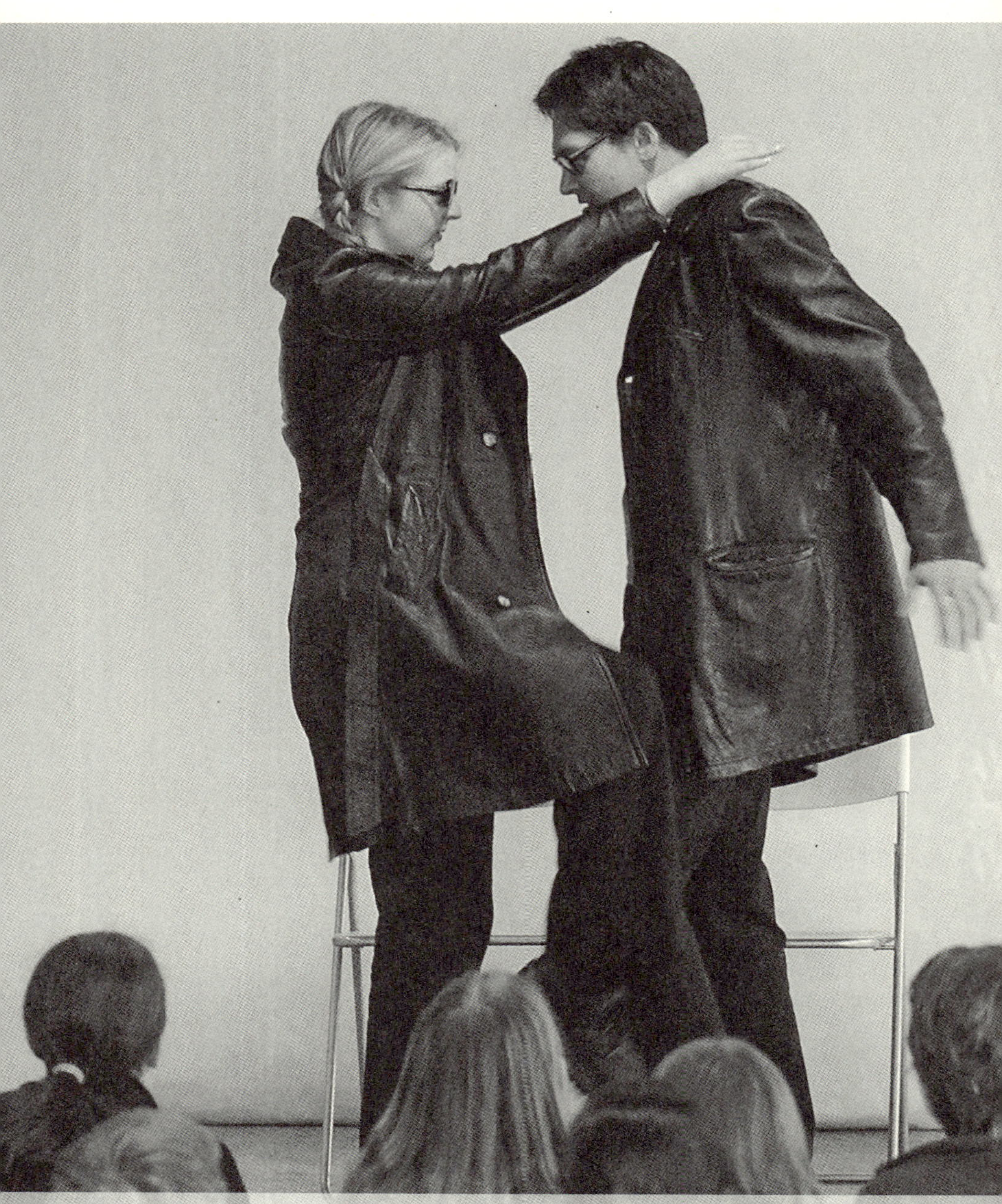

Feel the excitement, feel the thrill
Jana O'Connor and Jared Matsunaga-Turnbull, Concrete Theatre. *Photograph courtesy of Epic Photography.*

threefold: to acknowledge that it is difficult to bring up condom use with a partner, to have a brief glimpse of two gay characters who might have sex, and to have one brief wordless scene where it is clear the characters have had sex. One of the conundrums of a play on this topic, for this audience, in the schools, is how to talk about sex without ever showing sex, and how to include a representation of a gay sexual relationship. The first quick scene is between two boys. They are meeting for the first time and one asks the other how he feels about using condoms. Although the scene is very short, in the Concrete Theatre production one of the characters wears a rainbow scarf and that is enough, in addition to his question, to signal that the two boys are gay. It is too soon in the relationship to bring up condom use, states the instructor.

The scene with Ben and Fern, which is wordless, shows two characters in bed waking up, discovering themselves and the other person naked. The actions of the characters are a quick, accessible cartoon of a common situation that many humans experience: unprotected sex on a whim. The morning after, says the instructor, is too late to bring up condom use.

These two small short scenes set up the following scene ("Talking Protection"). In the scene, Carol Ann and Mac appear on stage thrashing under a blanket. Carol Ann stops the action and tries to bring up using a condom. She is unable to and escapes from the situation babbling a lame excuse. This method is declared by the instructor to be "too indirect."

"Talking Protection": Mac and Carol Ann (page 79)

> *It was just like how...the guy was trying to take this girl on a date and they wanted to have sex but she wasn't ready but she wanted to use a condom and that happens in everyday life. It was just real.*

The intention here is to ask the audience to practice talking about condom use with their partner, present and work through problems or blocks to condom use, and to provide information about where to get them. The scene assumes some audience members are already sexually active and that all of them are likely to be at some point. Both the male (Mac) and the female (Carol Ann) characters need advice from the audience. Carol Ann needs

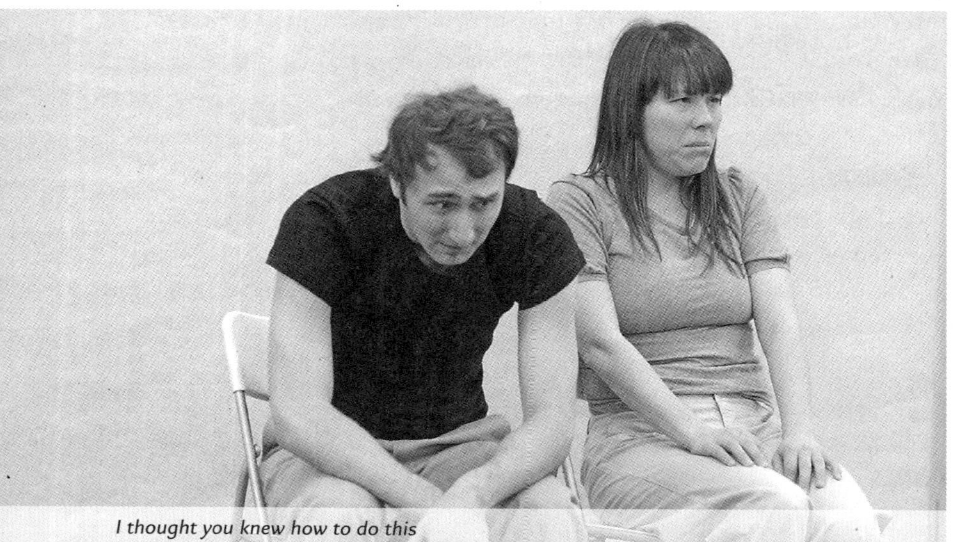

I thought you knew how to do this
Jeremy Baumung and Nadien Chu, Concrete Theatre. Photograph courtesy of Epic Photography.

advice about how to raise the topic, and Mac needs advice about how to overcome his fears and reluctance to use condoms.

The participation focuses on this sequence: if you are having sex, be safe, how to do that. The sequence is not: you had unsafe sex, what to do about the consequences. Everything in the show up until this point is underpinned with a strong message that young people can figure out how to make healthy sexual choices. The characters in the scenes up until this point (Marcel and Delphi, and Mac and Carol Ann) are rather idealized and the audience is able to help them avoid making a poor choice. In order to continue to be worthy of the audience's trust some of the very real issues of drunk and high sex, poor self-esteem, multiple partners, sexual assault, and others must now be explored.

"Dealing with Obstacles" (page 83)

> *[I liked] the first one, where the girl got sexually abused, I had an experience like that so I could relate to that. So yeah...I thanked her [actor] for it.*

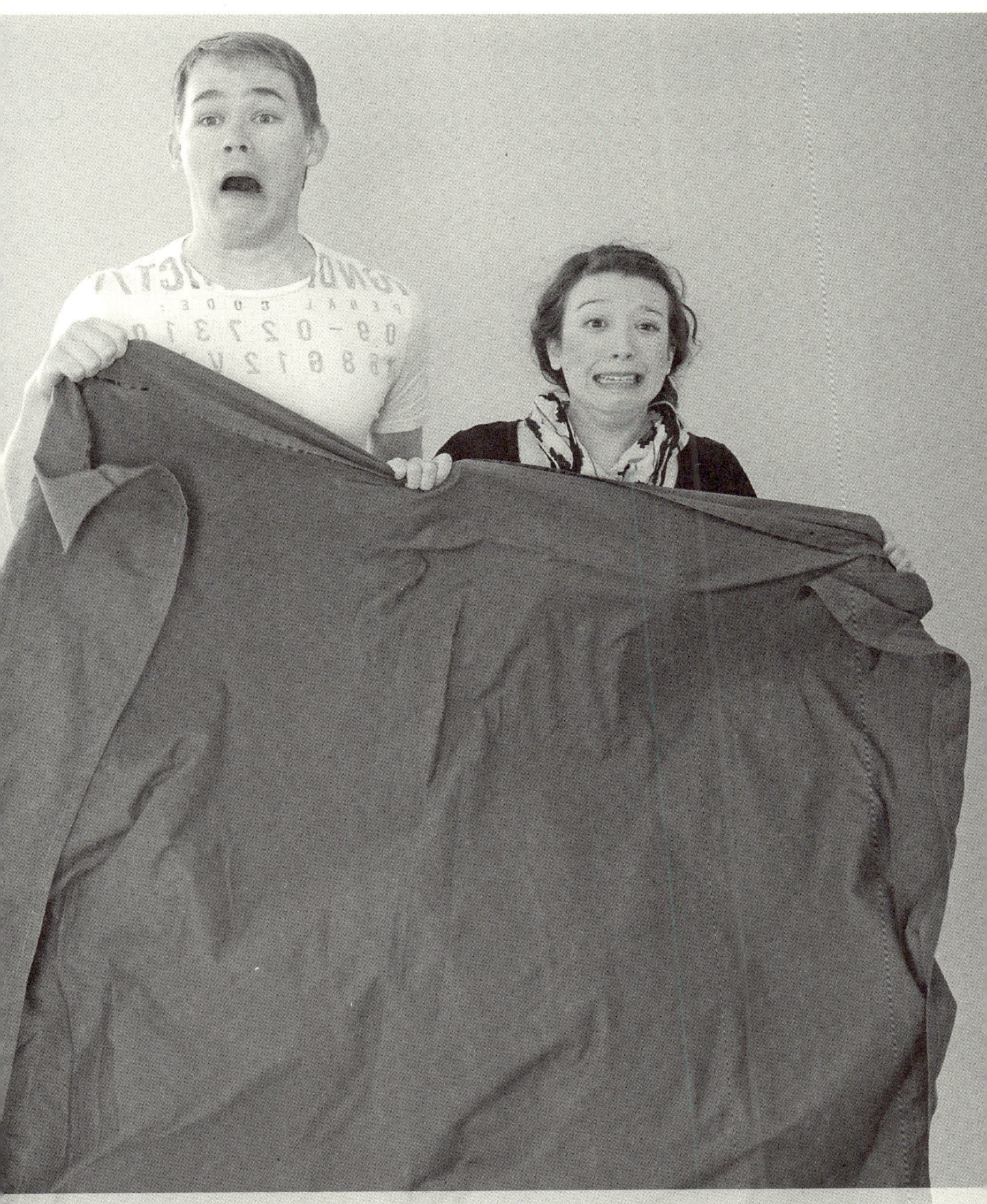

Too late
Cole Humeny and Ming Hudson, Concrete Theatre. Photograph courtesy of Epic Photography.

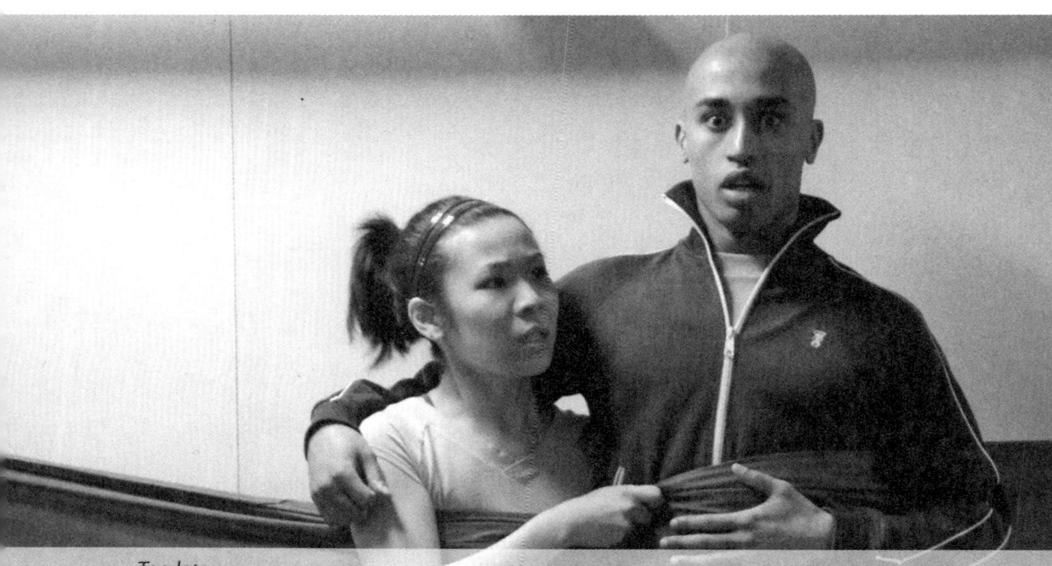

Too late
Evelyn Chu and Luc Roderique, Neworld Theatre. *Photograph courtesy of Tim Matheson.*

This part of the show is completely different in form, tone, and rhythm from everything before or after. If we think of the show as a piece of music, the melody is light and peppy with lots of trills and energetic, sunny swoops. The bass line is something else: the very real and terrible sexual experiences that some young people endure. The bass line is always present in the play, as it is in the culture, but until this point it is not named. This section is not participatory; it is a series of four stories about the consequences of some sexual choices. No character is pregnant, HIV-positive, or infected. This is a deliberate choice. The intention is not to ignore or underplay the unplanned pregnancy, sex=death, or disease scenario but to say mistakes happen and with help you can survive. This section also scoops up and speaks to the kids who have already had horrible sexual experiences and have yet to see anything in the show that acknowledges their pain. There is no participation here because it is the adults that must carry the risk, not the children. It is this section that is most likely to allow a student to approach an actor or the sexual health educator after the show and, it is hoped, seek help if these stories reflect their reality.

"Practice Your Skills": Living Clay (page 88)

> *Well, yeah because like kids at my age, we don't want to sit in a classroom. We just don't. So when you start getting like, people, moving and up and just...the motion of like just not being in a classroom you get the message across quite easier.*

There is an abrupt change in tone and pace as the show launches into the final section. The transition from the previous monologue section is short but crucial. The Alex character comes on to talk to the Instructor character for the last time. She is thoughtful and rather grave. The adult (the Instructor) gets one last chance to say keep learning and communicating, good sex takes a long time. Then we are back to participation and an opportunity to pull the previous participations together. The success of this sequence of participations depends on building ownership. The audience is invited to construct a character that is like someone they know and coach them through a relationship. Living Clay is the technique.

> *I got more comfortable with the subject; I think that was the biggest thing. It's just it's not as big a deal as it was. Yeah, it makes it easier to talk about it and yeah, accept it.*

"Step One: Stereotypes" (page 89)

The intention of this part of "Practice Your Skills" is to decentre and disrupt sexual/gender stereotypes. When the audience is asked to create an ideal fantasy character, they will (usually) create gender stereotypes. Boys create a stereotypical female and the girls create a stereotypical male. Each group acknowledges that the "ideal" is not very "realistic" and they then work with their own gender group to create a more real character. The intention is two-fold: one, to get the silly stuff cleared out and get more serious, and, two, to continue to build ownership. Each gender needs to feel that they are advising a friend that they like and that they invest in. Control over character traits, name, hobbies, flaws all introduce the proxy nature of the character.

Well, like, doing that clay molding. We gc crazy on that one...the boys made a Pocahontas and we made a Romeo so it's, so far-fetched from actual reality and nobody actually "wants" that because it's always like too perfect but it's fun just imagining the possibilities.

"Step Two: Real People" (page 90)

It was more fun when we actually created the real character, like not the glamorous character, the real character. Because we got to design a real person and like a real saying, and a real attitude and with real problems. So, it was kind of good.

In this section students are asked to create a more real teen, someone they could know, who might go to their school. By creating a character of their own, audiences invest in the character's dilemmas and problems. The character and the teen team create an alliance and work together on the next set of problems.

"Step Three: Meeting Someone" (page 91)

This stage is another step in building ownership and investment. The characters go back to their team regularly to get advice and quickly try it out. The problem is to meet someone but that is only the frame. The goal is to ask, hear, and try what the audience advises and to invest them with the power to direct the character. Characters take good advice, poor advice, and silly advice. Each actor works to use the exact words given to them and improvises with the other actor.

"Step Four: Asking Someone on a Date" (page 92)

Because these characters will eventually have a good strong relationship, another step is getting a date. In addition to continuing to build the ownership, the actors also ask the audience to go deeper. In some cases, they get poor or frivolous advice and the actor takes it into the scene. In this way, the consequences of bad advice are revealed. This works toward encouraging audiences to go beyond the superficial and take responsibility for the advice they give.

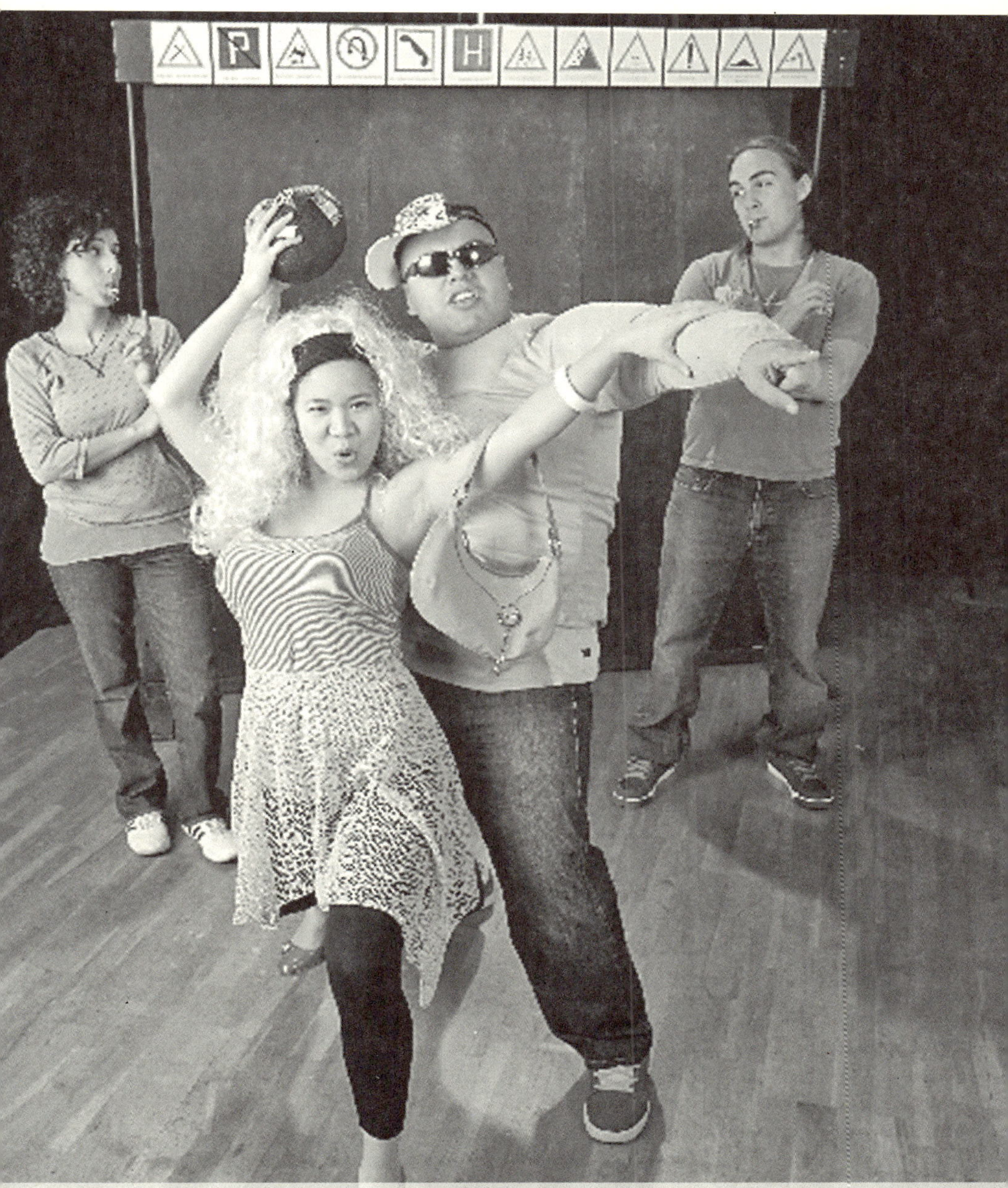

Stereotypes
Azin Sadr, Evelyn Chu, Pedro Chamale, and Raes Calvert, Neworld Theatre. Photograph courtesy of Tim Matheson.

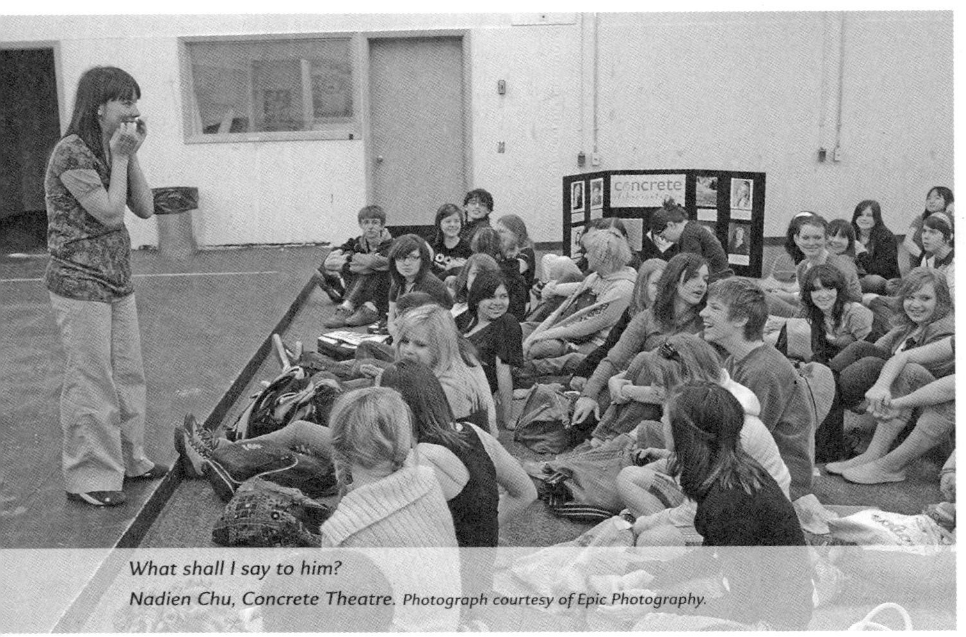

What shall I say to him?
Nadien Chu, Concrete Theatre. Photograph courtesy of Epic Photography.

> *Yeah, it was because you got to see, like what you said, how it would come into effect. Like if you said something negative you'd get to see how it play out but if you said something good you got to see what was the best thing and it was your ideas and all that so...*

"Step Five: Dealing with a Relationship Crisis" (page 92)

Having sex and changing your mind. The final part of this participation requires a serious, private talk between the character and their team. There is a crisis in the relationship and the characters have to get good advice. When they have told their story and got some advice, they begin the scene. The pattern of trying, checking with the team, trying something else, and having a success is repeated here but with the most serious and weighty emotional stakes.

> *Sex ed and health class...just becomes the same thing over and over again and you're learning...facts. You're not learning opinions, you're not learning how to deal with it...and you're not really getting...to how you would handle it. Like you might*

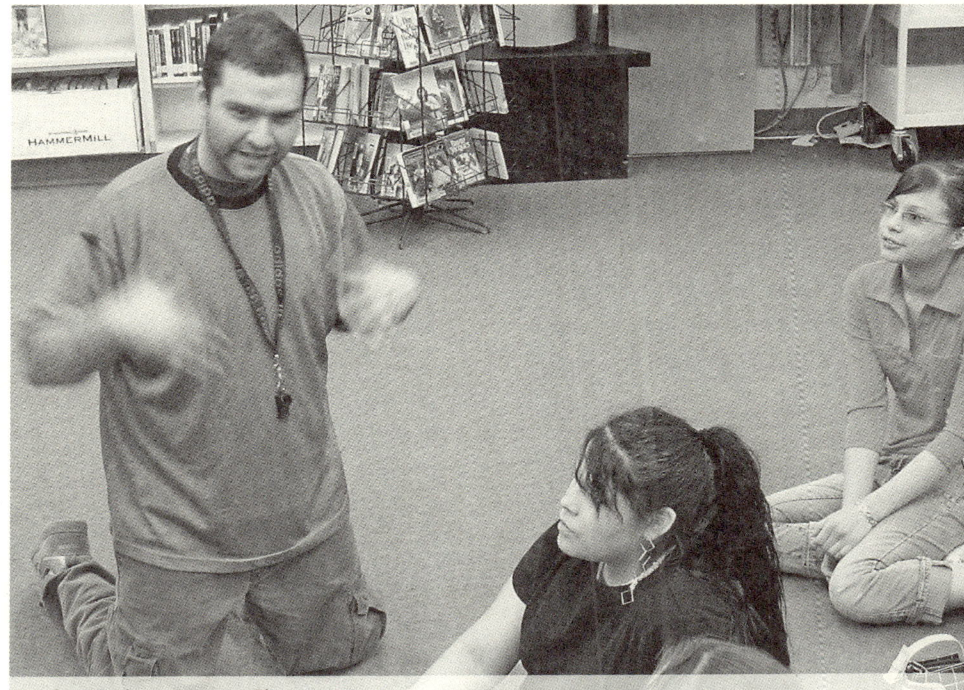

Nathan Cuckow, Concrete Theatre. Photograph courtesy of Epic Photography.

> *end up in a situation but all those classes...won't really help you because...they're not...telling you how to deal with it or how to say no or how to get around to talking about it. They're just telling you, you can get STDs, you can do this, that, and... it doesn't work.*

Once this section is complete, the show is over but not the participation. Actors revert to actors and begin the task of taking down the set or preparing for the next show. Each actor, stage manager, and sexual health educator maintains a relaxed and receptive demeanour. Audience members may approach someone with a question or comment or a disclosure. Disclosures are rare but they do occur, and this is one of the reasons to have a sexuality educator travel with the show. (See Chapter 6 on protocols for dealing with disclosures.)

Everyone is off shift when the last student leaves the room. Then actors, stage manager, and health educator discuss the show, especially the participations.

Debriefing after the show was incredibly important. Was it a good performance? Was it a bad performance? A discussion of was it a good performance for you as an actor, or was it a good performance for the audience? Because it's not the same thing. Are We There Yet? *is about the audience, and to keep that on track it, it all depends on the actor. So long as the actor knows that the show is outside of themselves, that is just a little reminder that they might need as the weeks go on.*

—*Gina Puntil,* AWTY *stage manager, Concrete Theatre*

NOTES

1. See Appendix 1.3 for a list of the goals provided to the program assessors.
2. Actually I do know why. If this program is so great, a lot more kids should get to see it, and if it stays a play many youth will be left out. If it was online, the impact would be so much greater, and isn't it just a bit elitist to insist on a live play only? I am waiting for the technology that can be both easily disseminated and genuinely "interactive," something like the holodeck. Interactivity at the moment is far too rigid for deep participation.
3. LGBTQ refers to Gay, Lesbian, Bisexual, Trans*, and Queer/Questioning.
4. All quotations in this section are from teen audience members.
5. See Chapter 7 for a discussion of slight variations in the definition of abstinence. The fine points of this definition must be in keeping with the health partner's practice.

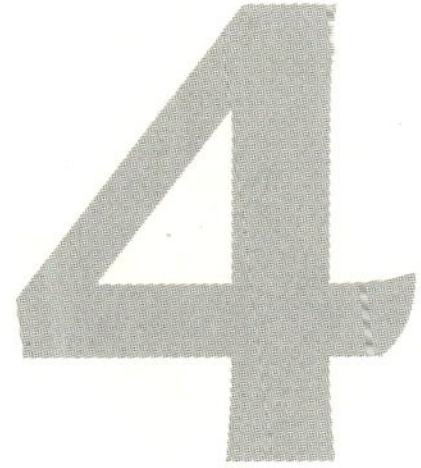

IN THE DRIVER'S SEAT

Participatory Theatre: Shared Knowledge Making

CONTENTS

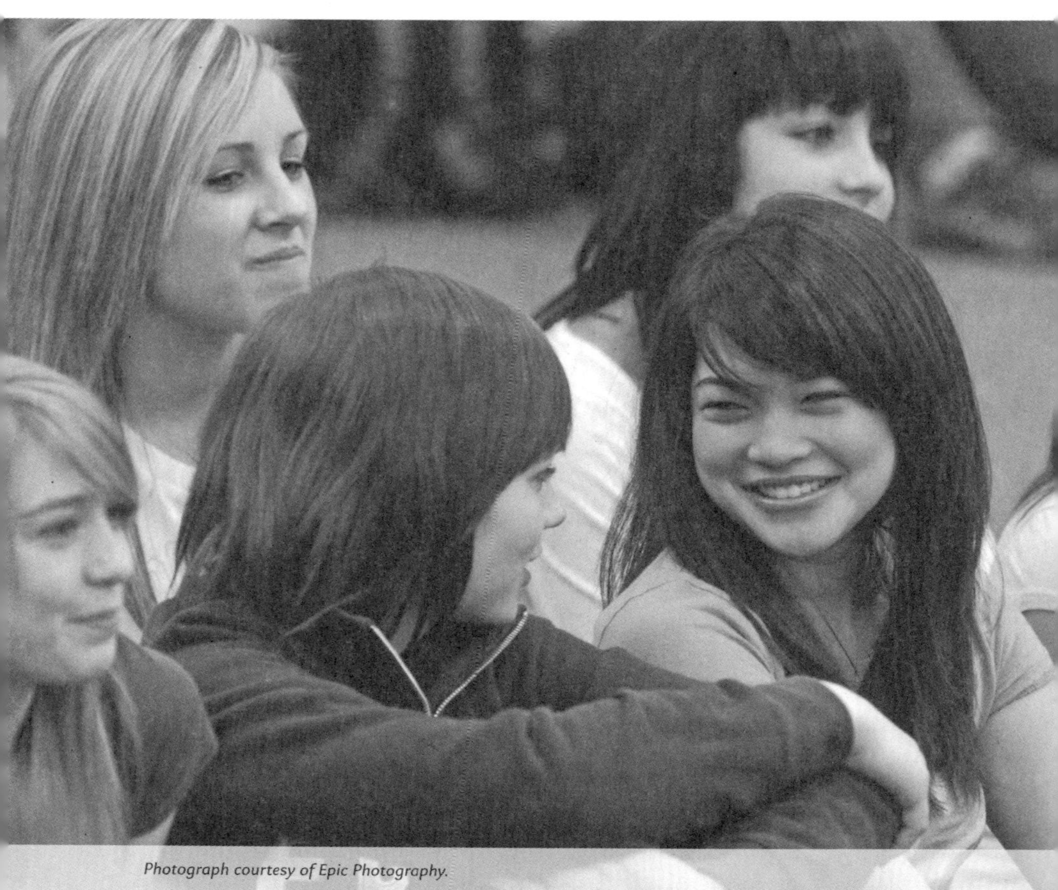

Photograph courtesy of Epic Photography.

This chapter provides in-depth discussion, tools, and strategies for actors and directors as they rehearse and perform this kind of participatory theatre.

> *You get to interact...like in class your opinion gets heard but I liked that they really used your stuff, like you can raise your hand and tell a teacher, this is what you could do, but you don't see how it would play out, and you don't see how it would be used in a real situation.*
>
> —AUDIENCE MEMBER

Yeah, like I definitely think that was one of the best things about the play was that the audience was able to participate and give the actors suggestions and stuff. So it wasn't just them acting and you're just kind of watching.

—Audience Member

Ignition: What Is It? Why Use It?

ALL THEATRE IS A TWO-WAY PROCESS between actors and audience, so all theatre is to some degree participatory. Actors and audience exchange air molecules, everyone is 3D, in the room together, and they impact each other by their presence. Audiences collectively and individually bring their own experiences, worldviews, and interpretations to what they see. Audiences and artists always create the meaning of a theatre event jointly. Participatory theatre, however, also has specific meaning, particularly when it is linked with youth and education.

Participatory theatre invites audiences to get involved verbally and sometimes physically in the action on stage. Generally, this is an unusual experience for theatre audiences in North America and Europe. Even those who have never seen theatre understand (perhaps from watching theatre performed in films) that the audience is expected to sit in the dark and the focus is on the people in the light. The notion that audiences should be still and listen became the norm because of the demands of certain kinds of theatre and theatre aesthetics: the nineteenth century saw the rise of naturalism and realism in the theatre and the theatre sought to create an experience for audiences based upon the invisible fourth wall and the willing suspension of disbelief. At that time and well into the twentieth century, an intense theatre experience was deemed to be one in which the audience peered into "real" people's lives in "real" rooms and willingly entered into this devised reality by forgetting they were in the theatre.

Breaking the Rules 1: A Brief History of Participatory Theatre

Outside and parallel to mainstream or bourgeoisie theatre, a less hierarchical more egalitarian and participatory theatre form developed, often in opposition to and in order to disrupt the intention of mainstream theatre and the assigned roles of actor and audience. Forms of participatory theatre such as street theatre, mumming, processional performance, and clown often occurred, and continue to be performed, outside the proscribed theatre building and outside the rules.

The oppositional and disruptive qualities of audience participation are inherently subversive and therefore always have political implications. For example, in the 1930s, workers' theatres in Europe and North America often used the power of participation to educate and empower audiences to rise up, demand their rights, and take action outside the theatre. Bertolt Brecht also put his considerable brain and talent to work to create forms and content that would politicize audiences and spark them to take action after the show was over.

Theatre practitioners during the 1960s and 1970s, responding to social, cultural, and political upheaval and building on Brecht's and workers' theatre, reinvented and revived audience participation. In Britain, Theatre in Education (TIE) artists and companies developed many significant participatory forms, particularly with and for youth. Examples of this kind of work include: Dorothy Heathcote's teacher-in-role work and her theory and practice of mantle of the expert; direct and improvisationally based audience–performer interaction such as hot seating; environmental participation such as in Catalyst Theatre's *Black Creek Project*, among many others. In the United States, artists such as Julian Beck and Judith Malina invited audiences to participate in happenings. And in Brazil, Augusto Boal began to develop his theory and practice of Theatre of the Oppressed.[1]

In most cases, the choice to use (invent or reinvent) participation is driven by trying to harmonize theatre practice with political practice. This is a difficult task littered with good intentions and appalling theatre. There is something libratory, celebratory, human, and anarchic about any theatre practice. At its best, it draws us in, draws us together, and engages us—heart, mind, and imagination. What chafes and goads are the hateful things about much theatre practice: elitism, rigid hierarchy, banality, wicked waste, and cowardly conservatism. For as long as there has been theatre for the centre there have been those who are galvanized by what the theatre can do and dissatisfied with what much of what it actually does. For many, that dissatisfaction is linked to a broader left wing ideology; for others, conventional and mainstream theatre is just too restrictive, too binding to accommodate their vision and imagination.

Theatre, Youth, Education, and Participation

When theatre, youth, and education are put together with participation it is almost always in order to make the theatre and the education emancipatory. It often sits within a larger, progressive political analysis and landscape. When youth, theatre, and education come together the fatal trap of didacticism opens up at the feet of the adults involved. When participation is added, it is to avoid falling into the pit. The best participation is not an attempt to sugar coat the pill or hide the message; it is the message.

The roots of the participatory form and content of *Are We There Yet?* are long and twisted. Two seminal influences were Brecht and Paulo Freire. These men, a playwright/director and an educator, sustained lifelong dialectical and dialogical praxis. Not the first and certainly not the last to ask how can education and the arts change the world, they tested their theories in practice and their practice changed their theory. Most importantly, they wrote about it.

Brecht

Brecht's writing is widely available, his plays continue to be produced, and theatre practitioners of all kinds throughout the world have encountered his key concepts. Most influential for the development of participation was his articulation of what the theatre needed to do in order to engage audiences in critical thinking. Brecht objected to theatre that engendered passivity in the audience. He worked to create theatre that disrupted the assigned roles and expectations of audiences and actors. Over his long career he experimented with many dramaturgical and production strategies to shake audiences out of the comfort of the familiar. He wrote his plays and developed his theories during the Depression, between the two world wars and after the end of the Second World War. It is not difficult to imagine how these social conditions and the pressures of economic and political upheaval demanded new forms and thinking from this passionate Marxist playwright. The urgency that he felt is clear in his plays and other writing but perhaps most in his poetry.

If Brecht attended theatre in the West today, he wouldn't see much change. Audiences sit quietly in the dark and give their attention to the actors living in the light. Brecht railed against the idea that theatre's job was to beguile audiences and entice them into a dream world so real that they forget they are in a theatre. Brecht did not want audiences to be transported. He wanted audiences to be sharp, aware, awake, and alive to the questions and contradictions in his plays. Audiences should not only know they are in a theatre, they should be reminded regularly, in case they are sliding back into passivity. Because Brecht was looking for ways to use theatre to make social change, he felt the first step was to honour the audience's intelligence. An active audience would be one engaged in critical thinking. Productions "marked a deliberate attempt to hold the spectator at arm's length, so that he would keep his critical judgment throughout" (Willett 1959, 176). Brecht and others used a wide variety of techniques to remind audiences they were in theatres, including direct address and asides (like many other playwrights). The machinery of the theatre was deliberately made visible. He wished his audience to be aware that they were in a theatre; "there would be no pretence of naturalistic imitation...he hoped to make the spectator see the play in objective repose instead of being bemused by what he deemed to be false glamour" (Clurman 1972, 58). Practitioners engaged in participatory theatre employ many of Brecht's dramaturgical and production theories, particularly direct address and revealing or dispensing with stage machinery, to achieve the same ends.

Critics charged that Brecht's alienation affect meant that he wanted to drain all the pleasure and magic out of theatre, that he intended theatre to be hard work and not emotionally engaging or fun. In some cases a rigid adherence to Brechtian principles has led to didactic, teachy preachy educational theatre, good *for* you, but not very good. Near the end of his life Brecht began to publicly address this perceived deficit and came to know what is common knowledge in the participatory theatre world: the best educational theatre is the hardest work combined with the most engagement and fun. In the early 1950s, in a note titled "On Poetry and Virtuosity," Brecht wrote,

> *We have almost given up examining works of art from their poetic or artistic aspect, and made do with works lacking any appeal as poetry and productions from which*

virtuosity is absent. Such works and performances may be effective on some level but it can hardly be a deep one, nor take a political direction. For it is a peculiarity of the means employed by the theatre, that they communicate insights and impulses in the form of pleasure: the depth of the latter corresponds with the depth of the former. ([1951] 1972)

Brecht's contribution to the theory and practice of theatre, education, social change, and hence participation, was enormous. He asked us to challenge some of the rules of the theatre and how audiences and actors should behave in the theatre. Brecht thought the theatre could teach, that the theatre could do more than entertain or present a moral lesson. All the elements of Brecht's theatre, scripts, acting style, and design were shaped to engage audiences emotionally and intellectually. He wanted audiences to be aware in the theatre in hopes that that state would spark change in the world outside the theatre. A key step toward change was to share power by revealing the workings of the theatre and acknowledging what most audiences know: it is possible to be totally engaged with the fiction on stage, to believe in the truth of it, and to simultaneously know you are in the theatre and thinking hard about what you see and feel.

Freire

Paulo Freire, educator and theorist, also puzzled over how to engender active critical audiences who could use education to take power in their lives. His audiences were adult literacy students and he approached teaching and learning with theoretical assumptions similar to Brecht. In the classroom that most students experience in North America most of the time, as in the theatre, the person at the front has the power and the knowledge; the audience or students wait passively for the teacher to pass the knowledge to them. Freire calls this the banking concept of education. Students are "containers... receptacles to be filled by the teacher...the scope of action allowed to the students extends only as far as receiving, filing and storing the deposits" (1983, 58). He maintains this kind of education keeps students passive and compliant but does not engender the activity both he and Brecht felt was necessary to make change: critical thinking.

Freire proposed another kind of education: education for liberation. "The teacher cannot think for his students, nor can he impose his thought on them. Authentic thinking...does not take place in ivory tower isolation, but only in communication" (1983, 64).

Participation in *AWTY* and other plays is shaped by these concepts of education, concepts that begin with the assertions that youth (in this case) are conscious beings, they hold expertise, and that both teachers and learners "are jointly responsible for a process in which all grow" (1983, 67). Freire practiced and wrote about a kind of education that involves the breaking of the power relationship between student and teacher and replacing it with a more equal relationship: teacher-student with students-teachers.

Of particular importance to participatory theatre (and the development of independent thinkers) is the building block of the relationship: dialogue. Freire developed a model of working with students that he called problem-posing education. The problems posed were related to the students themselves. He engaged them in dialogue about their own real-life problems in order to reveal their reality and make it a legitimate, worthy focus of study and learning. He felt this would establish the conditions under which students could reflect upon themselves and their world, and begin to think critically about the way they exist in the world in which they find themselves.

Critical reflection leads to the idea that reality is a process and transformable. The natural order of things, common sense, the ways things have always been, are revealed to be to be human constructs. Conditions and circumstances created by humans can be analyzed, challenged, and changed by humans. "Students, no longer docile listeners, are now critical co-investigators in dialogue with the teacher" (1983, 68) (and each other, we would add). The implications here are that the students have the tools to investigate and take action to solve their real problems, students teach teachers, teachers teach students, and no one knows the right answer beforehand. The process of posing problems, dialogue, critical reflection, and cognition can lead, Freire says, to creative transformation or change.

Boal

The publication of Augusto Boal's book *Theatre of the Oppressed* in English translation in 1979 was hugely influential and contributed a significant thread to participatory theory and practice. Boal emerged as a political activist and theatre practitioner in Brazil in the early 1970s. He combined Freire's inspirational educational theories with Brecht's theories and theatrical techniques and developed a suite of theatre-making approaches, theories, and methods. Boal developed his practice and theory in response to the military dictatorship in Brazil (Schutzman and Cohen-Cruz 1994, 2). He joined theatre artists around the world confronted with urgent questions about how theatre could be used to challenge oppression and empower people in their communities (Babbage 2004, 3).

Like Brecht, Boal was dissatisfied with conventional theatre practice that seemed to encourage passivity, and he built on Brecht's idea of inviting the audience to play an active role by questioning and critically analyzing the events that appear on stage. Boal moved to participation to find "ways of allowing the audience not only to think but to act for itself" (Fortier 1997, 140–41).

Boal developed a form by which spectators were also simultaneously actors, and he named this hybrid *spect-actors* (Boal 2002, xxvi). Spect-actors have agency, responsibility, and the ability to affect and transform the action on stage. For Boal, "all must act, all must be a 'rehearsal for revolution'" (1979, 122). He posits that theatre can become a weapon or a tool for people to examine and change their reality. Boal articulated key concepts about how participatory theatre, created from true events but placed in a fictional environment, could create ways to explore and address real-life issues (1979, 141). Like Brecht, his work strives to move the rehearsal that has happened in the theatre into real-life situations that audiences confront after the play is over (Schutzman and Cohen-Cruz 1994, 36).

Boal's most influential form is Forum Theatre. In this form, a scene is created and performed that contains a dilemma or problem for a character. The scene is then shown again exactly as before, but a control figure, the joker, invites audience members to yell "Stop!" any time they see someone being oppressed. The joker then invites the audience member to come on stage, step into the scene and become that character. The spect-actor then tries playing out a solution. Then someone else tries. In this way, many possible solutions to the problem or dilemma are generated and explored in a fictional, and therefore quite safe, environment. Practitioners of this technique hope the generation and development of solutions and strategies in the forum will provide real-life strategies that audience members will enact in reality (Boal 1979, 142).

Boal's work and the work of many Boal-inspired companies around the world have made a major contribution to the theory and practice of participatory theatre. While the theory, techniques, and goals are widely debated, Theatre of the Oppressed has impacted every theatre practitioner who seeks ways for audiences to take power in the theatre and think, discuss, debate, and learn collectively, creatively, and publically.

Breaking the Rules 2: Are We There Yet?

Participation may be the most extreme form of rule breaking in the theatre. Audiences are not only invited and encouraged to speak; if they don't, the play fails. This is a reversal of most people's expectation and learning about etiquette in the theatre. For teens/youth the rule of sitting quietly and giving all attention (power) to the people on stage is a challenge. In participatory theatre, the lights are on and the actors are talking to you right now, expecting you to talk back. Unlike the school touring production of *Romeo and Juliet* (which must rely on an authoritarian figure to keep the kids quiet or stop the show and threaten them), in participation you can blow a loud whistle and get everybody to focus and remind them of the task.

We discovered the power of the whistle while working with adults with mental disabilities. In that piece, *Stand Up for Your Rights*, we confronted one of the dilemmas of participation. On the one hand, you want audiences to participate, you want them to shout stuff out and argue and disagree; on the other hand, there may be many people and ideas and you need to have mechanisms to help them focus. The last thing we wanted with *Stand Up* was to have parents running into the room to grab their adult children because they were running riot and we didn't know what to do. Tony Hall devised a game frame for the show, which came with a number of metaphorical devices. The whistle, the referee, and red flags on the play were all used to shape the participations. We discovered that creating rules for participating as in a game, as opposed to being restrictive, was liberating. Stated up front and adhered to, the rules help everyone feel safe to participate and know that there are ways to get back on the rails when the show falls off. The possibility that the show might fall off the rails is key. It could happen, it isn't fixed, something might come up that has never come up before, and both audience and actors need to know there are ways to deal with that.

Are We There Yet? is participatory theatre. We use this form as a way to teach about sexuality, using Brechtian staging techniques and dramaturgy and Freireian problem-posing, dialogue, and the creation of critical co-learners. As a culture, it is in our best interest to educate youth about sexuality. We have a responsibility to help them to make informed, thoughtful, confident, healthy choices about sex. Participation can help in three ways: power, practice, and passion.

Power

An expert has power; and teens are experts on their own lives and feelings. Participation is the reverse of the usual paradigm in the classroom or the theatre. To create this reversal, participation democratizes the room. Not only does the audience know their own lives, they know that the decisions they make will affect them the most. The consequences of poor sexual choices are visited on the bodies and hearts of the teen audiences. The person who is most affected by the decisions has to have control or at least significant input into how, and when, and under what circumstances those decisions are made. Those most affected by a decision must speak and be heard. That's democracy.

Presented with a character like themselves who needs help right now, in a situation they recognize, they give advice as the experts they are. They talk to the character and debate with each other, and the character tries their advice. When the teen audience advises a character, they take responsibility for how the character thinks through his or her dilemma and the action he or she takes. Through the character, the audience takes power. Practice for taking power in their own lives.

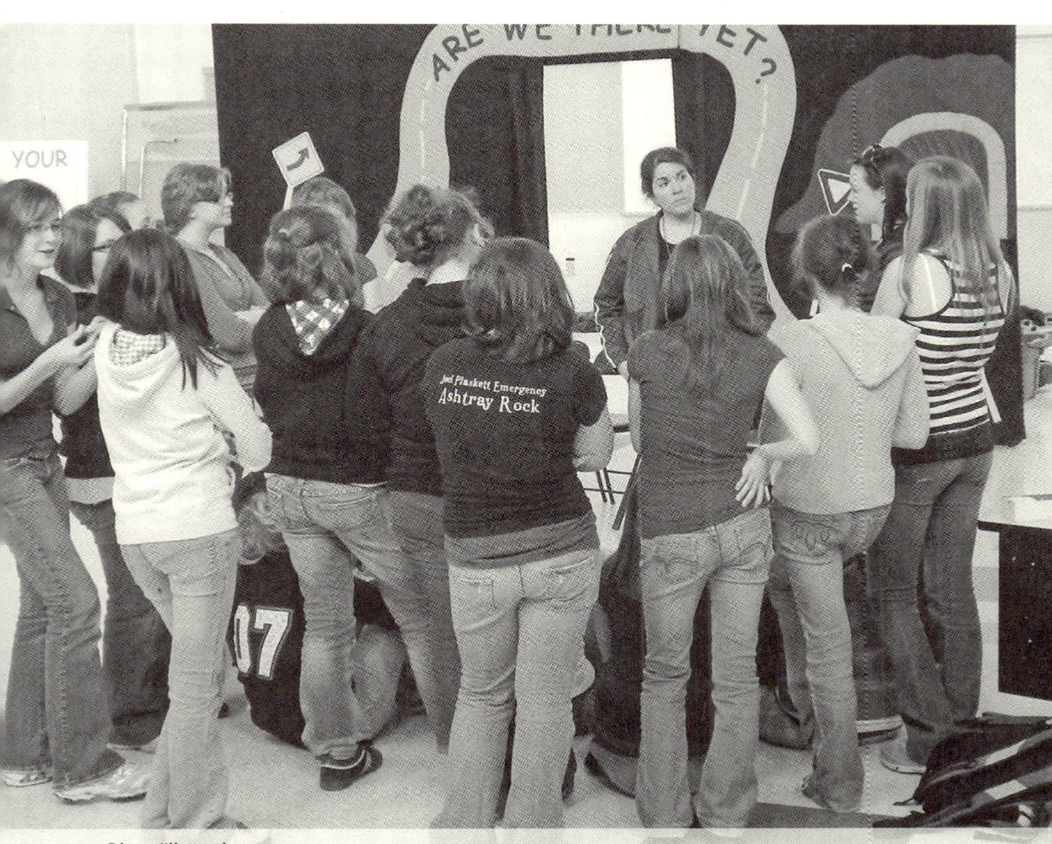

Okay, I'll try that
Natasha MacLellan, Mulgrave Road Theatre. Photograph courtesy of Emmy Alcorn.

Practice

The play creates the moments when we (the adults) are not there. The moment when a kid most needs help. When it's hot and heavy and emotions are running high and the pamphlet on STIS is at the bottom of a backpack. The theatre creates the moment and then actors ask the audience to help the characters through it. Sure it's magic. Your pals aren't there when you're about to have your first sexual experience, but it's practice. Practice in a safe environment with supportive adults all around and a chance to speak. Speak to a character, speak to a peer, and speak to yourself. Hear a character, hear a peer, hear yourself.

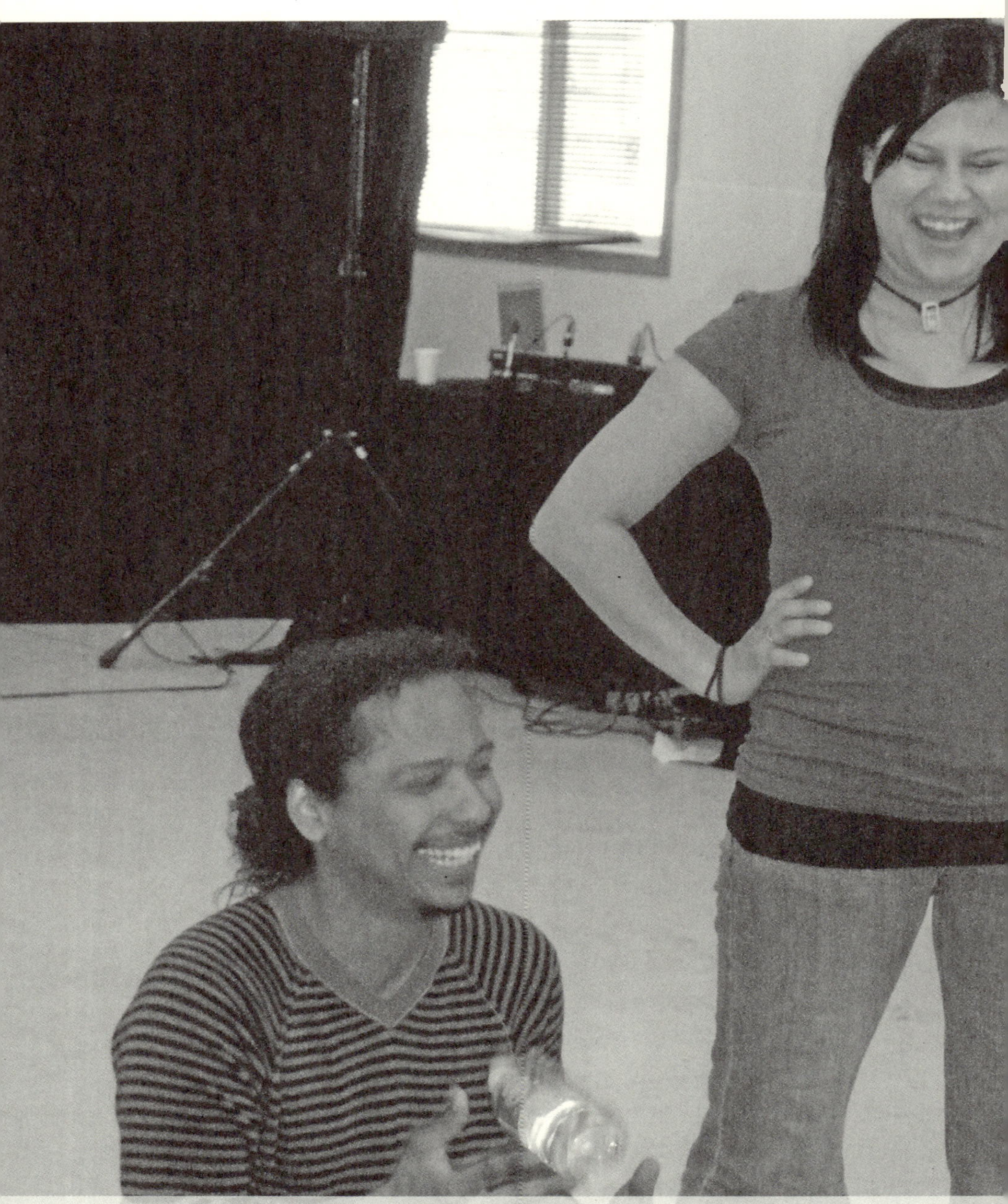

You really think I can say that?
Arron Naytowhow and Krystle Pederson, Saskatchewan Native Theatre Company. Photograph courtesy of Jane Heather.

Of particular importance is the public nature of the discussion and the action that emerges from it. The audience members, using the character as proxy and as a way to objectify the issue, practice talking to each other. They develop and rehearse language as they advise the character and hear what peers have to say. When the character tries out the advice, the audience gets to see some of the consequences. If the advice is poor or fails, they get to try again. Playing out poor or superficial advice is a great way to illicit practical advice that works and to deepen the emotional complexity of the dilemma.

Passion and Emotion

One of the pitfalls of participation is going after the apparently right answer or the easy solution. Each participation in the play has a correct answer that audiences often say and then sit back, safe in the knowledge that they got it right. However, part of the actor's job in participation is to deepen the analysis by animating from emotion. Most teens know "use a condom," that's easy. Talk to your partner about it? That's hard. Participation can encompass a key element often neglected in more conventional sexuality education: how it feels. Carol Ann doesn't need to be told to use a condom, she knows that already. She needs smart, blunt friends who can help her sort out how she feels, why it is hard to speak up, and how to talk to Mac about it.

Participation is a chance to think, speak, and feel. To feel anxiety, success, sympathy, pain, empathy, to feel what a character is going through and speak to them, give them advice, to shout out, "Get her to help you put on the condom!" "Do you want a baby in nine months?" "You're not ready! You have to talk!" It is a chance to feel trust that the adults in the room won't let you down. They aren't going to lie to you and they aren't going to get embarrassed or freaked out. To feel the power that comes from knowing that adults think you are capable and able and can make a good healthy decision about your sexual self. With help. From us. The adults.

Participation is messy. It's unpredictable and it's difficult. It can be terrifying. It takes training and a lot of love to do it right. A DVD or even a conventional play is a lot easier. But those are closed. Participation is open; it's democratic, practical, and emotional. Finally, it requires that we, the adults in the situation, share not just our knowledge but also our power with the kids.

> *So the students felt very important...there were several in there that in a classroom... they'd never volunteer. But in there, they seemed to know what to answer and it was like a totally different person that I saw answering questions and volunteering. I was amazed.*
>
> —*Teacher*

Blueprints for Making Participatory Theatre

Principles for Scene Building

Over many forays into creating and rehearsing participatory theatre, we articulated some core principles that are key to making theatre with significant, substantive impact.

Dramatic Scenes

Scenes are constructed so that characters who are like the audience ask for help and advice. Consider age, life circumstance, race, gender, experience, etc. This principle builds on the Freirian understanding in popular education and community development that top-down answers seldom work and seldom take into account the lived reality of participants. Problem solving for characters who are in wildly different situations from an audience has limited impact, and likely will result in magic fixes, that is, solutions that are not grounded in the full social, political, and personal contexts.

Production Note In *AWTY* teens assist teen characters to work through sexually charged dilemmas, where the brain may know what is safe, but the body and heart may not want to listen.

Dramaturgy

Characters go out to the audience after reaching a crisis, a point where they do not know what to do. For effective participation characters really have to need assistance. If a character actually knows the right answer (and how to enact it), then the participation becomes false; it is not theatrical, and why should audience members bother to engage and help? Further, the character must start where the core of the audience is, in terms of the crisis she is

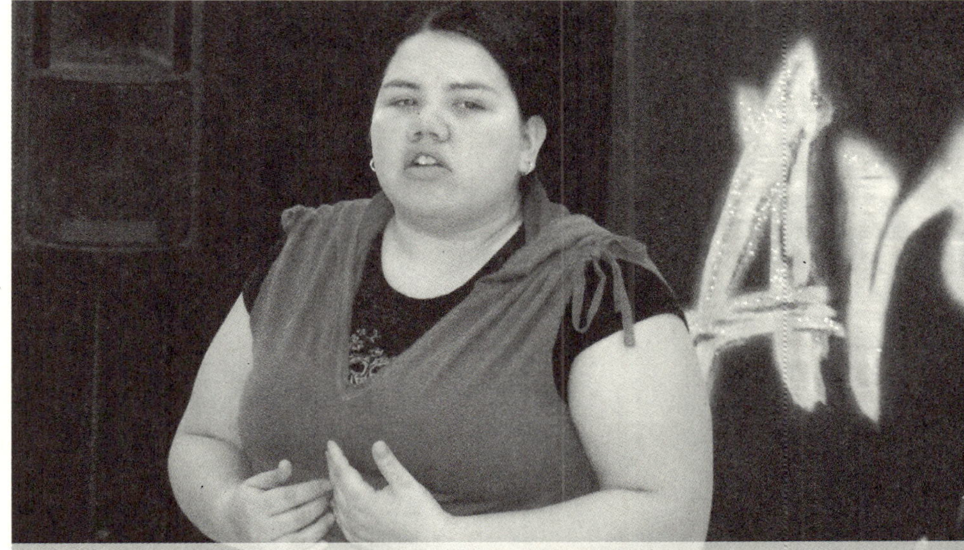

Now I don't know what to do
Jennifer Dawn Bishop, Saskatchewan Native Theatre Company. Photograph courtesy of Jane Heather.

facing; a character's questions should be the audience's questions, whether voiced yet or not. Deep participatory research makes it possible to create characters whose dilemmas are shared with its audience. Characters give voice to audience members' questions, and together they work on finding some answers.

Characters

Characters are based on current, relevant community research with people like the intended audience.

Production Note Actors in *AWTY* must immerse themselves in local teen culture and language. In varying parts of the country, the characters took on quite different tones, relationships, and ways of expressing themselves. Cultural differences led to substantially differing characterizations.

Characters ask for help in ways that are true to their character. Some ask for help directly; others engage with the audience from a position where they are sure they are right (even if they are wrong).

Production Note For example, in *AWTY* Mac confidently tells the audience that he and Carol Ann do not need to use a condom because neither person has had another sexual partner. Mac hopes against hope that the audience will agree with him, while the actor and writer hope the audience will challenge Mac's assertion.

In every case, the emotional life of the characters, their biases, vulnerabilities, desires, bravado, and rationalizations all need exploration if audience members are to dig into an issue (and its solutions) with the depth and complexity they deserve.

Production Note In the *AWTY* context, most audience members know about the importance of condoms; however, the social and emotional barriers to practicing safer sex are what is being pursued.

Participation

Characters interact with the audience and test out good and bad ideas theatrically, but with emotion and high stakes, in direct interaction with the audience and in improvised scenes where ideas are played out and then (re) considered.

> *You need to democratize the room, you want to make sure that everyone has a voice in this room, and so therefore the challenge is to make sure that you're playing to the people who are there on that day at that moment. And that's a really good way of making sure* that you're present and that you're engaged in a conversation with everyone.
>
> —*Jared Matsunaga-Turnbull,*
> AWTY *actor and director,*
> *Concrete Theatre*

What's Under the Hood? Tools and Techniques for Participation

While there are lots of ways that audiences are encouraged to participate in various kinds of theatrical events, we are interested here in participatory theatre that involves audiences in developing their knowledge, skills, and insights through active engagement with discovering their own solutions, solutions that are grounded in their lived experiences.

This kind of participatory theatre is based in several core techniques and relies on a number of tools. These are grounded in a commitment to engage with audiences openly, with interest and generosity. To empower and truly engage in emancipatory education, the event must really use and explore an audience's suggestions. A production needs to cut through the temptation to elicit right answers and move on; lip-service attention to audience ideas will not meet these goals. Indeed, often the exploration of apparently wrong answers leads to getting both myths and pat answers out in the open and more deeply understood.

While the following lists of techniques and tools may seem like a lot of things to remember and rather overwhelming, much of this work is incorporated quite naturally when a character's needs and wants are effectively aligned with the goals of the participatory sequence. Characters must need the help of their audience/confidants. When the point of a participation is aligned with a character's objective, a participatory sequence reads as true, honest, legitimate, and emotionally connected; theatre's power is used richly and actors don't lose their way.

Often characters in participatory plays appear only for a few minutes, so deep, community-based research and improvisation-based character development is important. (See also "To the Director: Rehearsing for Participatory Theatre" later in this chapter.)

The other key is deep curiosity. When a facilitator or an actor who is facilitating through character is truly curious about the ideas and perceptions of the participant/audience, much simply flows. Audience members sense and respond to this interest; they sense that their ideas are valued. Some might say you have to love your audience. Investment in open-hearted curiosity helps participations fly.

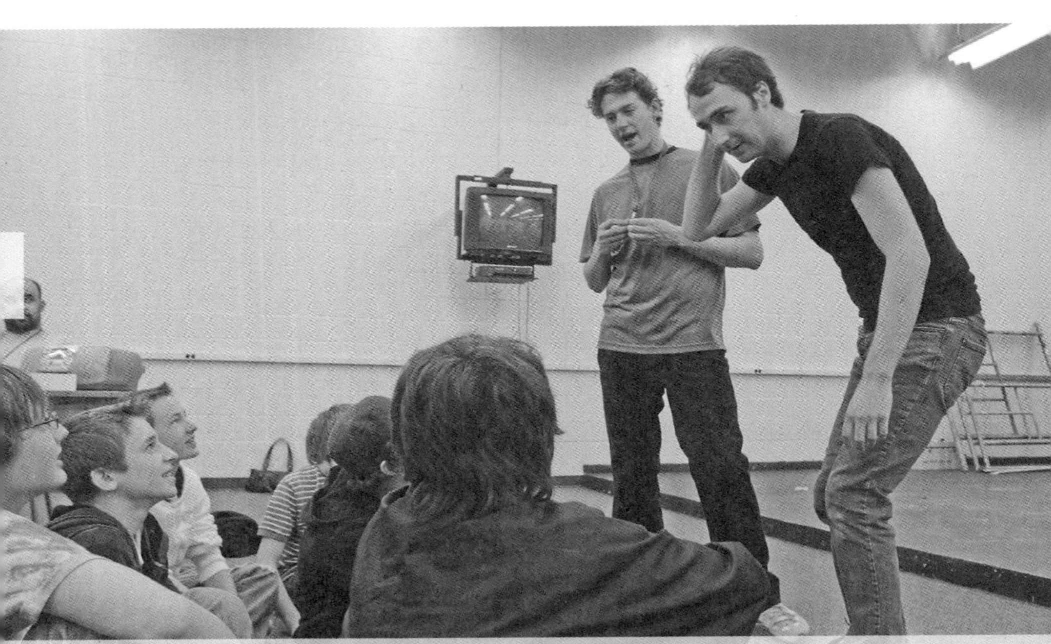

Character gathers ideas
Ryland Alexander and Jeremy Baumung, Concrete Theatre. *Photograph courtesy of Epic Photography.*

Principles for Performing Participatory Theatre

The techniques described below assist actors to meet some basic principles that are at the root of this kind of participatory theatre. First, in this work we set out to hear everyone, to encourage everyone to participate. This participation may take many forms: audience members may speak out, they may speak but only to their nearby friends, and they may speak via body language. Whatever form it takes, we aim to engage, see, and hear every person. Second, we set out to deepen and enrich the thinking, to expose and reflect on the complexity of an issue. The easy answer or knee-jerk attitude may get us started, get us through a few moments, but there is an opportunity with participatory theatre to challenge everyone to dig deeper, to see several sides of an issue, to understand more, to acknowledge some things are hard but important, to be brave, to look at something from many sides, then take action.

Techniques for Actors (and Facilitators)

This section is designed to work with the DVD that is part of this book. You will see these techniques and tools demonstrated and flagged in the DVD.

Gather

Gathering is the primary way to build involvement. It is a group brainstorm, with all the conditions that support effective brainstorming sessions: seek lots of ideas, no judgement, acknowledge and accept everything. Gathering is used early in participatory theatre events to signal that participation is easy and that everyone's ideas are welcome. It is also used when a new phase is started, to reinforce broad participation and to lay out the territory that can be explored in more depth.

To gather, a character or facilitator asks a question and wants lots of possible answers. One can gather from various starting points:

- Direct questions:
  What are some of the feelings people get when they hear the word "sex"? (Chapter 3, page 67)
- Interpretation questions:
  Okay, these two seem to be having trouble. Why do you think is happening? (Chapter 3, page 73)
  So their lines are in different places. What does this mean for them? (Chapter 3, page 76)
- Advice questions:
  Now I don't know what to do. I'm meeting Mac in a few minutes at the mall. What should I tell him? (Chapter 3, page 80)

To develop a gather, there are three basic attitudes that are useful. All can be translated into a specific character's language and approach to life:

- Yes and: "I have a problem." "What can I do?" "What else?" "Yes, good idea, what else?" "Any other ideas?" This is called the state of *Yes and*. It is the most straightforward approach to gathering.
- Yes but: "I have a problem, what can I do?" "Good idea, but I could never do that—any other ideas?" "Oh I wish I could do that but...!" "Is there something else I could do?" This is called the state of *Yes but*. The actor/character must invest in each part of *Yes but*. "Yes, then he will

understand, what a great idea!" and after sitting in "yes" only then moving to a realization, or a "but." "But, oh no, what if he thinks I'm a slut if I say that? Maybe he'll dump me!"

- No: "I have a problem and I don't know what to do." "Oh, I could never do that!" "Oh, my friends will disown me! What can I do?" "Oh, maybe you could do that but I could never...Couldn't I do something else?" This is called *No* or *blocking* (to get more ideas).

Each character or kind of facilitator will find that one of these approaches, or blends of them, is true to the situation and draws out lots of ideas.

Deepen

Of course, gathering is just the start, a way into thinking about a question or situation. The next challenge is to deepen the discussion. Deepen encompasses several things, including assessing (Would that really work?), dealing with barriers (I don't know how to do that), facing emotions (Wouldn't she be mad at me if I said that? or Whoa, maybe you could do that but I can't), and others. As theatre is used when educators, artists, and animators want to approach difficult subjects in-depth, when they want to encompass not only facts but also the humanity, emotions and social realities that are tied up in an issue, they aim to take an audience from their first impressions and ideas to deeper consideration of the challenges implied in a situation. Through deepening, theatre can uncover consequences and the costs, emotional and otherwise, of following good advice or risking taking a stand.

In the case of AWTY, which deals with embarrassing stuff about sex and sexual relationships, we know a lot of things that we should do (wear a condom, ask about partner's sexual health, talk about our boundaries, etc.) but these are not easy. With theatre, the complexities and risks of following the advice we know is good for us can be opened up. Maybe we shy away from these behaviours because they are scary, embarrassing, or confusing. We deepen the participatory experience to acknowledge the cost of things, the emotion behind things, the barriers to taking good advice from ourselves as well as others. If after deepening and acknowledging all this, and after facing the courage it might take, it is still the right thing to do or try or say, then we are really ready for action.

There are many ways to deepen a participatory moment, and theatre offers a rich set of ways to incorporate emotion, reveal complications and try out new ideas within a situation. In essence, one is asking audiences to take more layers of a situation into account.

To deepen, theatrical facilitators (such as the Instructor characters in AWTY) can use some or all of these approaches:

- Probe: Ask why, ask what that would it take, ask how, etc.
- Delve into an easy answer:

  Audience: "They should communicate!"

  Facilitator: "Right, now what should he actually say?"

  Yes but: Yes (that could work)...But (provide a complication).

  Ask if everyone agrees (and hear from those that don't).
- Test a possible solution: "How would he feel if she did that?...Is that good?"
- Explore a truism: For example, ask about the consequences of compromise for each person.

To see some examples of deepening by a Facilitator/Instructor, see the "Marcel and Delphi" section of the DVD.

To deepen the audience's consideration of an issue, characters (actors in role) can use many of those tools too. They can also use:

- Emote: "Won't she hate me if I do that?" "I wish I could do that but I just couldn't say that to my dad." "I'm afraid." "That's too hard!"
- Ask for more specifics: "But what would I say?"
- Dangle: Practice with the audience something that could be said to the other character, but trail off, asking them to fill in the blanks: "So then I'll just say to him, 'We need some...'" and wait for the audience to fill in the words.
- Leap to a wrong conclusion or take a suggestion farther than what was meant.
- *Yes but*: "Yes, I should just tell him what I think, like you say, yeah, great!... But wait a minute, then he'll probably hate me and break up with me and...I can't do that!"
- Block: Tell a story about how that approach didn't work before or how doing that made you feel. This will elicit more ideas or deepen a

discussion about how to navigate through the down sides of taking difficult but good advice.

- Compare: "Do you all agree?...What about the girls/guys?"
- Negotiate a version of an idea that this character can do: How does the idea need to be adjusted to suit this character and this situation?
- Play out an idea to see how the other character reacts: Playing out a suggestion can be theatrical and fun, including if it was a bad idea or if the character takes the idea too far.

To see some examples of these tools and deepening by a character in role, see the "Mac and Carol Ann" or "Living Clay" sections of the DVD.

Summarize

Another technique that is core to effective animation is the summary. Summarizing lets the audience know that you heard and remember what they said, what each person said, and that their participation is valued.

There are all sorts of byproducts of a summary. If you are gathering, a quick summary will help people remember what has been said so they can offer other ideas, or add something they think is missing. You demonstrate that you truly hear them. You offer the audience a chance for a quick reflection, and often they immediately extend the list and you have gathered more ideas or points of view. More individuals have had a chance to participate. If you are deepening, you encourage the audience to add to the analysis or address the barriers you mention. In either case, you are checking whether there is consensus. A summary also helps to refocus a group or remind them what a character is trying to accomplish.

A summary can be cool, simply as a list, or it can be laden with a character's attitude ("I like these, but these ones I don't think I could handle, but I did hear them, and this one, gee I'll need to give that one more thought...").

A summary can set up the animator to move on to a new stage, to decide which suggestion to try and to thank the audience.

Acknowledge the Audience For actors, the audience is your key playing partner. Audience members take risks to participate with you. As you are building their good will and willingness to participate in greater and greater depth, you need to acknowledge their contributions. How to do this? There are a lot of ways to say thank you and this should be done at the end of major participatory sections. As characters and facilitators take audience ideas into a situation, there are wonderful opportunities (and payoffs) for checking in ("Am I doing what you said?") and giving the nod to audiences or audience members whose idea you are using. Visual acknowledgement is central to the theatrical style of participation; there is no fourth wall, ever, and threads of connection are created and sustained in participatory sequences and the in scenes that follow. The most potent way to acknowledge the audience's efforts is to use what they advise. Use their ideas, use their strategies, use their words.

Use What the Audience Advises While sometimes it is tempting to leap on the right answer, get it done and move on, it is vital to approach the interaction honourably. Characters want help and if they do not take it or if they leap to something they wish they heard, there is a false participation and you have just reversed much of the company's efforts to gain trust and participatory engagement.

Tools Vital to Rich Participation

A variety of kinds of tools and strategies support facilitating interaction. Here are a few, and you will discover more! Many of these tools are demonstrated and flagged in the DVD.

Wait in Comfort

Sometimes an audience needs some time to think about a question or digest a scene they just saw. Don't panic! Silence does not mean they are not willing. When starting each unit of a participation sequence, have a question for the audience (often provided by the playwright) and a follow-up question. The second question can be a paraphrase of the first or a new way to ask the same thing. The rhythm often goes like this:

> First question...wait, watch...Second question...someone offers something.

Changing up the nature of the second question is often helpful. Sometimes using a situational example as a way to ask the second question is helpful.

Repeat and Paraphrase

Repeating is an easy and important tool. It lets others hear someone who is quiet, lets the participant know you heard them and got the point, leads to more and other ideas. You can also paraphrase answers, to repeat plus clarify, shorten, or again, to demonstrate you heard the point.

Paraphrasing and repeating also can build to a summary, a key technique discussed above.

The Closed/Open Question Combo

This one-two punch can lead a quiet audience to start talking more and elaborating on their ideas. It is key to deepening discussion. Ask something easy, low-risk, something that can be answered with a word, then ask for elaboration:

Character: Do you think I should tell him?
Audience: No!
Character: Why not?

Character: Do you think I should tell him?
Audience: Yes!
Character: What should I say?...or...Won't he be mad?

Use Character Need (Character and Objective Based)

Remembering all these tools can seem daunting, and they do take practice, in rehearsal and in performance. However, basing the work in character need can make more of it natural, almost inevitable. The character goes after what she needs, and this strategy in turn takes the actor and audience through the participation with truth and depth. In many cases, this approach can also help to avoid teachy theatre. We use theatre to ground issues and education in the full emotional and social lives of the audience. So, when a character who is like the audience is in a situation where he must grapple

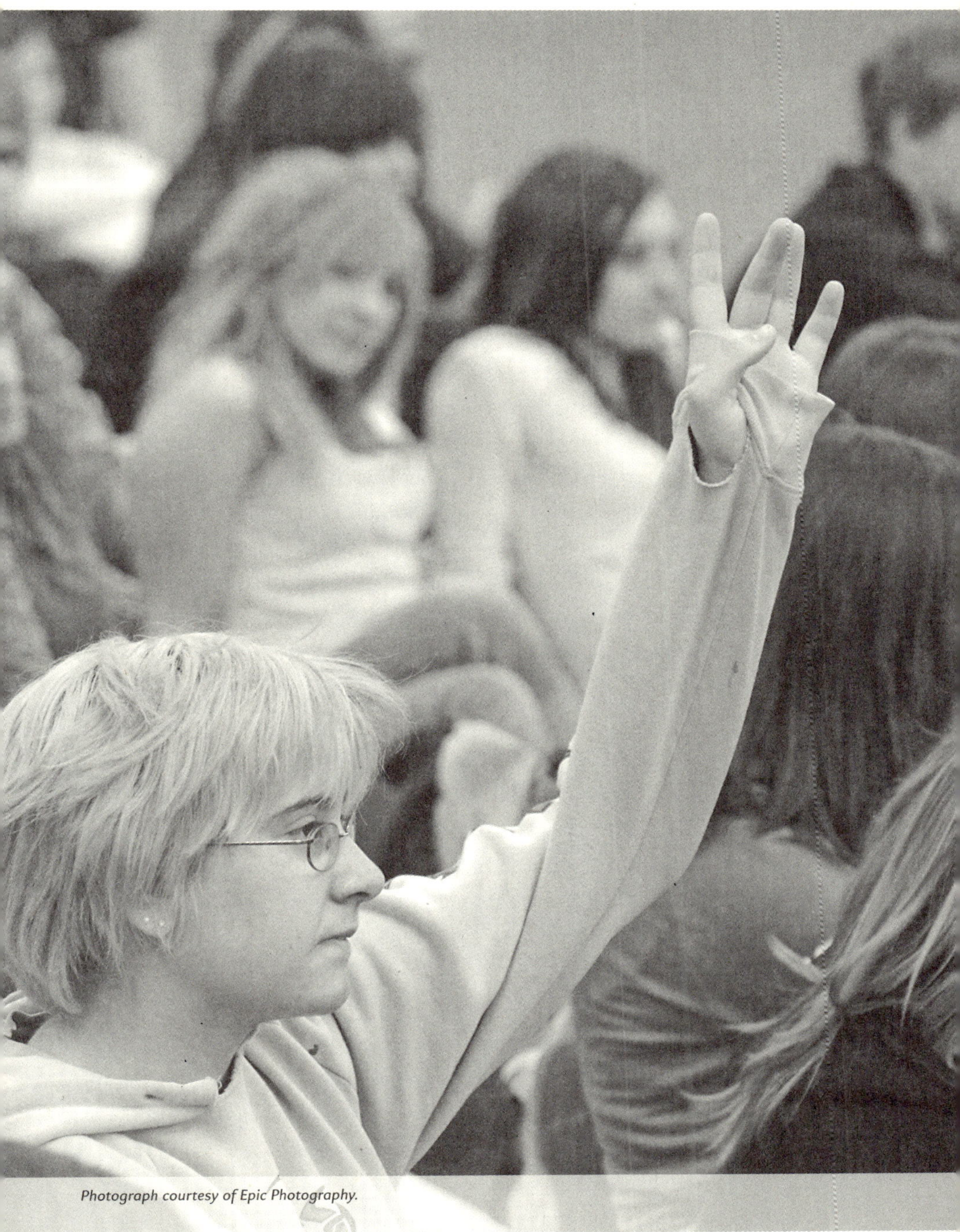

Photograph courtesy of Epic Photography.

with a dilemma or crisis, audiences are engaged, emotionally as well as intellectually. Then the character needs to solve the dilemma; his need drives the interaction with the audience. In essence, characters ask for their help, and the more they need it, the more deeply the participation is rooted. They need help. They look to the audience to get it. It is urgent. The stakes are high. This drives the energy of the participation forward, and audience members can experience feeling responsible for the characters' fates.

Payoffs from this approach are numerous. Firstly, the emotional engagement is built. We know that much of the impact of theatre rests with audience experience of engagement, involvement, and empathy for characters and their fates.[2] When the audience truly helps a character they care about achieve something she or he wants or needs, they feel successful. On the other hand, should characters get poor advice, they can try it out, fail then come back out to the audience for other ideas (to gather), or with questions (to deepen): "Why didn't that work?" Should an audience be fooling around and challenging you with deliberately bad advice, a character can challenge right back: "Don't mess with me, I need to figure out what to do, or..." The urgency and need can drive the investigation forward and encourage deeper thought by the audience. A character can learn something or discover something through the interaction with the audience; he can start unaware, think he needs something, and the audience can set him straight. Right in front of them, their interventions cause discovery—another wonderful payoff in the theatre. Similarly, a character can use good advice and still fail. Why? The audience again needs to think deeper and often they then ask the character to think about the other character in the scene: "Maybe it isn't what she wants?" All of these moments build involvement and deepen thought.

Invest in Curiosity

Another way to get on a flow with participation (rather than methodically applying each tool) is to invest in curiosity. The curious actor or facilitator wants to hear what audience members have to say; they engage honestly with the people who are their audience. Audience members can sense this. Curiosity helps to keep things fresh (you want to know what *these* people have to say, here and now). It motivates the interaction, and it heightens the pleasure in receiving ideas and exploring them. Curiosity helps actors to play in the moment with the audience. Just as actors strive to play in the moment in a realistic, scripted scene, so too they can play in the moment via curiosity about audience ideas. To see an example of curiosity in play, see the approach to the Instructor in "Marcel and Delphi" in the DVD.

Endow the Audience

As a character who is seeking advice from a group (the audience), endow the audience with a relationship to you. For example: Are they your best friend? Your conscience? Your provoker? The friend you never had? Do you (your character) think they are wiser than you? More experienced? The same? Endowing them with a position helps you to play to them honestly and openly, with authenticity. This relationship, as in regular scene work between characters, can change and grow as the participatory sequence goes on, with the audience becoming also culpable for the success of the advice they give.

Structure the Interaction

Usually, the point of a participatory sequence is not to go after the right answer but to extend options and explore some of them. A basic pattern to follow is:

- State the question (problem)
- Gather ideas
- Select one or more to probe in more depth to deepen discussion and insights
- Try out an idea or strategy
- Return to the audience for response/new ideas

Acknowledge the Audience

Say thank you! There are many ways to acknowledge audience participation and help. Here are a few:

- Say thanks: Say thanks as you end an interactive sequence, as your character leaves the stage, or when you succeed using their advice.
- Check-ins: Get some advice, go and try it in a scene, check back with a look or an aside, in essence saying, "Here I go" or "Am I doing what you said?" This invites audiences to continue to advise you and keeps the

connection between you and the audience alive, even when you are back in the world of the scene.

- Threads between actor and participants: As you play out some of their advice in a situation, keep a thread of connection with the audience. Use quick looks, let them in on how you are feeling as you try to follow their advice. Think of them as your partner, your best friend, your confidante, your conscience. Build that relationship as you play out their ideas.
- Really hear them: Use all the ways you know to be an active listener: acknowledging, checking in, repeating/paraphrasing, reacting (positively or negatively) to their advice.
- Do exactly what is suggested: Use the ideas exactly, use the exact words, do just what they say. This builds their sense of power and responsibility.
- Keep visual and emotional links (via body language).
- Huddle to check in: Use physical as well as verbal cues to build their sense of being on your team. Move around, get near to them, gather them together, share a confidence.
- I did what you said but: Build audience responsibility for their ideas. Ask them to figure out what worked and what didn't and why/why not.

Acknowledging the audience's role in your character's fate helps them to invest in the participatory sequences and feel engaged and responsible. Ideally, they come to feel a character's successes and defeats keenly, so they dig all the deeper and engage all the more in the upcoming participations. Research shows that those who participate the most also report the most impact later.[3]

Manage the Room

Often there is one of you (the actor) and a lot of them (the audience). There are two particular challenges: too much or too little participation. In both cases, some of the strategies that work involve using the space, moving around to change up your position.

If an audience is quiet, get nearer to them. Watch for small tells that let you know someone is thinking but not yet speaking an idea or point of view. Walk over, let them speak quietly, just to you. Often they want to help but they do not want to shout it out. Maybe they are shy. Maybe they are not yet

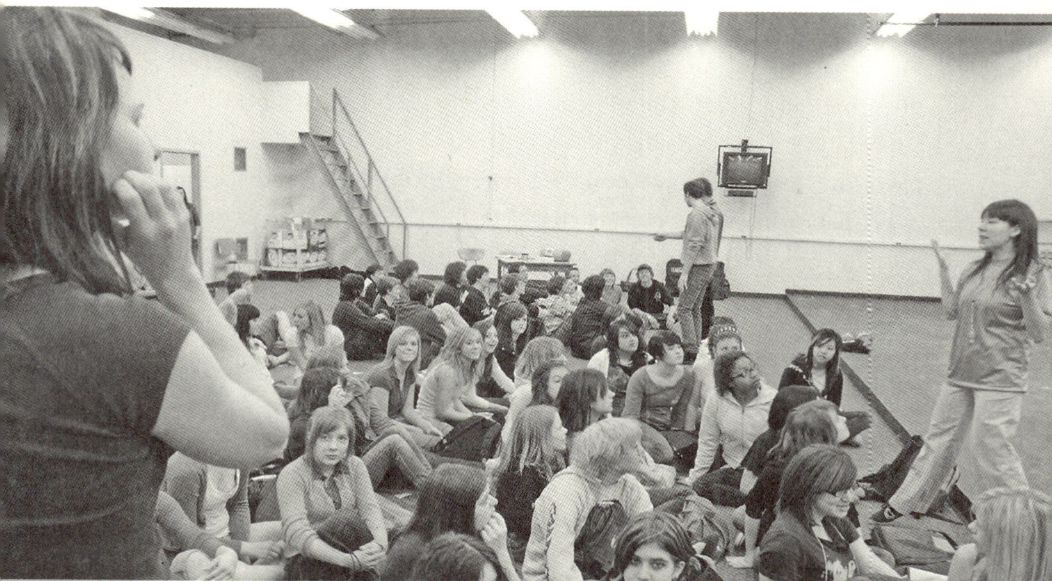
Kristi Hansen and Nadien Chu with Jeremy Baumung and Ryland Alexander, Concrete Theatre.
Photograph courtesy of Epic Photography.

sure that it will be fun rather than dangerous to speak. You can always paraphrase and repeat for others to hear, as appropriate. Other techniques, such as the closed/open question sequence helps here, as does paraphrasing your initial question and being willing to wait.

While silence can strike panic into an actor, the chaos of many people all with something to say can swamp you. Physical techniques are again important. For example, stand on one side of the room, hear someone near you and repeat what they say so all else can hear. You are the centre and the leader. Conversely, stand on one side and give your focus to someone far on the other side; you and she create the focus. She will speak up to allow you to hear across all those others and so the full group is involved.

Sometimes an audience has many, many things to say. You manage them with mini summaries and also through the character. A character can say, for example, "Whoa, I'm confused, what shall I do first?" Sometimes an audience loses track of what you are working on. A character can restate or refocus the question; remind the audience of what you need.

Play Out Suggestions

In this participatory form, characters leave a scene in a moment of crisis or dilemma and go out to the audience for advice on how to handle the situation. Much of this can be explored, character with audience. But the real payoff and testing ground comes when a character puts the advice into action in a situation involving another character. She or he takes the advice back into the scene and everyone sees how it works.

A few strategies help to make the most of this moment. First, you may have received lots of advice; make sure they know what you are going to try just before going into the scene. Tell them. This helps the audience watch for how particular strategies work. In the case of a long, involved discussion, also make sure they remember what your primary objective is and what your stakes are.

A number of these strategies can be seen in the DVD exchange between Mac and Carol Ann.

Count on your scene partner. You may have decided to try out bad advice. Believe it might work. Go try it out in the scene with full commitment; your character is convinced it might work. If it is truly bad advice, your scene partner will reject it, reject you, or even leave. You try and fail. Then you can go back to the audience for better advice: "So now what?" or "Thanks a lot guys." This is entertaining, energizing, theatrical, and leads to some new ideas. The audience sees they have power and takes it on. Or quieter members of the audience see their comments are needed now and may offer a quite different strategy.

Sometimes it is not bad advice but it is advice that does not take in the other side of the equation, the other person. Let things go wrong, then return to your advisors. Why did that happen? The audience will tell you and give you some new strategies.

To see some examples of actors directly playing out and testing suggestions, see the DVD "Mac and Carol Ann" participations, as well as the "Living Clay" sequences.

Playing out suggestions is the most immediate feedback on audience ideas. They advise and advice is tested immediately, in real-life situations.

Moments of returning to the audience are ripe for theatrical, entertaining, and meaningful moments. You can build the connections and

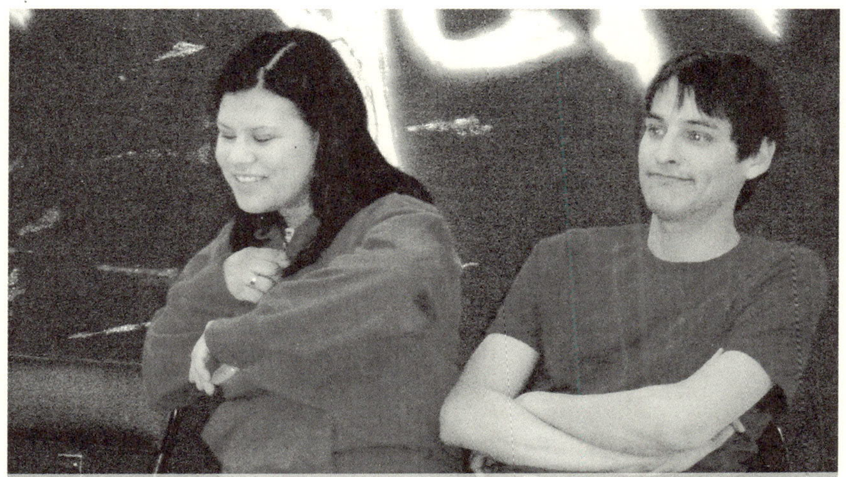

Trying out audience advice
Krystle Pederson and Clifford Cardinal, Saskatchewan Native Theatre Company. Photograph courtesy of Jane Heather.

relationships with audiences in these moments. It is a moment to be real. You can congratulate or gripe about the advice you received, challenge them or thank them. You can establish a character who will say thanks for help or for what happened in their very own way and each audience will respond differently.

To the Director: Rehearsing for Participatory Theatre

Directors of interactive plays need to build a layered process that devotes considerable focus to developing core participatory skills and the play's specific participatory sequences. Normally, actors are not trained in participatory techniques, so rehearsals usually need basic skill building as well as several steps of rehearsal for the show itself.

Skill Building

It is useful to identify and practice the core techniques—gather, deepen, and summarize—as well as the basic tools, particularly wait in comfort, repeat/

paraphrase, and acknowledge. Develop these skills as a foundation; rushing into the specific participatory sequences without these core skills tends to encourage actors to seek the most straightforward and apparently right answers so they can succeed and move on, rather than invest in the audience's deeper exploration. On the other hand, actors who have some core skills can more easily move to enjoyment and, as one actor advises, to a state of comfort with audiences:

> *Relax. Be there with your audience, ride with the audience. See and hear and listen to them, not just expect something from an audience.*
>
> —*Pedro Chamale,* AWTY *actor,*
> *Neworld Theatre*

Simple exercises in the core techniques and tools set actors up to be able to reach this comfort. Working on these skills without the overload of playing a scene pays off later. A few examples of many possibilities are described here:

> *Marcus Youssef, who directed our first production...did a facilitation workshop where his focus was really on being present—really coming out and just standing in front of the audience, and we are the audience for each other, and just being there...It's what is required, just to be in a room and listen to the room and see where it takes you...It's a counterpoint to, "I'm coming out here to perform for you, and you're going to watch me."*
>
> —*Adrienne Wong,*
> AWTY *director, Neworld Theatre's*
> *2010 production*

Other exercises in reaching all members of an audience, in hearing and remembering (summarizing), and in delving deeper into topics (practicing asking *why?* and *what do you mean?*) are also useful. Exploring and playing out moments of discovery in response to audience ideas is an advanced exercise that is extremely helpful because it will translate well into the animation in role that much of *Are We There Yet?* asks of actors.

Research

Meanwhile, researching the audience is vital. In this kind of participatory work, characters, like the audience, are caught in dilemmas so that audiences can explore their own options and actions within situations that are relevant to their lives. While the script is built from such research, actors new to a piece need to particularize character choices in light of who their audiences will be. Research needs to include hanging out among groups similar to those who will be the audience; reading what they read; listening to what they listen to; discovering their slang, their interests, and priorities; and watching how they interrelate.

Stages of Rehearsal

1. Rehearse the scene that leads to a participation sequence.

Usually scenes that lead to participation end with a character (or characters) in a crisis or dilemma: scenes end hot. How hot can the scene end? What are the building blocks? What are the subtext and backstories that both assist the heat and provide clues and interpretive spaces for audiences?

> *The kids are picking up a lot of information that's not just in the text that's spoken; it's in what's happening in the dynamic between the characters. Body language and all those kinds of things. The kids really engage with the characters and feel what they're feeling, which is a lot, because of course when you're talking about sexuality, there are so many feelings there. When you can see those feelings played out on stage it has a huge impact.*
>
> —*Caroline Howarth,*
> AWTY *director, Concrete Theatre*

2. Explore intention and structure of each participatory sequence.

After developing the theatrical vocabulary of the core principles and techniques of participation, it is important to take a close look at the structure of a participation. Given the intentions, what are the key steps and landmarks? What is the journey through a participatory sequence? This investigation is not dissimilar to the ways we explore and unpack the development of a dramatic scene. A classic formation of a participatory sequence is:

- Character has a dilemma/problem and wonders what to do; needs advice or insights from the audience
- Gathers ideas from the audience (gets lots of ideas from lots of people)
- Probes an easy answer, thus deepening the investigation (How do I do that? What would she say if I did that? Why should I do that?)
- Asks for more/other ideas
- Chooses one of the audience's ideas and tries it out, tests it in practice, improvising a scene; discovers a complication, returns to the audience
- With the audience's help, character learns/discovers, adjusts, tries again with more success
- Acknowledges the audience. Because of their help, the character can move on

Each step should be practiced. Solid confidence in the structure, or architecture, of a sequence assists an actor when in the overload of audience participation. Actors also continue to develop and extend their techniques skills at this point.

3. Link character and intention.

In this kind of theatre, as a company explores possible scene and character interpretations, selecting options that most parallel and support the project's intention for the audience is vital.

For example, in the participation sequences with the characters Marcel and Delphi (Chapter 3, page 73), the intention is: "to encourage clear communication (verbal and non-verbal) about sexual boundaries." So, while this scene can be played a variety of ways, the most useful choices have the characters wanting desperately to be together but confronting strong obstacles to meeting these desires. The obstacles include their inability to communicate clearly and lead to a crisis between them. The stakes must be high (they need to work out the problems or they will lose each other). They need the audience's help to figure out what went wrong; then they need the audience's help to deal with their very different personal boundaries. They need to talk so that they can work things out so they can stay together. The obstacles are intense; the audience's help is needed to name these obstacles and discover ways to overcome them.

The audience has the most to work with when the subtext of the scene leads to body language that expresses the characters' care for each other, desires, hopes, insecurities, passions, and confusions. Stakes are high (so it is worth their while) and obstacles are intense (it is a difficult knot to untie). As a result, discussion is rich, varied, complex, and therefore about humanity. The conversation is about living rather than about teaching points.

> *I don't have experience teaching people how to be facilitators; I've never done that before. So it was useful [to have] ways of thinking about the facilitation at different stages...starting with the objectives and overall structure and finding comfort within that and then being able to go deeper into the question of the character's need. Those were principles I found I kept coming back to.*
>
> —*Adrienne Wong*

4. *Develop characters.*

Characters should be developed based in a combination of the participatory research with your future audience and the understanding of the play/scene and participatory sequences. Often scenes give only a little character information, but the success of the participation relies on building a rich sense of character and character history, with history and traits based on in-depth research with the audience. Develop a backstory to support the scene. Characters may use their histories directly in the participation, with stories that block to deepen easy answers. The characters need immediate histories, which motor the scene, and they need backstories that assist in ramping up the stakes (the character's need to meet their objective). Often, actors and the director need to build a common set of events and interactions as well as wider individual histories. Hot seat interviews for history and character development as well as improvisations, discussion, and, ultimately, careful selection are important. Discoveries in rehearsal need to be tested against their usefulness in animating the participations.

5. Rehearse participation.

It is vital to rehearse participation sequences in as full and layered a process as you would a scene. For this you need to ask anyone and everyone in the rehearsal hall to play audience. Later it will be vital to work with test audiences, as the audience is the scene partner in these parts of the play.

For an extended participatory sequence, first rehearse the structure, solidifying the stages and linking these with the goals of the sequence. After the basic structure is known and rehearsed, with a focus on incorporating the core principles and techniques, it is important to work also on variations:

- What if audiences don't follow your expectations?
- How can you get comfortable with playing sequences out in varying orders, depending upon the audience's responses?
- What blocks can be used to deepen audience thought and engagement?

Some of the answers are linked to a strategic development of character: if a character has a strong and appropriate objective, you have a spine to work with in whatever order or pace a particular audience responds. The character's dilemma and journey toward dealing with that dilemma will drive the scene and lead to the intended participatory exploration. Similarly, a richly drawn character will give an actor ways to ask the audience the key questions (such as, "What should I do?") but in a character's vernacular. Well-researched and developed characters also provide ways to block in order to deepen the audience's exploration ("Great idea, but I don't think I can do that, maybe you could but I never could.")

Once the basic participatory sequence is deeply rehearsed, it is important to try variations and special problems presented by audiences:

- What about shy, very quiet audiences?
- Rowdy groups?
- Situations where only a few audience members dominate the interaction?

All of these can be simulated in rehearsal, prior to testing your work.

6. Test audiences.

Because the audience is, in essence, actors' scene partners, it is important to work with audiences prior to opening and to go back to rehearsal to respond to these experiences. First groups should be friends, there to support the actors as they try out the participatory material. It is ideal to have a test audience situation where you can do some stop/start work or replay a sequence after some quick notes, so a workshop format is helpful.

After work with friends, where actors can try lots of things out and rehearse interacting with varying kinds of audiences, test audiences should also include groups who are as much like the intended audience as possible. The key here is to have opportunities to try a draft plan, then have time back in rehearsal to work on issues that emerge.

> *Our first preview audience was...[in] the third week. We just did the participation sections. We had about seventy-five minutes in the classroom. I moderated and set it up as, "this is our rehearsal." I made it really clear: we did some things over; I interrupted the scene, sometimes just to interrupt the scene to show it's rehearsal. Then we experimented with different ways of doing the participation, and came back and debriefed with lots of conversation.*
>
> —*Adrienne Wong*

> *I tend to start with a small test audience, maybe in the rehearsal hall, just bring a few adults in...There's often a lot of fears, that the kids won't talk, the kids'll talk too much. So then a slightly larger audience of peers of the actors or university students. But then you have to move to test audiences with school kids, thirty or so, just to get that feeling of how do you work with that group. And once the actors are in the room with those young people, that's when all the bells start to ring and you start to say, yes, this is how this really, really works.*
>
> —*Caroline Howarth*

Often experiences with test audiences can ready a group to discuss and develop opportunities for managing large groups. They provide opportunities to alter strategies and to get over the tendency to seek the right answer then rush onwards. Actors need a chance to have an aha moment about riding the wave of an audience. They need a moment where they can relax and trust the journey. They need a moment where they discover how to fall in love with audiences.

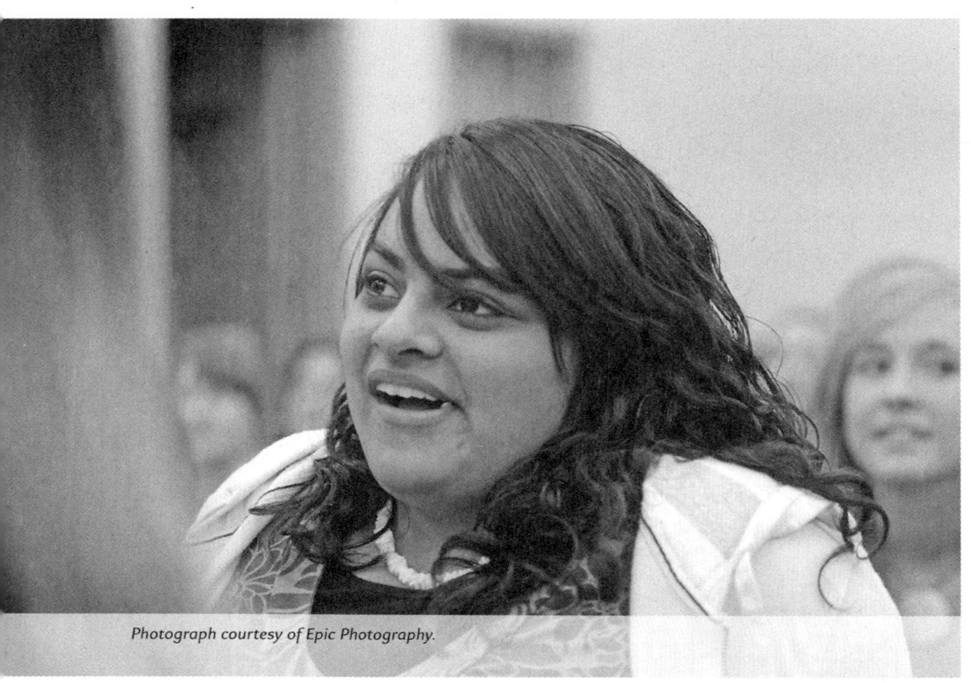

Photograph courtesy of Epic Photography.

Actors also need to keep working to discover how their character can truly and overtly learn and discover things (strategies, insights, or the courage to address their crises) from their audience.

7. Participation on the road.

Because one of the scene partners is the audience, the show is truly discovered on tour. Actors need the groundwork from rehearsals and permission to continue to discover and confront how the play works as they work with real audiences. After solid foundation work is established and once conditions are created where a team discussion is welcome, Concrete Theatre holds weekly debrief meetings while the show is on tour. Normally, the health partner, actors, and stage manager attend, and often the director joins the group. These sessions are important so actors can explore ways that they can handle certain kinds of moments, for everyone to debrief emotive or difficult moments or groups, and to continue to grow the participatory aspects of the performance.

You're asking actors to trust their own instincts and then also building an atmosphere of trust within the group. They become experts in their sections so that they can know when it's not working and have the confidence to ask somebody else whether they're doing it wrong. Then [the company] can brainstorm: Well, what do I say if this guy challenges me in this way? What could I have done differently? Then you end up with three or four different suggestions of how to navigate it. When something comes up, instead of getting one new way of doing it you're getting four.

—*Adrienne Wong*

A company philosophy and protocols for ways to talk and exchange ideas need to be in place to enable all to voice experiences and concerns openly, particularly given the improvisatory, interactive approach to such a sensitive and button-pushing topic. Because these discussions necessarily involve actors talking with other actors during the run, the director and the full company need to establish the approach and ground rules explicitly during rehearsal.

Gearing Up: Stages of Participation

Theatre audiences do not expect to participate actively in a play. They anticipate arriving, settling back and enjoying a story and an emotional ride provided by actors. They may presume they will have a communal experience in that they will be a member of a group, an audience, and take the journey along side others, but they also may presume that they will have a private intellectual and emotional journey in response to the production.

Plays that ask more of the audience, such as those with direct participation and interaction with characters and events, need to move an audience from their assumptions and expectation of relative anonymity to a sense of enjoyment and pleasure in overt and more public interaction. For success, the play script and the production itself should support a journey into the play and build a sense of pleasure in the experience of participation.

The DVD gives you a sense of the audience's increasing levels of participation. As actors use specific tools and techniques to build a participatory atmosphere they are identified and flagged.

In AWTY, the performers build the levels of participation from the moment audiences enter the playing space.[4] Actors greet audience members as they arrive, informally chatting, handing them cards with resource information on them, seating them and chatting. Already the audience experience is altered as the actors are out among the audience rather than awaiting the start back stage. This approach pays off throughout the performance; AWTY actors observe that often those who they speak with directly at the top of the show are first to volunteer later, when actors look for active participation during the performance. In essence, actors are building a foundation for interaction, giving their audiences a sense of comfort and easy communication. They set themselves up to be approachable, interested in the audience, and relaxed. This atmosphere is important for later, when the play invites audience members to deal with a sensitive subject in increasing depth.

In-depth participatory theatre asks audience members to advise characters that are similar to themselves and provide advice to the characters while in the midst of experiencing intense situations that could happen to that audience. Characters face crises, problems or dilemmas and turn to the audience for assistance. In advising characters, audiences are, in essence, advising one another and themselves. In AWTY characters deal with dilemmas about sex and sexual relationships, topics that few are willing to speak about comfortably and in public. Well-handled participatory theatre makes these important conversations possible.

Are We There Yet? Building Levels of Participation

> *By the end they had everyone participating and that was great because, um, yeah, not all of our students would do that in a classroom situation, usually.*
>
> —*Teacher*

The following section discusses the major building blocks used to establish intensive and rich interactions between actors and audience members. It is meant to be read while referencing the AWTY script and the DVD, which provides an example of each of the major participatory sequences in performance with teen audiences.

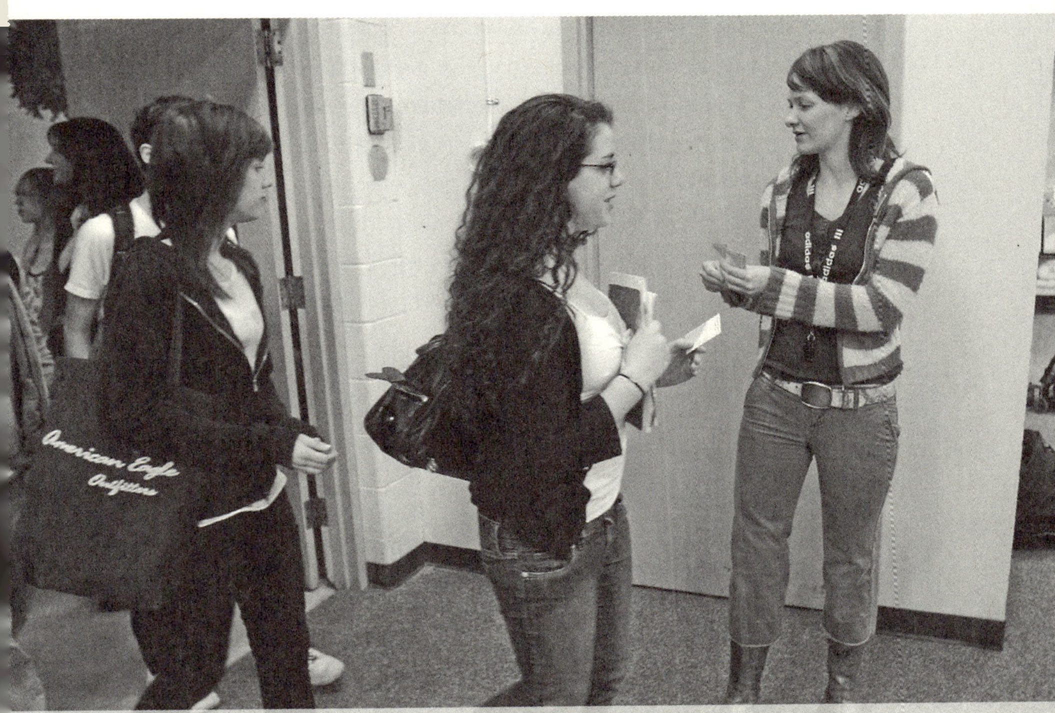

Greeting the audience
Kristi Hansen, Concrete Theatre. Photograph courtesy of Epic Photography.

1. Arrival: Relationship Building

Chapter 3, page 67

Actors chat with audience members as they arrive, building rapport and getting to know what they may be like. Identifying audience differences from performance to performance will affect how the actor interacts and asks for advice later; this is a key opportunity to read the audience, get a feel for the group, and sense their cultures. While showing the audience where to sit and handing out resource cards, actors signal that this is a performance with a difference; they are setting up the two-way communication and their interest in the teen audience. In rehearsal, actors prepare for this arrival period by developing some questions and topics that the teens find easy to answer; it helps to have these available to use as needed. Actors might ask, for example,

"What class are you missing to come to the play?" They might chat about the resource card and ask, "Have you heard of this great website?" etc.

During the rehearsal period, this stage, and others in the play, are assisted by live research with this age group (fourteen to sixteen years) and in their milieu (school, recreation, and teen popular culture). During the tour, this preparation is enhanced on a day-by-day basis by observations as actors arrive at the school and start to interact in the hallways and as the audiences arrive at the show. Open-hearted interest in the audience is key.

2. *"Just a Minute": Actors Risk Lots, Audience Risks Just a Little*

Chapter 3, page 68

- Participation is Fun
- Raising the Topic (Sex)

This high-energy introductory section asks for a deliberately low-risk and easy level of participation that has a fun payoff. Audience members are asked for single words; it is a brainstorm on feelings people have when they think of the word sex. Actors risk more than the audience: whereas the audience throws out single words in a brainstorm atmosphere, the actors improvise stories based on these words. Actors demonstrate that they are here to deal openly with the risky subject of the emotions felt about sex. In this section, actors also signal to the audience that participation is easy and fun, that participating will not necessarily lead to being singled out, that the audience has the power to affect how the play goes, and that the actors will work with whatever is thrown at them, no holds barred. Some words that audiences often offer: *nervous, warm, hot, happy, shy, excited.*

> *I think the perfect story for "Just A Minute" is usually a story that has a little bit of risk and risqué-ness to it. The kids are going, "oh, I can't quite believe that person said that." But also actors maybe incorporate a first time experience. A lot of times actors will draw on things that happened to them when they were in junior high. I think a "first time" story is great because it has a sense of excitement and "oh, I really want to try this out," but there's also a lot of peril involved, and danger, potential humiliation or embarrassment, so I think those stories are great, rich, fertile ground to look for a story*

that can capture all the words that the kids throw out, from excited to horny to disappointed to...

—*Mieko Ouchi,* AWTY *director, Concrete Theatre*

Techniques:[5] Gather
Tools:[6] Yes! Yes And, Second Question, Situation Prompt, Use a Story, Repeat, Summarize

3. Marcel and Delphi: Problem Solving for Characters Like the Audience

Scene: "Signs and Signals" (Chapter 3, page 72)

- Participation about Characters in Crisis
- Participation with a Facilitator (Instructor Two)
- Going past the First/Easy Answers

The power of *AWTY* is in its focus on assisting audiences to apply information and knowledge that they have but may not necessarily use within emotionally charged situations. The situations are recognizable and meaningful to them, and have high stakes. Using information and knowledge and acting on things that we know are important can be hard. For example, we know honest communication is important in a relationship, but actually doing that around a sensitive topic such as sex is difficult. Or we want to enjoy being physically close to someone we care about, but how close? How intimate? How soon? What does he/she want? How do we speak about what we want?

In this sequence, the audience is asked to move up a level in their participation and talk about what two characters are experiencing and how they could deal with the difficulties they are having with their relationship. The audience watches a scene of a young couple who wants to be together but keeps getting in trouble when they try to express themselves physically. The scene has an important backstory and is rich with subtext and body language; characters think and feel things they do not say. The scene develops to a crisis point and an actor/facilitator (Instructor Two) stops the scene and then asks the audience why the couple is having trouble.

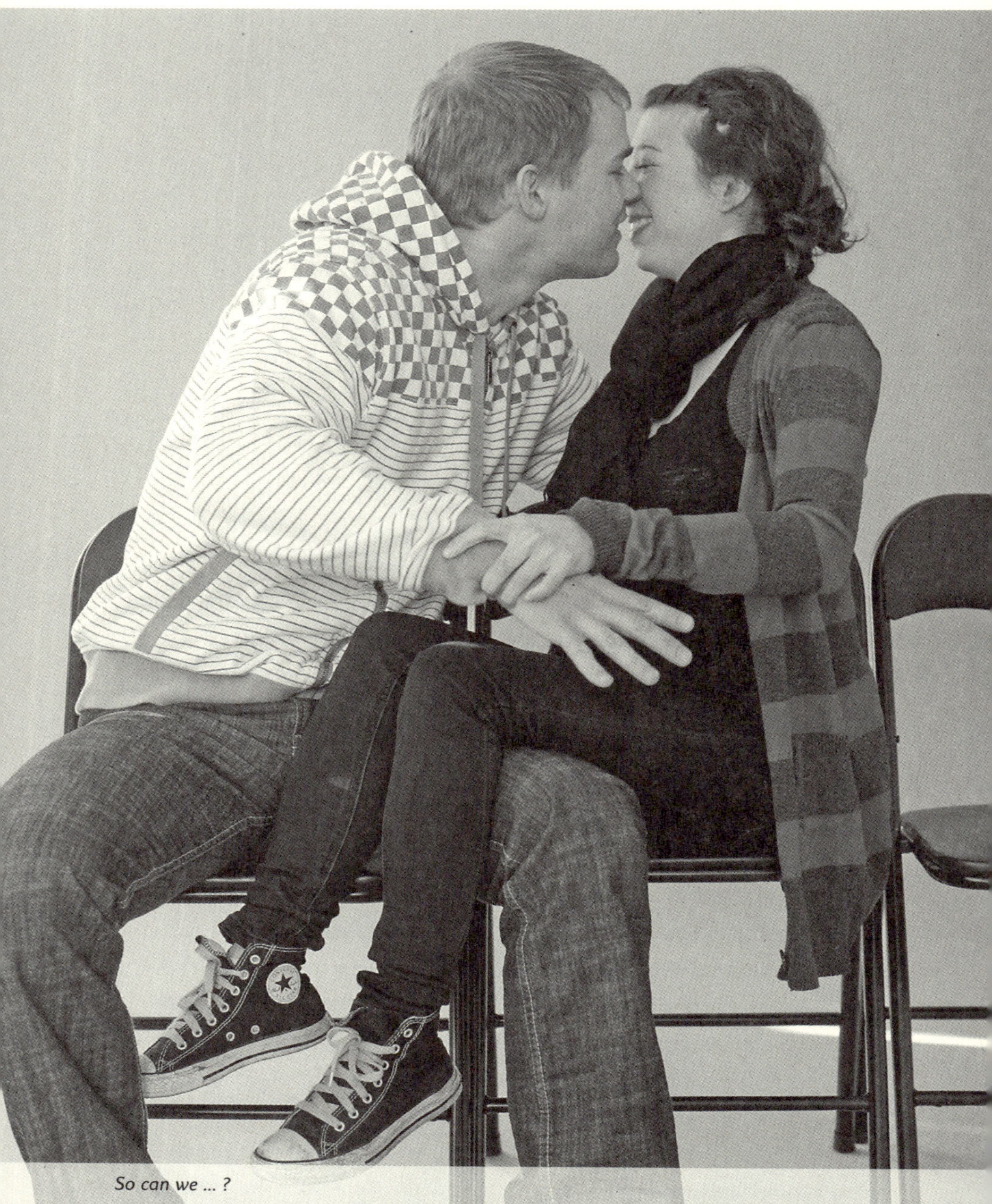

So can we ... ?
Cole Humeny and Ming Hudson, Concrete Theatre. Photograph courtesy of Epic Photography.

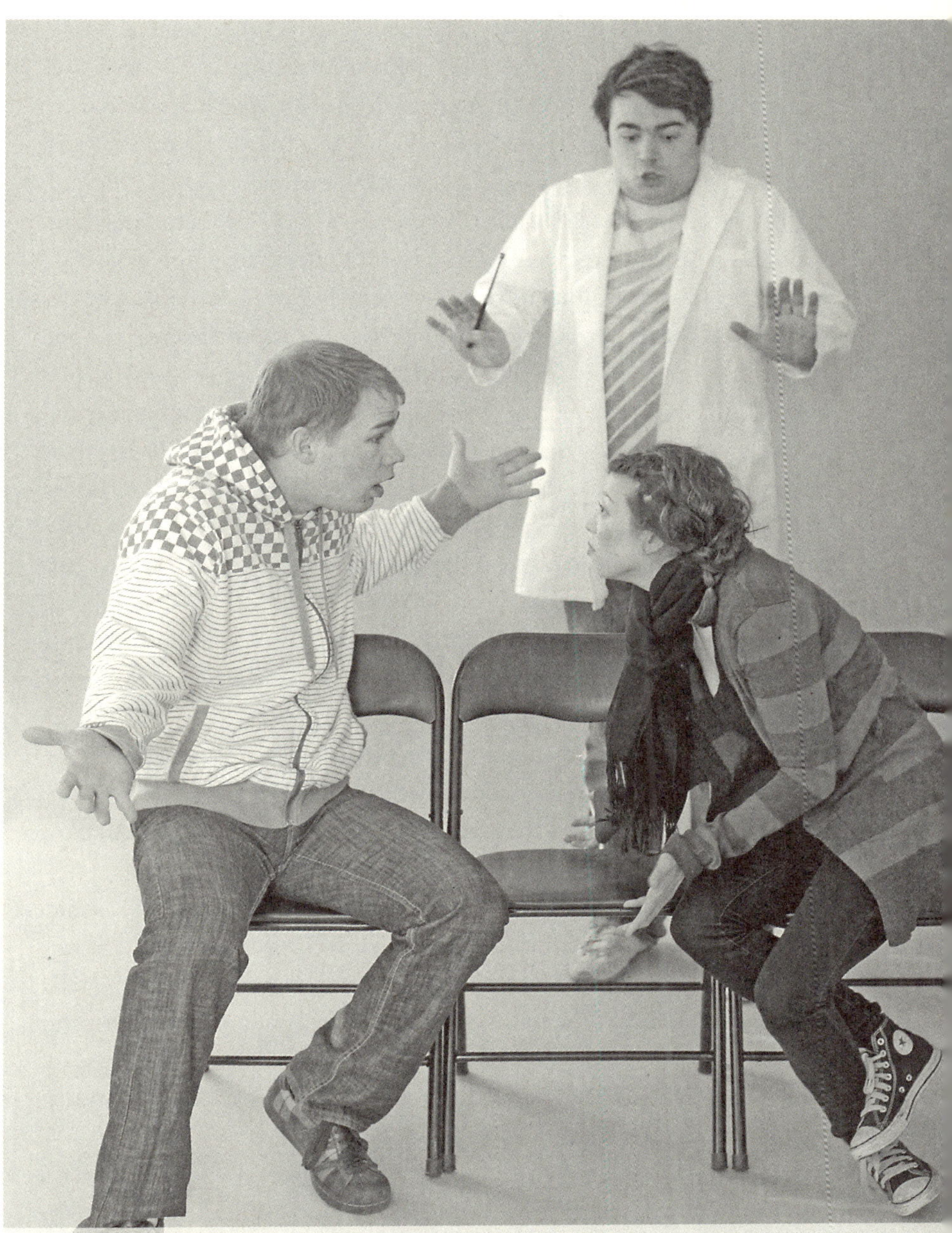

I don't know what you want
Cole Humeny, Garett Spelliscy, and Ming Hudson, Concrete Theatre. Photograph courtesy of Epic Photography.

At this stage of the play, using a facilitator enables the audience to talk about but not to the characters, characters that have similarities with the audience. Audience members identify with one or both characters and recognize the situation. The facilitator helps them to assess what they just saw (and felt). He *GATHERS* ideas then CHECKS IN with characters.[7] The gather approach continues to build an atmosphere where all ideas are valued; after all, there are many interpretations and points of view on why and how human relations are difficult! The actor/facilitator wants to encourage lots of people to take this step and offer their ideas, and the gather stage is important to encourage many voices, to signal that everyone's ideas are welcome, and to signal that this is a play where the point is to explore situations and consider options rather than seek one correct answer. It is important that the actor/facilitator uses this stage to continue to draw out a variety of voices and signal that participation is valued and not too scary. There is a state of *Yes and* in the facilitation; in essence, the facilitator is saying, "*Yes* (what a great contribution), *and* are there any more ideas?"

Here the facilitator is helped by sitting in a place of deep curiosity. He is curious about the scene (the situation) and curious about the audience members' views of how and why it went wrong.

After audience members are asked to say what they see in the scene and to interpret what may be going on, the facilitator CHECKS IN with the characters to find out how they see things. This provides a prompt to move to the next level: despite these problems, the characters do not want to break up, so what do they need to do? This question comes back out to the audience (Chapter 3, page 74), and the discussion is moved beyond observation and opinion and toward ideas for action. As audience members think and talk about how the characters could improve their communication and relationship, they start to name values and approaches they do, can, or will use in their own relationships. They identify some of their own ideas and strategies and hear those of others.

The actor/facilitator's role here is as a guide through a process of reflecting on and interpreting the characters' behaviours (What happened? What is going wrong? Why?) and then, with the help of a check in with the characters (they say they don't want to break up), DEEPENING the audience's discussion by moving them to consider actions these characters could take (What

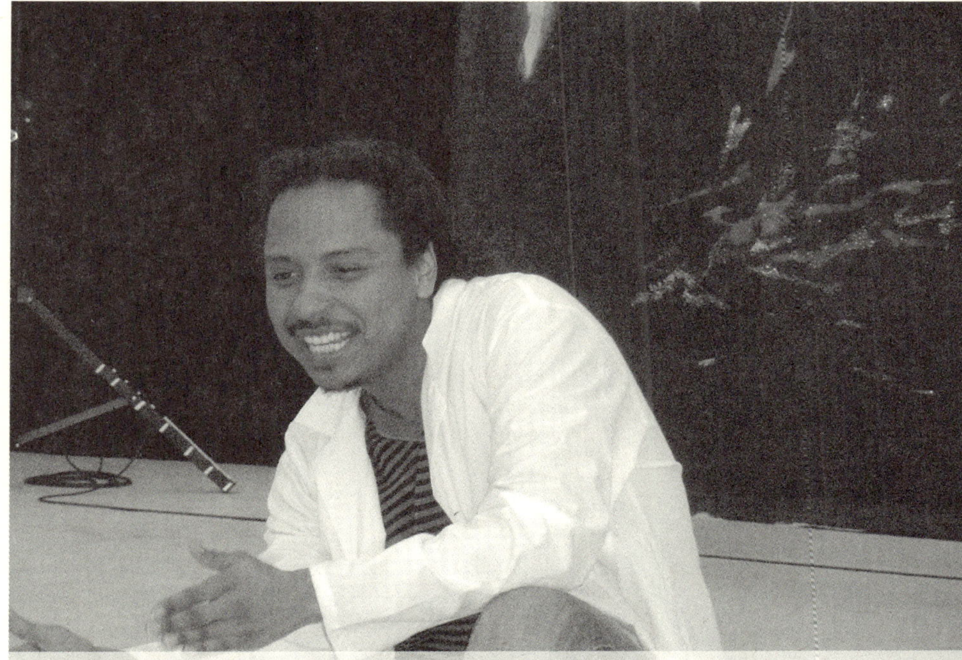

What does this mean for these two?
Arron Naytowhow, Saskatchewan North Theatre Company. *Photograph courtesy of Jane Heather*

can they do?). A process is started here, one that is developed much further in later participatory sections, where, while all ideas are welcome, there are complications. While all ideas may be good ideas in theory, the element of character is added to the mix. For example, while some in the audience may think that Marcel and Delphi's relationship is so problematic that they should break up, these two characters don't want to. The answer was not wrong but in this situation, with these two people, this option will not be taken. Plays can offer this complexity; there are good answers that must be mixed in with real life, as people and characters are not all built the same. And that is okay.

Instructor Two is used to prompt the audience, to gather ideas and demonstrate respect for ideas and insights. He charts the course of the participation. After building an atmosphere where ideas are valued, he starts to probe and deepen the discussion. The discussion is in terms of real

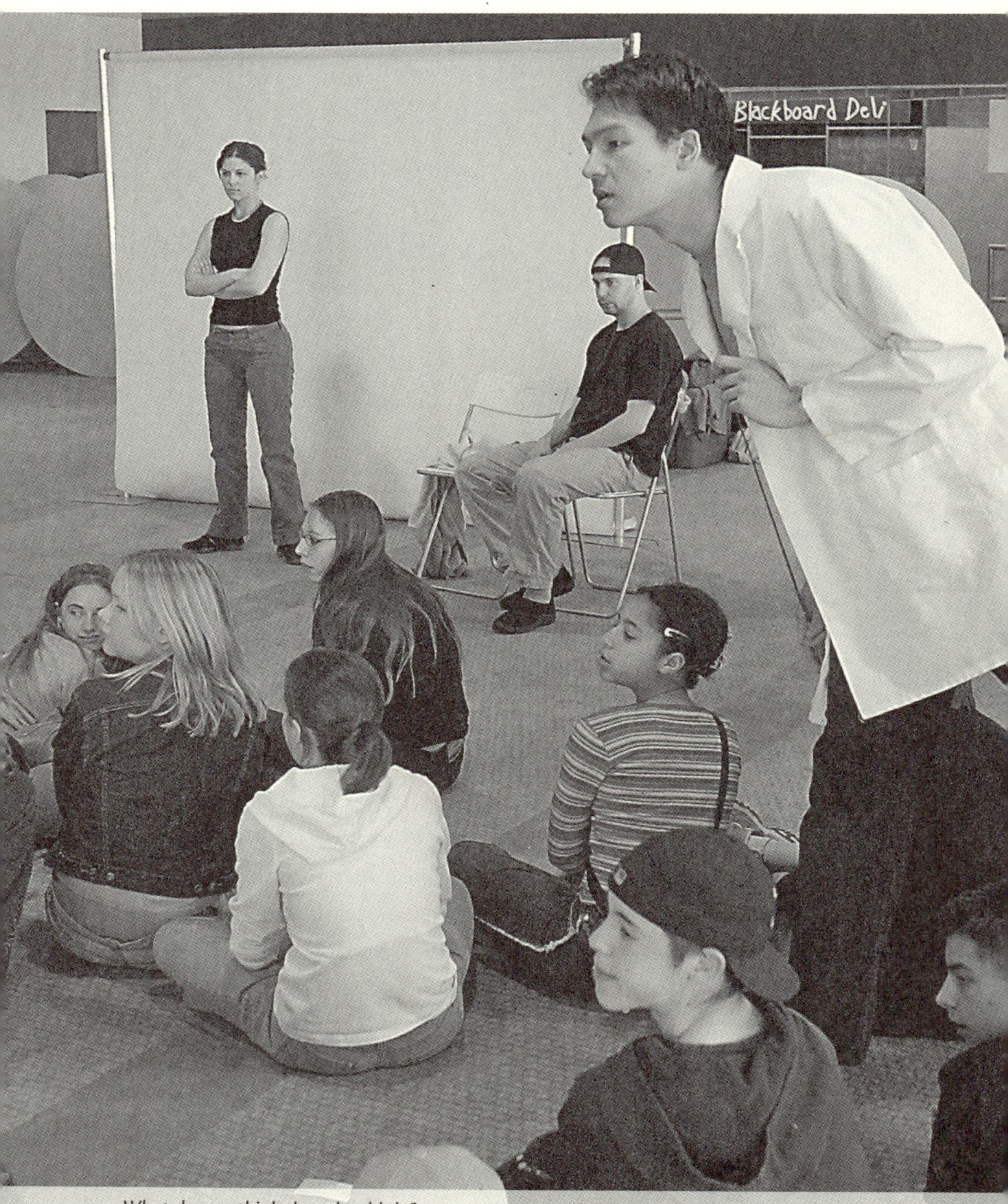

What do you think they should do?
Jared Matsunaga-Turnbull with Shannon Larson and Bob Rasko, Concrete Theatre. *Photograph courtesy of Epic Photography.*

characters, who are in a difficult situation. Audience members are asked to interpret and take into account a full and complex situation. Easy answers are probed and apparently right answers may or may not work for these specific characters. The facilitator role is also used in this sequence because, in this early stage of the play, there is a need to teach some vocabulary and skills. One of the barriers to clear communication is the lack of language that is comfortable enough to use in speaking about sex. An exercise for identifying sexual boundaries is introduced to the characters and the audience (Chapter 3, page 75), and this again moves the participatory discussion to a new level.

> *The approach I took with Instructor Two is "I have some knowledge on this but I'm not sure exactly what to do in this situation, maybe we can talk this out together." As soon as you build the relationship of togetherness and "we're gonna work through something, we're gonna work on this in a collaborative fashion," then I think we can get further along.*
>
> —*Ryland Alexander,* AWTY *actor,*
> *Concrete Theatre, August 29, 2010*

As suggestions come from the audience, the facilitator's job is to PROBE some of these ideas. For example, a common answer to "Since they have different boundaries, what should they do?" is "compromise." This idea, while attractive, has some problems when it comes to respecting a partner's sexual boundaries, and in this project, it is vital to probe this idea in-depth. The facilitator unpacks this idea with the audience. (Chapter 3, page 76; Appendix 1.5)

A very personal set of discussions has taken place by providing the audience with characters and a situation to assess. They advise, watch, and interact via a facilitator. Easy answers, such as "communicate," are unpacked and probed (What should she say? Why do you think he doesn't tell her?), language for talking about a sensitive subject is offered, and with the help of the facilitator and the audience, the characters move forward, develop skills and go off to try to apply them.

> *I think something that can't be underestimated in* Are We There Yet? *is the skills that you learn as you accumulate performances, and one of the things I really notice about the Instructor in "Marcel and Delphi" is, as people get more confident with the show and more confident with that role, we start to get to the kind of jazz of it. They move beyond the "I have to hit these five points in order to get to the end of the scene." They can have a bit more fun, and realize you don't have to do things in the same order. Maybe the kids take you in a roundabout way. You know where you're going, and you have to have the confidence, and that comes with experience, of knowing that you will get there.*
>
> —*Mieko Ouchi*

Techniques: Gather, Deepen
Tools: Paraphrase, Summarize, Check In with Characters, Probe, Investigate, Test Out Ideas

4. Mac and Carol Ann: Problem Solving for and with Characters

Scene: "Talking Protection" (Chapter 3, page 79)

- Working with Characters to Guide Them through a Crisis
- Facilitating in Character
- Acknowledging Attitudes
- Dealing with Emotion and Personality: One Answer Does Not Fit All
- Testing Out Strategies

The audience is ready to move to a new level of participation, one that builds their connections with characters who are in dilemmas that are recognizable to the audience. In this sequence, audience members give advice directly to teen characters and the characters try to use advice they are given. Some advice is successful, other advice may be good advice for some people but the particular character cannot use it at this point, and other advice complicates things even more. In this participatory sequence, the audience in effect becomes responsible for their suggestions; characters need their help if they are to find their way through obstacles in their relationship, and some pieces of advice work out better than others.

The characters need help. They need the audience's insights, wisdom, and thoughts. They need to explore their feelings and they need to learn how to

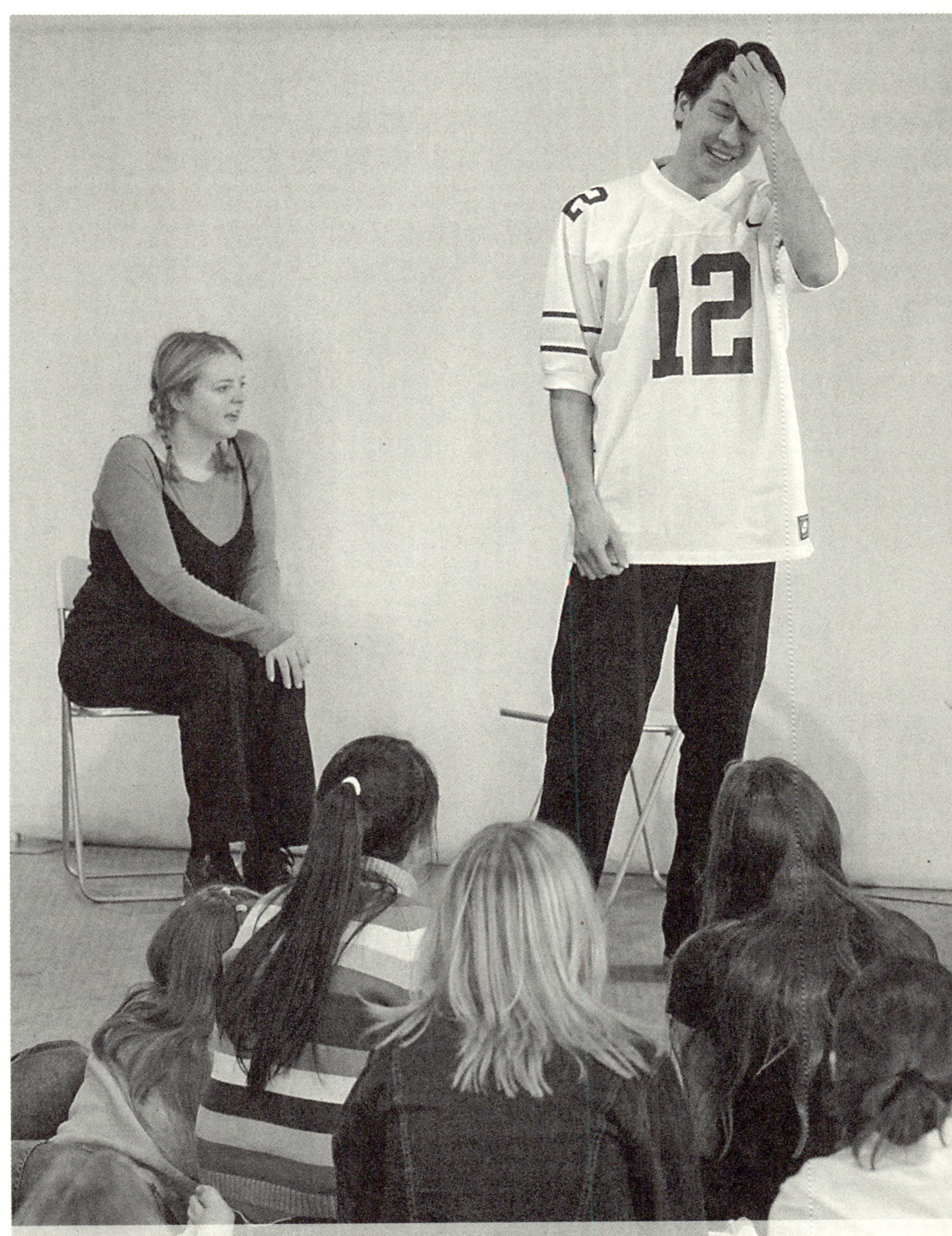

I should have thought of that
Jana O'Connor and Jared Matsunaga-Turnbull, Concrete Theatre. *Photograph courtesy of Epic Photography.*

approach a difficult, complex situation with their partner. They don't know what to do or how to deal with their feelings. It is through this need that the audience is drawn to participate and think through the dilemmas the characters face. There are no easy answers: the characters are complex, the situation is difficult, and strategies that may be theoretically correct (such as "just tell him what you think" or "be honest") are not necessarily easy or possible for a specific person in a specific situation at a specific time.

On one hand, the audience is dealing with real-life situations in all their complexity. On the other hand, this is theatre, and there is permission to try out all sorts of ideas, ones that might not be offered in real-life situations. Audience members can challenge characters to try bad ideas, ask characters to try out ideas they would not use but are curious about, blurt out things, uncensored, and discover strategies they have not thought about before. In essence, because it is theatre, there is permission to speak about things they may not speak about in their lives; areas of silence can be voiced; tentative ideas can be explored and tested in this safe situation. It is play in the deepest sense of the word.

When characters directly interact with the audience there is an opportunity to personalize a situation, build emotional involvement with a character (and their fate), and convince an audience that this is not a lecture-demo but something connected to their direct experience. The actor endows the audience with being wise, insightful, and full of ideas that are important. In essence, they are a character's best friends, with all the complexity that allows. Friends can be intimate and can also challenge. They can offer good and bad advice. They can play the fool or can operate as bosom buddies.

> *[As Carol Ann] I think it's really important to be emotionally invested and make sure they know how hard this is to say, how much you like him, how much you want to make it work, and that you're ready for this big step of having sex and wanting to do it right and how important that is to you. So the audience is going to absolutely sympathize with you if your emotional need is that great. They're going to want to help you. You can really appreciate when someone's being so honest with you, and you can't really dismiss them. You can't really dismiss that emotional need.*
>
> —*Kristi Hansen,* AWTY *actor,*
> *Concrete Theatre, August 27, 2010*

Theatre allows yet a further step. Characters can say things to their audience/confidantes that people may or may not say in real life, not even to their friends. They can admit fears and ignorance. Admit mistakes. Ask for help unabashedly. They work from a character base, not an instructor base. The teaching and learning occurs because the dramatic situation deals with vital moments in characters' and audience members' lives, moments where they need to learn about and use a myriad of skills and information and name their values and intentions. The characters seek help in getting what they want, but in varying ways. Each character works differently, in their own vernacular, in their own terms. Some ask for help openly, vulnerably, whereas other characters challenge their audience buddies. (In the DVD, note that Carol Ann interacts with the audience in different ways than Mac, but both work from a position of a fully formed character, with a history, a personality and a set of wants and needs. Over many productions, we have seen extremely different, and effective, approaches to these characterizations.)

Actors are most effective when they develop complex characters with histories that relate to their dilemmas, rich emotional lives that they can reveal, and lots of obstacles between them and solving the situation they are in. The audience is needed to help them work through the land mines of the situation and the conflicts and contradictions inherent in the characters.

In this sequence, the characters try out some good ideas that do not work. This strategy deepens the discussion and asks audience members to look more deeply at the situation. Carol Ann may be told to tell Mac why she ran away and that they need to use condoms; she enters the situation thinking this will work. However, Mac is too angry or worried to hear any of this; soon Carol Ann is back out with the audience, trying to figure out why that great advice did not work and what she should do now. Sometimes characters try out a bad idea. In this moment, the audience learns several things: they have power (the actor does what the audience member suggests); this is an honest enterprise (participation is invited and suggestions are taken seriously, not ignored); the audience is responsible for a character's fate (the bad idea may get the character into only hotter water and more difficulties); it is theatre (we can have some fun while we investigate serious matters). Once the actor builds a good and honest rapport with the audience, characters can relate

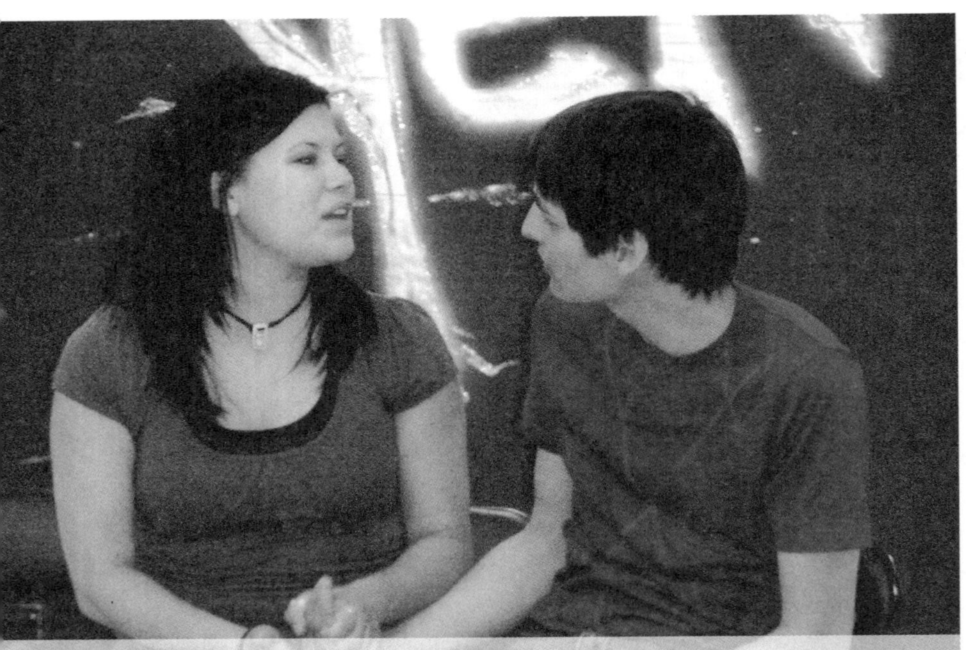

It'll be okay
Krystle Pederson and Clifford Cardinal, Saskatchewan Native Theatre Company. *Photograph courtesy of Jane Heather.*

to audiences with a wide range of emotions and approaches, from intimate confessions, to blasting them (for bad advice), to panic, to gratitude.

Theatre also allows the writer and characters to say things a person who is like the character might never say in real life in order to plunge even deeper into the issue. For example, Mac expresses some of his underlying fears about condom use and his sexual capacity: "What if she sees you and you aren't...what she expected? What if everything just...fades away? What if she laughs?" Here a character can say the unsayable and move to a new level of honesty and vulnerability with the audience.

Animating in role offers a very rich, in-depth kind of participation, asking for a range of emotional experiences and insights as well as specific strategies and knowledge. The themes of the play are explored in the context of flesh-and-blood characters who must deal with their own emotions and relationships as well as those of others. The audience is invited to explore an issue or topic in a lived complexity, before applying knowledge, skills, language, insights, and strategies in their own lives.

Techniques: Animate in Role, Gather, Deepen, Play Out Audience Suggestions
Tools: Paraphrase, Summarize, Dangle, Story Tell, Block, Probe, Investigate, Test Out Ideas in Scenes, Keep a Thread between Audience and Character, Play Out Bad Advice/Good Advice, Try to Take Advice and Fail or Succeed, Thank the Audience

5. Clay: Ownership and Applying Insights

Scene: "Practice Your Skills" (Chapter 3, page 88)

- Building a Team
- Building Audience Ownership (of a Character's Fate)
- Applying Principles and Knowledge in a New and Difficult Situation
- Building the Stakes
- Enjoying Success (No Magic Though!)
- Confronting a Problem: Using the Huddle, Threads of Connection, Accountability

This section is the least scripted and the most participatory. The audience is divided into gender-based teams and invited to build a character that they will guide through several stages of a relationship. The intent is to build a very high level of ownership in each team, so that the audience feels entwined in the character's fate. Stakes are high and the audience is engaged and responsible for the characters' approaches, wants, and foibles. With this degree of ownership established, the characters face a major relationship crisis and the audience assists them to renegotiate their sexual boundaries.

"Step One: Stereotypes" (Chapter 3, page 89)

First the team is built, and the new ways of working are introduced. Stereotype characters are created by the teams and a scene where they meet is played out with high exaggeration. This section sets up the ground rules and procedures; a coach (actor/facilitator) and Clay (an actor who will take on the character traits the group proposes) guide the group process. In addition to introducing the rules of the game, the stereotype sequence lightly

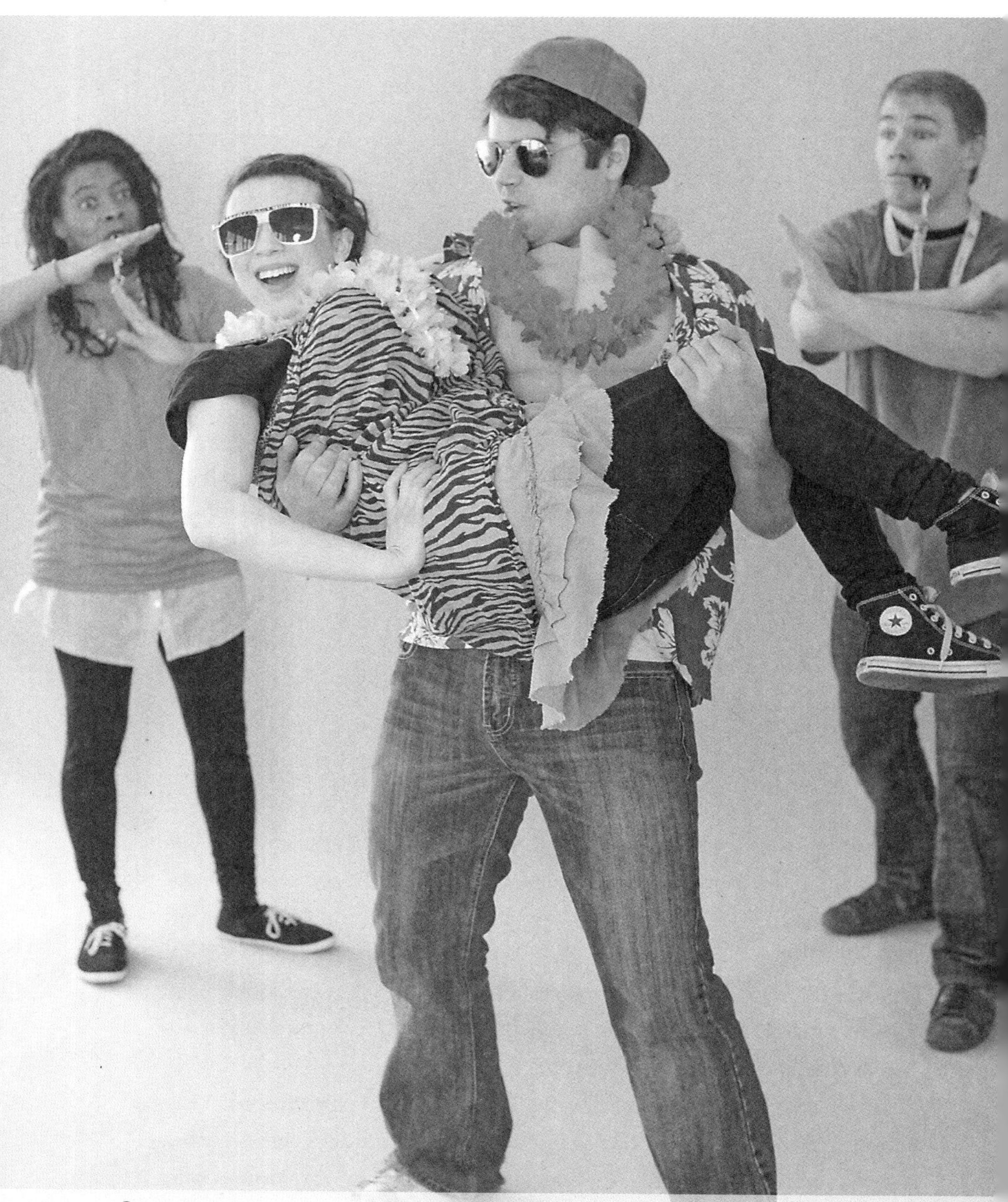

Stereotypes
Monice Peter, Ming Hudson, Garett Spelliscy, and Cole Humeny, Concrete Theatre. Photograph courtesy of Epic Photography.

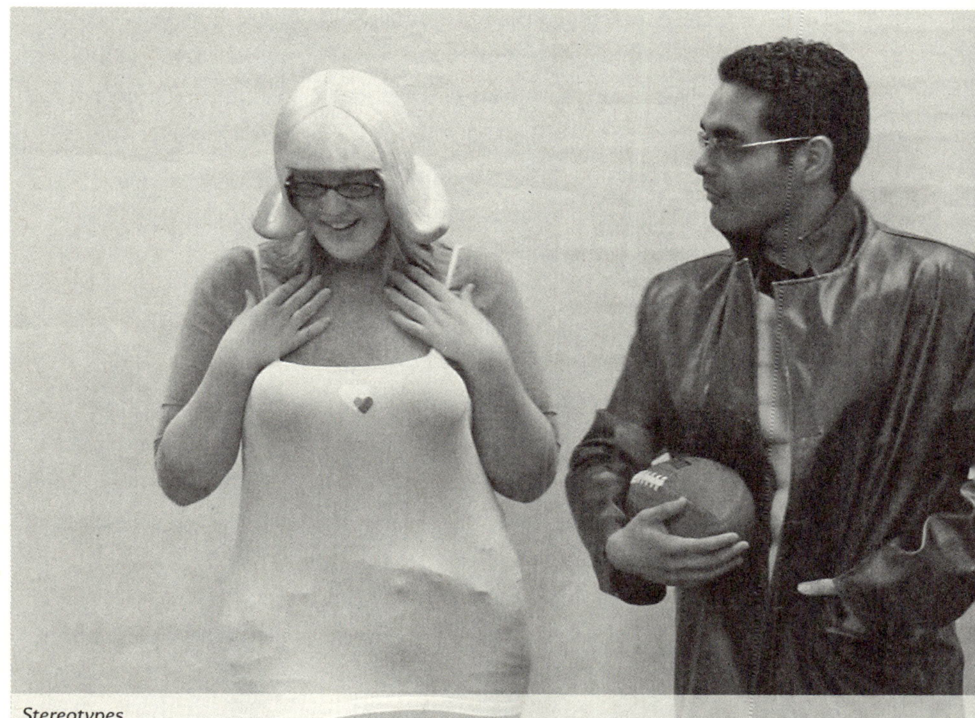

Stereotypes
Jana O'Connor and Gilly Urra, Concrete Theatre. Photograph courtesy of Epic Photography.

dispenses with the unreal life of media, pop videos, and advertising; now the groups are ready to create characters "that could be someone they go to school with."

"Step Two: Real People" (*Chapter 3, page 90*)

The actors build as much involvement as possible from as many as possible, and normally many who have yet to speak up do so now. Several things help to build this level of participation: involvement grows, entertainment is high, and a sense of a private huddle is created. As the new, more familiar and realistic character is created, the process again develops from brainstorming lots of ideas (a GATHER) to selecting from this long list. The Coach and Clay both elicit suggestions so they can reach a lot of the group. Audiences develop alliance and engagement with their character as the character is developed and later as the character confronts moments where they need advice. Often from a position of engagement and investment and a sense of high stakes, participants see their strategies tested. They get immediate feedback on things that work and things that don't work for their character, who is grappling with a relationship with another specific character and particular situation. It is not a play about rules; it is a play about developing skills, agency, and confidence to take action.

"Step Three: Meeting Someone" (Chapter 3, page 91) *and* *"Step Four: Asking Someone on a Date"* (Chapter 3, page 92)

These two scenes establish the characters, build the team ownership of their character, and establish theatrical conventions where the team both advises in a huddle with the character and coaches them while they are in the scenes (see DVD for several examples). Audience members can live out each moment, coaching characters through foibles, mistakes, and difficulties; involvement and engagement is very high. Meanwhile, actors take as much advice and side coaching as possible, establish strong threads between their team and their actions, build a sense of responsibility with the group, and in the scenes, establish that the characters care a lot for each other.

In the interests of shortening the show for specific school situations, companies have explored collapsing these scenes together. Although this is a good strategy when schools cannot accommodate the show's optimal length of eighty-five to ninety minutes, artists observe that this strategy leads to a loss in participants' ownership and depth of responsibility for characters' fates.

"Step Five: Dealing with a Relationship Crisis" (Chapter 3, page 92)

The previous scenes lay the groundwork for confronting a major crisis in the growing relationship. Audiences can see (and feel) that the characters care a lot for each other. Involvement with their character sets the stage for rich engagement in working through a new and challenging problem. In this final scene, audience members confront a new level of challenge and are intrinsically invited to apply tools developed over the rest of the play (for example, "Defining Your Boundaries," Chapter 3, page 75). Because the crisis goes beyond early issues, they also discover and test new strategies.

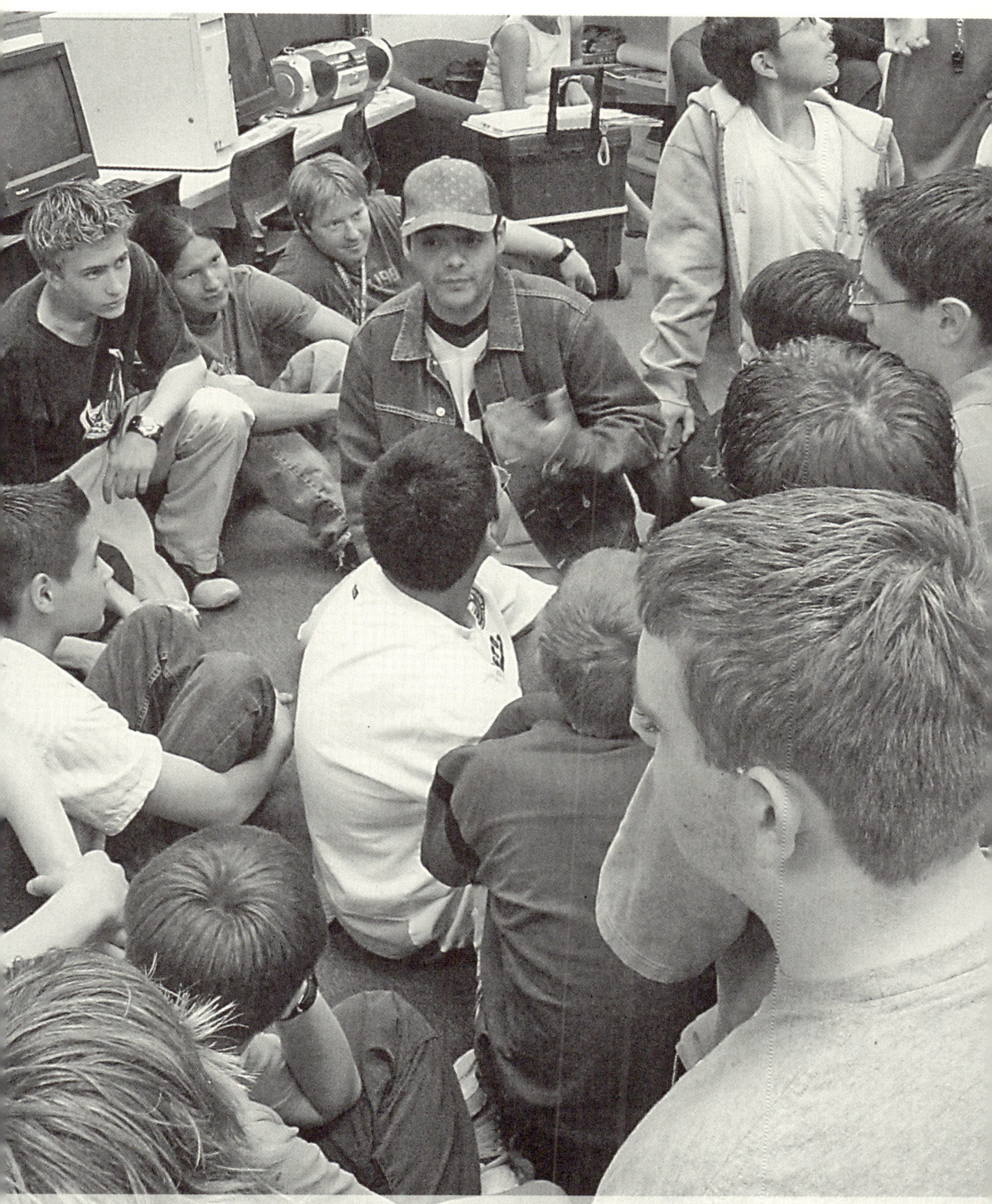

Character seeks advice
Gilly Urra (in hat), Concrete Theatre. *Photograph courtesy of Epic Photography.*

The scene is started with a huddle, an intimate and honest story about the characters' relationship crisis. The character establishes a new tone; it is very serious. Then the character asks for help sorting out what to say and do.

By this point in the performance, usually levels of participation have grown from little, one-word comments through to in-depth, intense involvement in coaching and problem solving for characters that are in complex and challenging situations that could happen to audience members, now or in the future.

Techniques: Audience Creates the Character, Facilitator (Coach) and Character Animate, Animate in Role, Gather, Deepen, Play Out Audience Suggestions, Struggle with a Complex Problem

Tools: Paraphrase, Summarize, Block, Probe, Test Out Ideas in Scenes, Keep a Thread between Audience and Character, Build a Team, The Team Huddle, Play Out Bad Advice/Good Advice, Try to Take Advice and Fail/Succeed, Side Coaching, Time Out

6. After the Play: Being There

Given this high degree of investment by many in the audience, around a highly sensitive topic, after the play it is vital that all members of the company are available for individuals to speak with. Some want to chat in groups, and sometimes individuals need a one-on-one. This is a kind of relevant art that builds responsibility for audiences, and companies need to stay accessible and also have a strategy in place for handling intense responses. While the play does not set out to elicit disclosures of abuse or other power, violence, or relationship problems, it can do so, and companies plan and practice how they will respond when such a situation arises. (See Chapter 6 on the role of the health educator.)

This kind of play builds an audience's sense of connection with the artists, a connection seldom so vitally and directly experienced in other forms of theatre.

> *Just remember it's about the kids. I think you're going to get a huge reward if you just focus on that. Each class is different, each group is different.*
>
> —*Evelyn Chu,* AWTY *actor,*
> *Neworld Theatre*

NOTES

1. For clear and extensive examinations of the history of participation, theatre, and education, see Jackson (2007) and Nicholson (2009).
2. See Chapter 9 for information about how audience engagement affects levels of impact.
3. See Chapter 9 for insights into how participation levels affect audience change.
4. Because Concrete Theatre originally commissioned and produced the play, production descriptions, unless otherwise noted, refer to Concrete's approaches to staging the play.
5. Techniques: Theatrical participation is facilitated through several key techniques. These are discussed in "What's under the Hood?"
6. Tools: There are a variety of useful methods for accomplishing the techniques of theatrical participation. These are defined and discussed in "What's under the Hood?"
7. Techniques and tools in are demonstrated on the DVD.

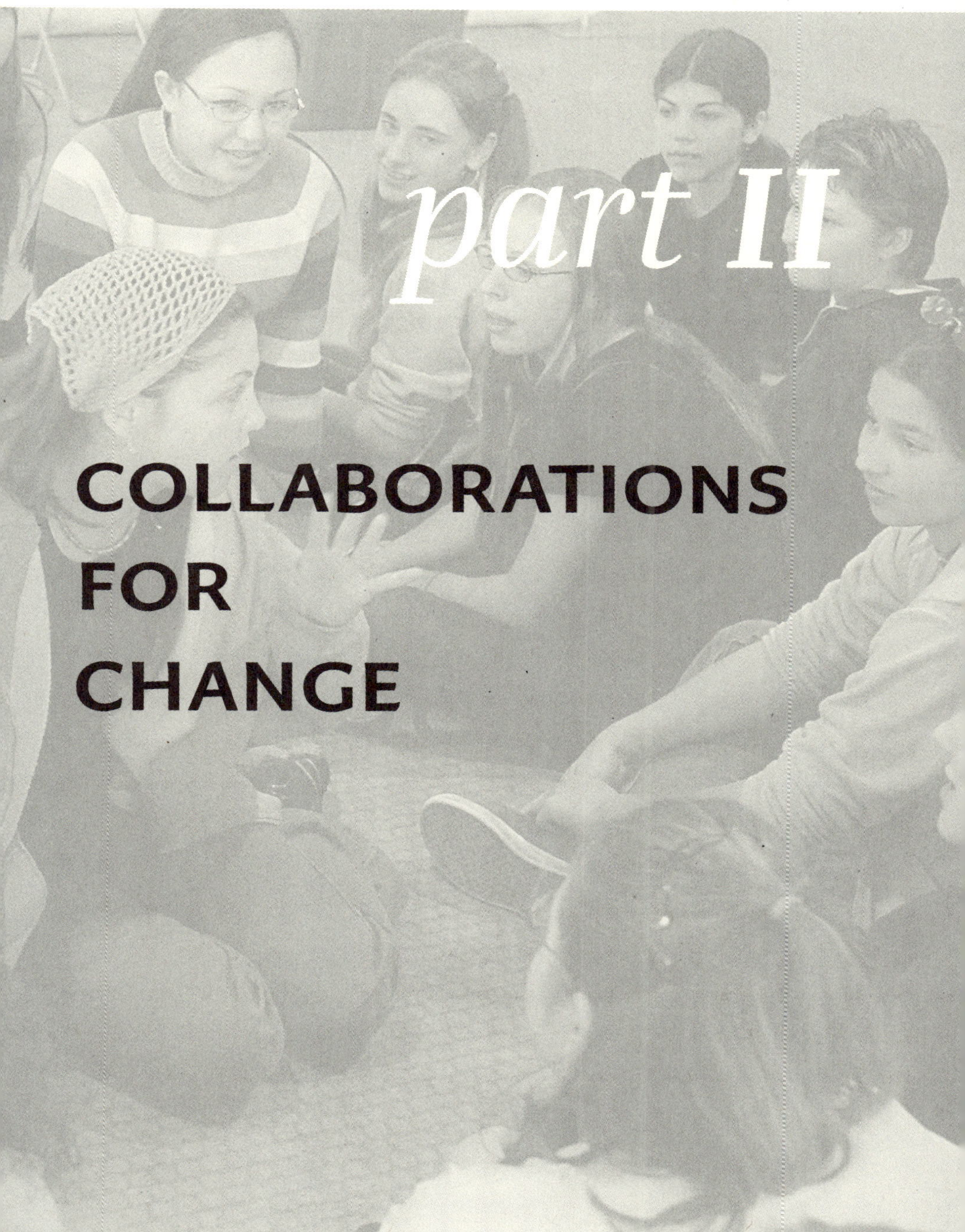

part II

COLLABORATIONS FOR CHANGE

The Importance of Partnerships

THE ARE WE THERE YET? PROGRAM relies upon an important partnership between a theatre company and a sexual health organization to achieve its goals. The idea of a partnership between a theatre and a human service agency, non-government agency (NGO), or community organization, where each partner contributes its own expertise, culture, and resources toward a common goal, is not new. In the 1970s and 1980s, practitioners working in popular theatre and theatre for social change regularly worked with organizations in the community to avoid the practice of hit-and-run theatre. Theatre practitioners and development workers recognized that the educational and social impact of the theatre dissipated when not supported and accompanied by an established community agency or organization with a congruent intentions and mandate. Adult educator and popular theatre organizer Ross Kidd (1987) vigorously advocated partnerships and influenced many theatre artists' community practice: "Theatre on its own can bring people together and create a forum for awareness-raising and discussion, but it cannot create the conditions for organized action. Without links to local organizations or to a process for organizing people around the issues, the experience normally ends with the end of the theatre activity." Theatre can be a significant catalyst for change, and can deeply link insights and information with motivating impulses and emotive connectors. On the other hand, the impact of one theatre event, however insightful and powerful, may not create lasting change in and of itself, amidst all the noise of contemporary life, advertising, political, social, and economic factors, and competing messages. Theatre can stir up audience engagement and concerns, which can be a force for change, if integrated with organizational, educational, and action strategies. It can also raise issues for people who then look for ways to make use of their insights and seek some kinds of support, organization, or group opportunity.

Linkages can be accomplished in various ways, but in Canada they are most often achieved via partnerships between a theatre company and an organization that is tied to the issue, topic, or initiative, and is set up for long-term action. Partner organizations include development-focused NGOs, citizens' action groups, neighbourhood organizations, education-based agencies, unions, public health organizations, and government agencies. Examples of such partnerships include:

- Catalyst Theatre partnered with Alberta Alcohol and Drug Abuse Commission (AADAC) for many years to build community awareness about the impacts of abuse on families and supports for recovery processes (*Drinks before Dinner*) and to support teen resiliency programs (*What's up Chuck?*, *The Black Creek Project*, *Talk is Cheap*, *Zeke and the Indoor Plants*, and others)
- Great Canadian Theatre Company partnered with playwright Andrew Kushnir and Project: Humanity, a non-profit organization that raises awareness about social issues through arts
- Headlines Theatre partnered with British Columbia's Social Planning and Research Council (SPARC) and used theatre to develop broad-based citizen dialogue to form new policy on housing (*After Homelessness*)
- Second Look Community Arts partnered with the Canadian Red Cross to write a play about anti-personnel landmines, which was performed by schools and youth groups across Canada
- The Law Society of Alberta partnered with Catalyst Theatre for an initiative that developed awareness and actions around the legal rights of mentally handicapped adults and their families (*Stand up for Your Rights*)
- Ground Zero partnered with Ontario Council of Hospital Unions to raise public awareness of the threat to public health care during the deficit-slashing era of the 1990s. Union representatives and theatre workers

allied to produce a series of events ranging from media opportunities such as a MASH tent on the lawn of the Ontario legislature through to an extended tour to union locals throughout the province

In some cases, the theatre company becomes the ongoing, issue-specific organization, building all of its theatre activities around a specific community, issue, or initiative. Some examples of this approach are:

- Cardboard Citizens, UK, on homelessness
- The Lawnmowers, UK, on issues of concern to people with learning disabilities
- Cornerstone Theater, USA, on the urban experience of living in Los Angeles, which works in community residencies to have community members identify issues, create the play, and perform with the company
- Geese Theatre, UK, on prison issues

In these cases, the theatre companies are both long-term and action-based in and of themselves. As issue-based leaders, they often become important players in alliances with other social organizations.

In other cases, a public health or other kind of development or public education organization builds theatre expertise and activity internally, to integrate with much of their ongoing programming:

- Ottawa Planned Parenthood annually offers Insight Theatre, a "non-profit, public education theatre program created by, for, and about youth. Every year, a group of senior levels students from schools all over the city face the challenge of creating, directing and acting in their own show about sexual and reproductive health, and presenting it to their peers" (Ottawa Planned Parenthood 2009).
- Forum for African Women Educationalists (FAWE) is a pan-African NGO that works "to empower girls and women through gender-responsive education" in thirty-two African countries. One of their programs is *Tuseme* (Let Us Speak Out), which uses theatre-for-development techniques to address concerns that hinder girls' social and academic development. It "trains girls to identify and understand the problems that affect them, articulate these problems and take action to solve

them. Through drama, song and creative arts, girls learn negotiation skills, how to speak out, self-confidence, decision-making and leadership skills" (FAWE 2009). FAWE works with a range of partners, including NGOs and education ministries to achieve gender equity and equality in education.

Depending upon the context, education- and action-based partner organizations may play a number of roles. During the production and pre-production period, partners may determine an ongoing action strategy (within which the theatre event(s) play a role), provide up-to-date research and expertise on an issue, prepare a community/audience for a theatre event, facilitate bridges between audiences and others involved in the issue, and support the theatre event itself. Partner organizations can also ensure that the effect of the performance is felt after the performance concludes by linking audiences with resources for education and action, providing infrastructure and ongoing consultation and/or leadership for audience members, and generally responding to the heightened engagement and desire for action that emanates from a strong theatre intervention. Conversely, theatre artists can play many roles for socially activist organizations, including: raising issues in a popular way; connecting ideas, information, and analysis with issues' impact on people (individuals and groups); providing engaging ways to pose and solve problems in the community; imbuing issues and action with humour, pleasure, and creativity; creating skill-building opportunities; stirring people to want to take action, and more. Theatre creates opportunity for reaching out to people via story. Theatre can respond quickly and evolve to fit changing circumstances.

The trick is to find mutually supportive ways for each partner to assist the other. The theatre company will of course know the most about the potential of theatre and theatre components of a program, as the partner organization will know best methods to shape and deliver other aspects of the initiative. Often this includes providing insights and organization for longer-term interventions, education, and action, and demonstrating how their organization can be accessed in the short-term and over time. Each must work closely with the other and this intensive interaction can be a challenge. Both kinds of organizations have separate areas of expertise but, to be most successful, they must share common values and commit to common principles. In the case of *Are We There Yet?*, for example, partnerships are strongest and most effective when both partners (theatre and sex education/ health organizations) are:

- Committed to the idea that a partnership between a theatre and a health organization enhances the capacity of the program to make positive change in a young person's life
- Sex positive[1]
- Respectful and committed to developing knowledge of the working methods, aims, organizational structure, and culture of their counterpart
- Committed to strong communication and timely problem solving
- Anti-racist, anti-homophobic, anti-sexist, and pro-choice

Some topics, including sexuality, are provocative and raise issues and questions that must be addressed, either immediately or in the long term. The alliance between theatre and human services continues to demonstrate efficacy with hot issues such as HIV/AIDS (Theatre for Life, South Africa), homelessness (LAPD, Los Angeles), domestic violence (Certain Curtain, UK), and addictions and mental health (Workman Arts, Toronto).

Are We There Yet? was founded by a particular partnership between a theatre company and a sexual health organization. As the play was adapted in varying communities, so too the nature of the theatre–health organizational partnership was revised and transformed. The principles we extracted from the original AWTY collaboration were applied to each new situation and context with surprising results.

NOTE

1. "Sex-positivity allows for and in fact celebrates sexual diversity, differing desires and relationship structures, and individual choices based on consent" (Queen and Comella 2008, 275).

5

CAR POOLING

Community Partners and Alliances

CONTENTS

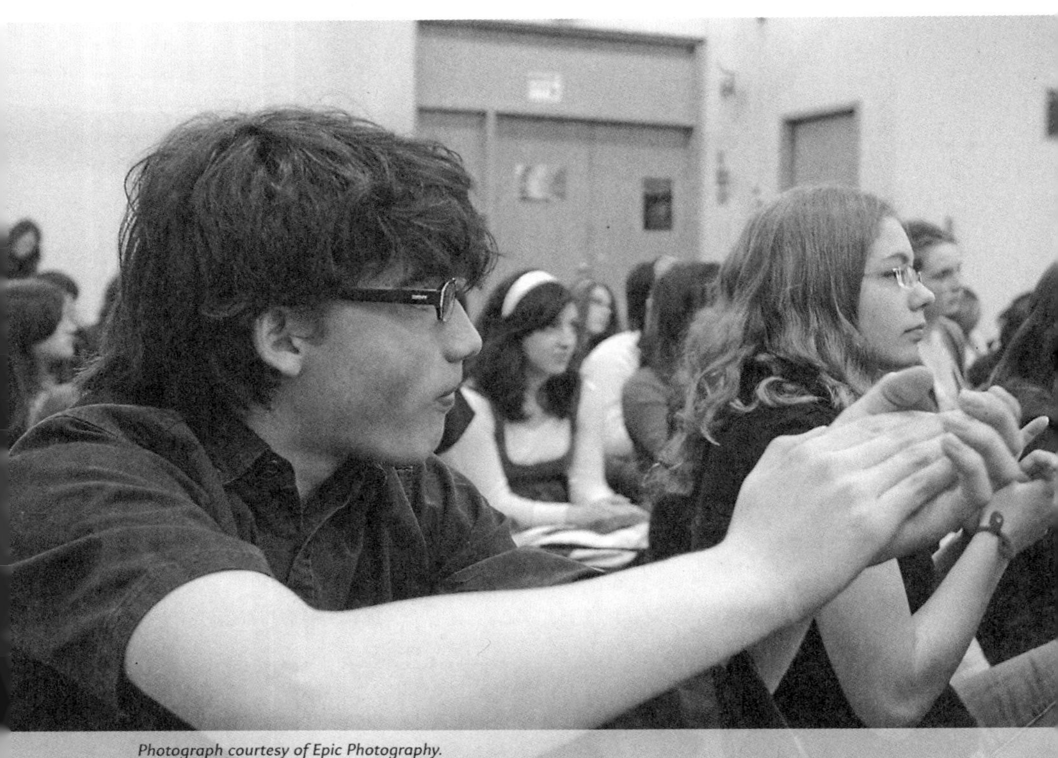

Photograph courtesy of Epic Photography.

Theatre for change is made more powerful when linked meaningfully with organizations that pursue the initiative long after the theatre component is complete. Several models for collaboration were forged as the Are We There Yet? Program was adapted for new settings.

> *So my thing was capacity building in each of those communities so when you leave with the play, who are they left connecting with?...Now they have that face...there's that safe person that they can go talk to and work through how they can get information or access to things like birth control or condoms... So that was the key for me. Somebody left there afterwards that they can come to, better than some stranger who's going to pop in and leave.*
>
> —LEONA PURCELL, PUBLIC HEALTH NURSE AND CO-ORDINATOR, GUYSBOROUGH YOUTH HEALTH AND SERVICES CENTRE, GUYSBOROUGH, NOVA SCOTIA

It's a phenomenal experience. I can't say enough positive things about the project itself. To be involved in a project like this is very exciting, very enjoyable. We have fun doing it as well, not just the youth. We have fun in getting that information to them as well. I also hope that we're able to get more nurses or more educators involved in the program here so we can continuously increase the number of schools or students we reach.

—Brett Dow, public health nurse,
Sexual Health Program, Saskatoon
Health Region

The Are We There Yet? Collaboration

INITIALLY, CONCRETE THEATRE PARTNERED with Planned Parenthood (now Options) to design and deliver the Are We There Yet? Program. In the original form, the AWTY sexual health partner provides a workshop, usually one week after students have seen the play. In addition to this workshop, a sexual health educator attends every show. They are introduced in the play, describe their role or agency, help define abstinence, do "myth busting," and are available for audience questions. This involvement is significant in a variety of ways: they are an important resource for the audience; they are also introduced in the fun and open atmosphere that is created by the play; and they are made familiar to the audience. The health organization also plays an important role in orienting the theatre company—a vital contribution, given the complex and personal topic of sexuality.

The AWTY Program requires a meaningful partnership between theatre practitioners and health educators. While various collaborative models are used, the partnership is central to this program's success. We maintain that it is the combination of the theatre performance followed by the health workshop that generates the most complete and powerful vehicle for sexual education. In the theatre event, all of the questions are debated and discussed in public; the workshop allows for some private and anonymous questions and comments. Theatre is best at placing audiences in a situation in which they both observe and participate. They feel and think simultaneously, always around characters and their dilemmas. However, theatre is not the best way to teach mechanics (for example, what a female condom looks

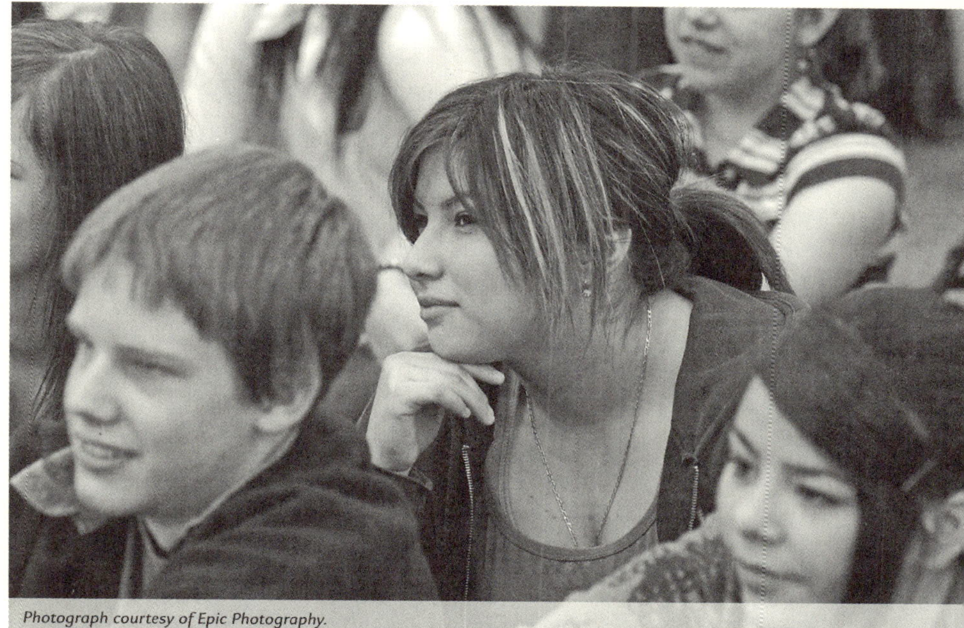

Photograph courtesy of Epic Photography.

like or how to open and put on a condom). The workshop is best for providing information, methods, and statistics, such as outlining different birth control and disease control methods and the effectiveness of each. Further, when well handled, the workshop reinforces ideas and further engages teens with developing personal and interpersonal awareness, healthy attitudes, and strategies and skills that emerge via the performance. The workshop encourages the spectators to further reflect on the play's content and its implications for themselves. Beyond this, the health organization can become a longstanding resource for this audience; located in the community, it can serve these citizens over time, as their needs and interests change.

Such a partnership was foundational to the conception of the AWTY Program. From the start, the need was identified and the program structure designed with a partnership in mind: Concrete Theatre was to create an interactive theatre piece, and Planned Parenthood Edmonton built on ongoing workshops used in schools to design and deliver a program-specific follow-up workshop. Planned Parenthood provided some of the core research material and suggested themes for segments of the play,[1] expert response to the play as it developed over time, and insights into the sexuality education field as it relates to various age groups. As the project developed, the two organizations enriched this model with substantial collaboration during rehearsals and weekly debriefing throughout each run of the play. In short, the core model entwined the two organizations' approaches, allowing each to do what they do best: the theatre company to create and deliver excellent dramatic experiences based in participatory community research and knowledge of their audiences, and the sexual health organization to train theatre participants in sexual health information, build comfort with talking openly about sexuality issues, support and educate youth as they explored these issues, and, very significantly, provide support and resources for schools and teens long after the theatre had moved on.[2]

To be effective, partnership models must be built recognizing both organizations' roles, history, organizational structure, capacity for change, relationship to the community, and more. In this field, we too often pay lip service to these considerations but do not necessarily have effective strategies for revealing and working with our differences. The very advantages that collaborations provide, such as differing and complementary areas of expertise and relationships to the community, also create complexity and challenges in partnering.

> *Well, I think just, you know, getting to know each other. The partnership itself growing, I mean it's almost like a family kinda thing and you know family, all families, have growing pains and different struggles but I don't think there was anything major that stood in the way of building that partnership.*
>
> —*Brett Dow*

One of the key AWTY Community-University Research Alliance (CURA) research project goals was to adapt the script and the program as a whole for various communities. Recreating the project in several circumstances assisted us to take a close look at varying partnership strategies; each community approached the health–theatre partnership differently, usually in response to quite varying community and organizational conditions. Indeed, one of our findings was that, in some respects, the partnership models, and their ways of creating and delivering this program, were more adapted than the actual play text or the workshop content. One of the program's strengths is its flexibility and non-prescriptive nature. In some urban areas, a sexual health agency such as Options delivers the workshop component of the program. In rural areas, nurses working from local health clinics attended the shows and led the workshop. In Aboriginal communities, health jurisdictions are very complex. A new model of communication and collaboration between several health agencies and regions was developed to suit these circumstances.

Four Communities, Four Partnership Models

The AWTY Program was presented via four quite different partnership models in Edmonton, Saskatchewan, Nova Scotia, and Vancouver.

In Edmonton, Concrete Theatre, which specializes in theatre for young audiences, and Options Sexual Health (formerly Planned Parenthood Association of Edmonton), an independent, not-for-profit sexual health agency, form the partnership. Together, they are co-founders of the AWTY Program and are two of the original partners in the research program. They had experience with previous collaboration with one another and with other organizations.

The basic partnership model is:

- Theatre company produces and tours the play with actors contracted, trained, and rehearsed by the theatre;
- Sexual health organization provides sexual health educator, who attends and participates in some rehearsals, is in the play at all performances, and leads follow-up workshops about a week later. Often this role is taken on by more than one sex educator, as the tour plus workshops create a very intense schedule.

This foundational model evolved and in some ways deepened over time to include the following additional levels of collaboration:

- Sexual health agency provides an orientation workshop for actors, director, and stage manager during rehearsal, where they explore their own attitudes to various sex-related questions, clarify the sex-positive intentions of the program, learn about contraception methods, STIs, and other sexuality topics, and hear about the kinds of questions teens have about sex and sexual issues (when they are offered opportunities for asking questions anonymously).

- Toward the end of rehearsal, the sexual health educator and actors practice how they will deal with disclosures should they occur, as well as other audience responses. In Edmonton, this involves working out a safe and responsive way for actors to interact with teens and respond to their comments after the show. They discuss ways to identify a teen's desire to disclose difficult experiences or seek complex advice on a personal situation and practice safe and respectful ways to connect the teen to the sex educator. While such disclosures are unusual, the topic is charged, and this is a vital preparation point. Actors, stage manager, and sex educator practice a hand-off to the sex educator who supports the teen. Recognizing that the student may have approached the person they feel most comfortable with, the actors and other participants also recognize that they need to get the trained expert involved as soon as feasible.
- On tour, there is a weekly debrief meeting with the sex educators and the artistic team. Topics include specific encounters, kinds of audiences, reflection on handling certain comments during participatory sequences, hitting the right level for each audience, etc.

As the play is booked by Concrete Theatre to play beyond Edmonton and environs, Options provides training in a variety of ways for other regions' sexual health educators. In other cases, where a local sexual health organization is comfortable in the role, they take it all on, after participating in rehearsal and orientation. This is feasible when the theatre company (as with Concrete Theatre) is highly informed about the play's intentions and the issues, and when the partner organization is already active in teen sexuality education programming and available to participate in rehearsals and test audience sessions.[3]

In Saskatchewan (Saskatoon and northern communities, on and off reserve), the Saskatchewan Native Theatre Company (SNTC), an Aboriginal theatre company that creates and performs theatre for urban, reserve, and

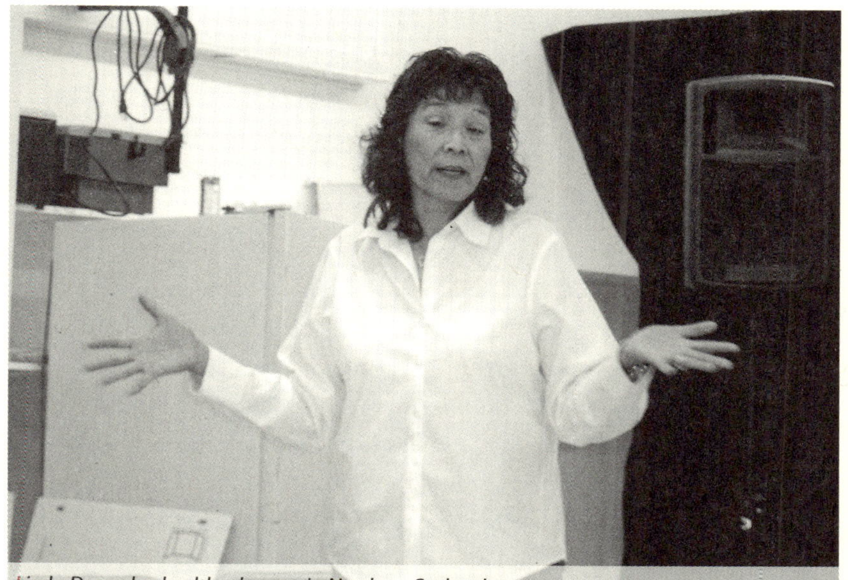

Linda Desroche, health educator in Northern Saskatchewan. *Photograph courtesy of Jane Heather.*

off-reserve audiences, produced the play. SNTC provides cultural and theatre education for youth and young adults and is also experienced with creating theatre for specific audiences around specific issues (for example, for health conferences).

Several health organizations, including Saskatoon Health Region, Northern Inter-Tribal Health Authority, Mamawetan Churchill River Health Region, and community-based health providers in northern Saskatchewan Aboriginal communities formed partnerships to support the program. As there are several health jurisdictions in this region, building participation was complex, and there were multiple sexual health educators and organizations involved. Ultimately, the key to forging these partnerships was individual sexual health educators' commitments to the project. While this was a powerful way to connect, training and integration proved difficult when the tour went outside of these individuals' districts. Jurisdictional issues, isolation, distances between communities in the region, and lack of expertise in sexual health education were all challenges to be addressed.

An Aboriginal elder, who supports the young Aboriginal actors, builds connections with each community and ensures a cultural perspective worked within all stages of the program. Over time, *Are We There Yet?* ran in Saskatchewan with and without an elder in this role. All involved believe the elder role is vital.

Within the rural context, which included many quite isolated reserve and non-reserve communities, the collaborators tried several models for building expertise that was rooted in the community. These included providing training and orientation centrally, which local health educators and nurses could access prior to the project arriving in their community. However, while this worked for some, the most consistently powerful method we discovered in this context was to have a sexual health educator who was experienced in working with Aboriginal teens travel with the show and create links between her and each local health nurse or health provider. This created, in a sense, the best of all worlds. Continuity and expertise were provided to actors and audiences and knowledge and experience among health workers was built at each local level. This model ensured expertise and connection was readily available for teens long after the play had left the community.

> *It gives them the opportunity and the freedom to ask questions later and I see the play being able to do that for kids who may never get that talk in their homes. It becomes a place where they can have the freedom, the chance to connect with the resources available within their community, and to normalize the feeling that they might be having.*
>
> *—Kenji Maeda, sexual health educator*

In Nova Scotia, a partnership was formed with the Mulgrave Road Theatre Company. While it normally does not produce theatre for young audiences, this partner's mission is to create theatre that is inspired by the Atlantic Canadian experience. Guysborough Youth Health and Services Centre, health rather than sex education specialists, partnered in this initiative.

This model had centralized leadership, provided by Leona Purcell, public health nurse and co-ordinator of the Guysborough Youth Health and Services Centre. Public health nurses from each community met by conference call as the project developed, then travelled to participate in two training sessions to prepare for the project. As the play toured to their town, each worker hosted the project in the school, participated in the play, and led the follow-up workshops. It is a strong model: it provided professional development for public health nurses in sex education work with teens, which augmented the already strong integration of the health nurses with the school, the teens, and their community.

As part of the project, Mulgrave Road Theatre met with members of the school board and visited every school to introduce the project and answer questions about the content and the organizational needs of the production.

> *I was brand new at this...I was really nervous about going up and talking to a principal or another adult about sex...I recognized that it was a great project but even in the early days when we were in the office, "OK we're doing a project about* (sotto voce) *sex." And I thought, "If I have barriers myself to even broach the subject with someone, then the show was really important to do." Yeah, there are barriers and it's really important to break them down and I had to break them down for myself first.*
>
> —*Emmy Alcorn, artistic director, Mulgrave Road Theatre*

Neworld Theatre is committed to exploring Vancouver's diversity by investigating borders between styles, cultures, and disciplines. Its work is normally not focused on youth. Vancouver Coastal Health, represented by Kenji Maeda, who has extensive teen-focused sexual health education experience as well as interest and engagement with theatre, is also a partner.

This model involved the health educator participating full time throughout the rehearsal and tour period, as well as building the tour via connections with health teachers at the schools. The team also presented the piece (as information, professional development, and promotion) to health providers throughout the region. This model created opportunities for exploring the level of involvement of the sexual health expert in the play and levels of engagement with each school.

Principles for Building and Adapting Partnerships for Specific Communities

Each model has its strengths and each model had to grow out of the specific community's conditions. Another community with other conditions would spawn yet another model. While one model cannot fit all, a few principles are evident.

1. The spirit of the project is to link a theatre company that is dedicated to theatre for education and development with a health agency that has sexual health expertise and that provides local, long-term resources for the participants. In other development projects that deal with different topics or issues, this principle could be readily generalized. A partnership should be formed to ensure there is ongoing support, organization, and resources in the community; collaborate with a community; and support future education, knowledge, and resource needs long after one theatre project is complete. With sensitive issues such as sexuality, training, orientation, and self-knowledge are needed for all involved in the project. Members of each organization need to develop clarity about the goals and the capacity to communicate about the topic and the project. For example, in this project schools ask about the message (often wondering whether the project promotes abstinence), as do community leaders, some parents, and local health personnel. Any point of contact (theatres, artists, administrative staff as well as health providers) need to be able to respond with clarity, explanations, and confidence.
2. Sexual health personnel need to have opportunities to share their expertise with the theatre artists; rehearse their roles in the play; develop protocols for discussion of issues that arise; prepare for a follow-up workshop (which makes use of the play); and build teens' knowledge of sources of support in the community. They need to ensure they are prepared for responding to immediate as well as longer-term needs.
3. Theatre companies/artists need opportunities to clarify what conditions are necessary for effective preparation and rehearsal; scheduling that is viable for the performance group; feedback/reflection/support on tour; and conditions required of performance venues.

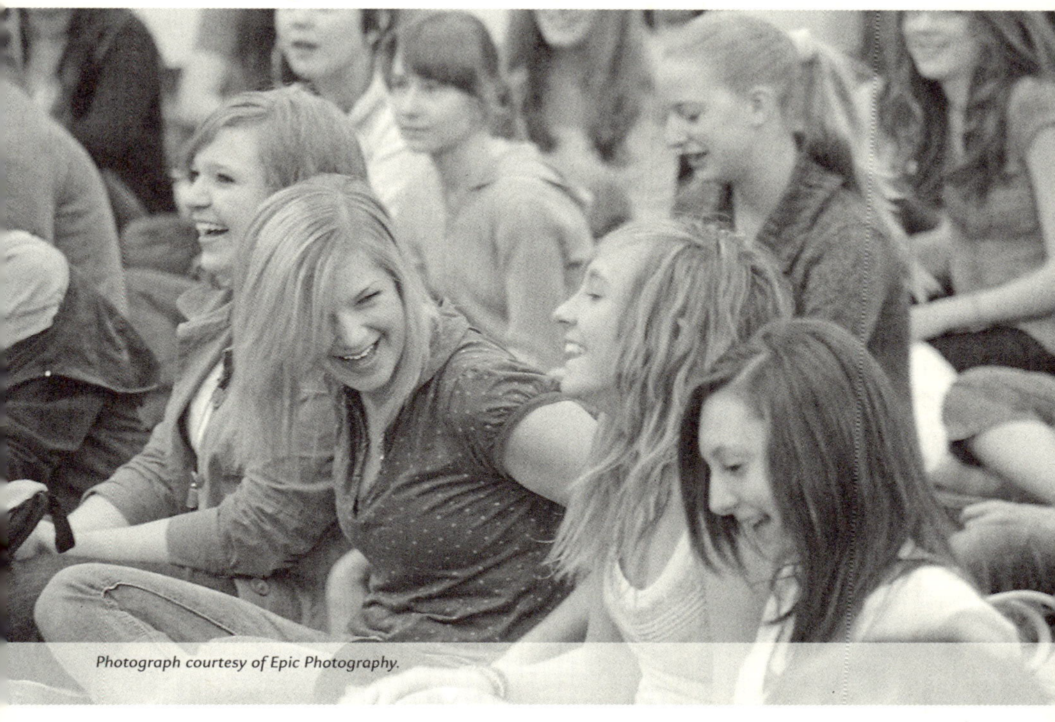
Photograph courtesy of Epic Photography.

4. All organizations need to be clear early on about time, costs, and conditions required for each organization to thrive and for the project to move forward.
5. Partner organizations need to be clear about who will promote, contact audiences (in this case via schools), and book the play, workshop, and other related activities. They need to have the information and agreements in place when representing one another to the wider community. With this project, the school and/or education region is the tertiary partner and building effective relations with these organizations is also important to its success.
6. While infrastructure and capacity will guide partnership models and the division of roles and responsibilities among partners to a large extent, another relevant consideration is the relative relationships with other community partners. For example, in this project partners booked the show and workshops in varying ways, often as a result of identifying who

already had working relationships with schools and/or with the intended audiences (in this case, teens). For other topics and issues, many of these principles and roles apply.

Forming and Sustaining Partnerships

Collaboration between very different organizations is worthwhile, even vital in work such as this, but it is not easy. While they may share a particular project goal, such as commitment to improving teens' sexual health and capacities for respectful, safer expression of their sexuality, theatre and health organizations tend to operate very differently, with contrasting agendas, rhythms, funding models, and cultures. Effective collaboration requires both sides to make major commitments to communication as well as building common understandings and insights into each other's approaches.

Most organizations have little or no experience with this kind of partnership. Larry Brockman, executive director of Options for many of the years during its AWTY involvement, points out some advantages and challenges for public health organizations who consider this kind of liaison and approach to their education mandates:

> *As a human service organization, the government is keen on partnerships; any time you ask for money they want to know who your partners are, who are your community partners, who are your business partners? We need more specific terms, as partnership has become too broad a term. If you go into the corporate world, there is a very clear definition of partnership but in the human service world it's a very amorphous thing.*
>
> —*Larry Brockman, executive director,*
> *Options Sexual Health Association,*
> *Edmonton*

Brockman states that if the organizations intend to partner for a long time, a commonly understood project infrastructure is important: "Where there is interdependence and inter-reliance there needs to be infrastructure." It is important to "figure out how you're going to live together for a while." Based on the observation that there have been "very high quality people from both partner organizations" over the course of Edmonton's AWTY Program, he proposes that a framework for negotiation and partnering is key, noting that "frameworks need to be in place because staff changes, people change" (Brockman, interview).

The following chapters discuss the health partner's role in *Are We There Yet?*

NOTES

1. See Chapter 8 for more on the playwright's research and development process as she created AWTY, the play.
2. Options's and other health organizations' roles are described in more detail in Chapter 6.
3. See Chapter 4, "To the Director: Rehearsing for Participatory Theatre," for stages of rehearsal and the use of test audiences during the rehearsal period.

6

DUAL DRIVE

The Are We There Yet? Sexual Health Partner Roles

CONTENTS

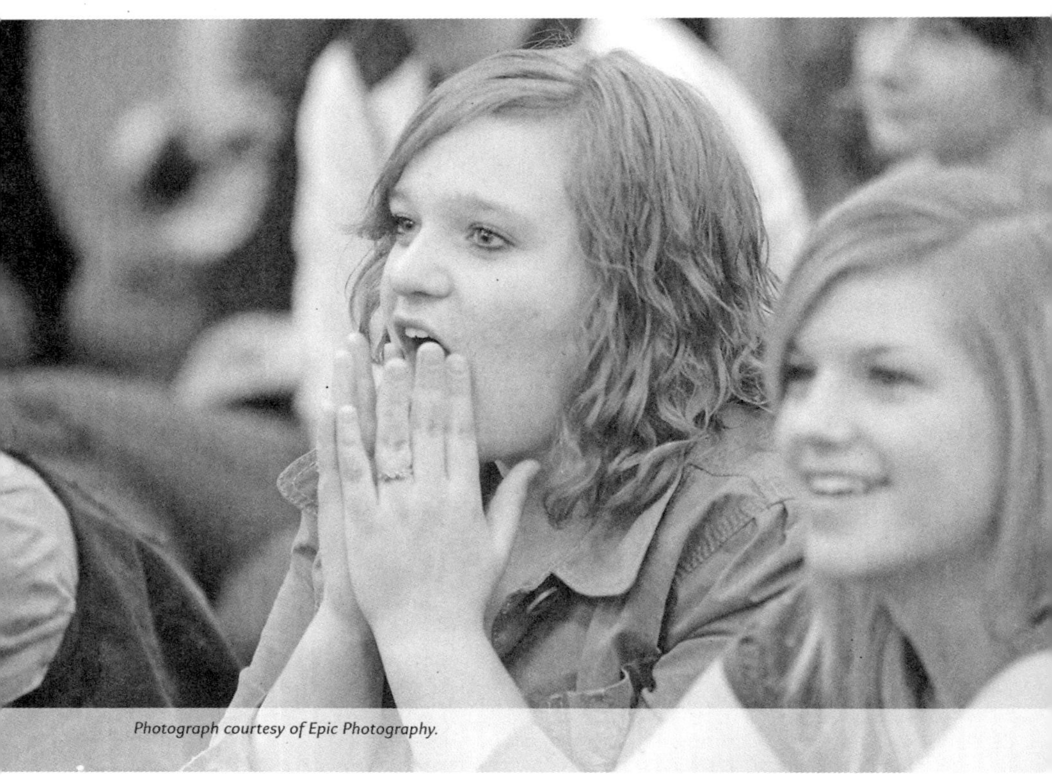

Photograph courtesy of Epic Photography.

Sexual health educators who partnered with theatre companies across the country discuss the project. Brian Parker of Options Sexual Health Association, Edmonton, who worked with Are We There Yet? for many years and trained educators across the country, describes the sexual health workshops that he provides.

> *It is about connecting with youth. By just talking about the medical parts of things, we don't really engage the youth. No matter what we do, we need to engage the youth in a way that they feel listened to. This is one of those shows that can do that. It's tried, tested, it's true, it works...It's work to be a partner, but the purpose of a...health organization is about the clients and the people that they serve. If they want to serve them properly, then this is a show that would be a great one.*
>
> —KENJI MAEDA,
> SEXUAL HEALTH EDUCATOR

We have a hypersexualized culture: in the music, the Internet, on the TV on prime time. Society has inundated these kids with sexuality, with sexual imagery, and suggestiveness. Yet kids can't ask about it or express that. It's too hard to reveal any ignorance. They're supposed to know it all.

—Leona Purcell, public health nurse and co-ordinator, Guysborough Youth Health and Services Centre

PUBLIC HEALTH NURSES AS WELL AS educators who specialize in sexuality have been very successful Are We There Yet? health partners. The AWTY health partner has several roles: he or she participates in the play performances; leads the follow-up workshop; provides expertise for the theatre company in rehearsal and support the tour of the play by participating in a regular debriefing process. In some cases, the health partner also books the play as they are most connected with local schools, school boards, and health programs. Some health partners link the play into an ongoing curriculum component that they provide.

There's a certain rapport that I build with the group because we're a team together. During the rehearsal I provide a one-day full workshop about sexual health components. Because the comfort is there, the cast, stage manager and I can really talk about all things that come up during the process—during rehearsal, during the runs. Being part of the rehearsal process really helped me to figure out how the artistic elements and educational components intersected and where one or the other was deemed more important or critical.

—Kenji Maeda

Different regions have established different kinds of partnerships. In urban areas, a sexual health agency such as Options delivers the workshop component of the program. In rural areas, nurses working from regional health clinics attended the shows and led the workshop. In Vancouver, a sexual health expert associated with an agency joined the theatre company to book the show with schools the agency already served and participated fully in rehearsals. In Aboriginal communities, where health jurisdictions are very complex, we developed a new model of communication and collaboration between several health agencies and regions to suit these circumstances. These adaptations are further discussed in the next chapter.

Why a Partnership

Health educators in every region that presented *AWTY* state emphatically that the partnership and the role of the sexuality educator in the performances are crucial for the teens and to the positive outcomes health educators are aiming for. The play puts sex on the table. The actors perform and leave. Teens with questions, situations, or dilemmas to solve, or just in need of someone to talk to, need more than a website or a phone number. A live human from their community, who saw the show with them stood up and identified themselves with the play and answered questions, becomes "the safe person they can go talk to and work through" (Purcell, interview).

For sexual health educators and organizations, being part of the play is like an advertisement to promote a local resource and help teens "identify who in the community is responsible for the role of teaching about sexual health" (Brockman, interview). Health partners in rural areas also felt the health partner role was vital:

> *Who's the go-to person? That's really important, where you can go, identifying people that you can feel free to talk to about these things, sometimes it's not so easy to get to the clinics.*
>
> —*Leslie Brooks, communicable disease control nurse, Northern Inter-Tribal Health Authority, May 16, 2007*

With the Aboriginal adaptation, race and culture was also seen as an important factor.

> *It's not a group of white nurses—with limited experience teaching [sex education]—coming and talking about how to put a condom on a wooden goody—that never worked.*
>
> —*Leslie Brooks, May 16, 2007*

The person or organization that can help teens with questions, resources, and advice after the show is over was seen as critical. Health professionals were also aware that the show might provoke a memory or trigger a disclosure, and for the safety of the teens and the theatre personnel (who are often the first contact for the youth), a health professional on site was also identified as key.

> *Some of the issues in some of these communities...are big, when somebody blurts out something you can't ignore it, you can't just leave that hanging in the air, you have to be in a position to address it honestly and respectfully in that moment.*
>
> —*Leslie Brooks, May 16, 2007*

Being part of this project is rewarding but also demanding for health organizations. Larry Brockman reflects on the advantages to the health partners. He finds that that the play deeply embraces current thinking about effective sex education; he remarks, ""it certainly reinforced the power of addressing the affect. In the IMB (Information Motivation Behaviour) model you need the cogitation, the affect, and the behavioural. One without the others won't do it." (See Chapter 2 for more on the IMB approach to sexuality education.) Brockman points out that AWTY offers organizations:

> *an innovative approach to outreach and education with teens, builds comfort levels and openness with sex and sexuality, creates an opportunity to amplify creativity and dynamism in educational approach, and establishes the organization as being able to connect to youth in the way that youth feel comfortable in speaking up and coming forward with their issues.*
>
> —*Larry Brockman, executive director,*
> *Options Sexual Health Association,*
> *Edmonton*

For a full-time sexuality education organization, the play:

> *gets you back to youth on a regular basis. Even if the play is only running for four to six weeks, it impacts our life a minimum of three months...It's the interaction with the*

schools and young people—it helps in that tug of war between hands-on and administrative work, it helps balance that out.

—Larry Brockman

Brockman also suggests that, for his organization, more engagement with the school board would have been useful in the long term to build beyond long-standing relationships with specific schools to a deeper, long-term commitment to the project from the school system. The Nova Scotia adaptation reports their increased liaison with the school system as one of their project's positive outcomes.

I think having a health partner in conjunction with the play is absolutely imperative... The health partner within that community is identified in the play...[We] rehearsed with the actors, and [are] there to show the youth that "in your community it is this person that you need to contact, with regard to any of these issues that are brought up in the play"...And doing the follow-up workshops is important, so that there's a debriefing of the play.

—Wendy McPhail, sexual wellness co-ordinator, Mamawetan Churchill River Health Region

Getting Ready: Training for Health Partners

While some health partners will already be sexual health experts, others will be people in public health who do not specialize in this area. Both starting points make for valuable and viable partners in this program.

In Nova Scotia and Saskatchewan, every effort was made to train and prepare the health educators for their role in the play and the workshop. There was a wide range of previous sexuality education experience among these partners. The AWTY community-university research project provided meaningful opportunities for project development and for extending the range of sex ed work in each community. In Saskatchewan, orientation was provided in year one, and when the program was remounted in subsequent years, training and orientation were provided by those who participated in the first year. Based on adapting and disseminating the program in several communities and with several kinds of health partners, Brian Parker of Options developed a useful manual and DVD to support future AWTY health partners, as well as those interested in developing other theatre-based sexual health programming.[1]

> *Fantastic...for [public health nurses] to have an opportunity to have a workshop on sexual health only, that was really open and explored lots of topics...It was fun. Really healthy. The best day they spent in twenty years, some of them said...And the opportunity to be involved in this play, which is fun, which the kids see as positive in the school.*
>
> *—Leona Purcell*

Part of the training for health partners (and theatre personnel) is an examination of one's personal morals, beliefs, and values around sexuality. Parker stresses the importance of being sex positive and approachable. He highlights the importance of acknowledging one's personal views and of clarifying one's professional roles.

> *It was really positive to have Brian (Parker) down to do some work with nurses as a team around sexual health education. Even to look at their own stuff and be able to park that in order to be the educator you need to be.*
>
> *—Leona Purcell*

Sexuality is a minefield and sexuality with youth even more volatile. For example, two issues that Parker identifies as particularly important to discuss during orientation and training are responses to homosexuality and abortions.

> *Brian Parker from Planned Parenthood was there, and gave us a rundown on what the project was and what had been done with it at that point in time and what the goal was in terms of the adaptation with Sask Native Theatre Company and the objectives of the play were. We did some workshops with Brian, which was very comfortable and*

very relaxing because it gave us a real great insight into where the project came from, what the hopes were and the goals in terms of what youth get out of the project, and it was a great experience to do that.

—*Brett Dow, public health nurse,*
Sexual Health Program,
Saskatoon Health Region

In addition to preparing for their own role, health educators who want to employ theatre's power need to engage with the theatre artists.

It is particularly important for the actors to be really connected to the health educator, to build trust and to reinforce that the health educator does know their stuff. I think it's important to have at least a half-day training together and training separately. They should come together at some point too. Both are important.

—*Brian Parker, sexual health educator,*
Options Sexual Health Association

Participating in the Play

The health partner has an important role within the performance of the play. He or she is introduced as part of the play and identified as the sexual health expert in the room. The health partner corrects any misperceptions or misinformation that arises about pregnancy, birth control, and disease prevention. (Chapter 3, pages 75 and 83 and the accompanying description of each scene, which includes commentary on the health partner roles and functions in each scene.) While these interventions during the play are important in and of themselves, they also serve to link the sexual health educator with an enjoyable, engaging, and straightforward approach to sexuality education for the teenage audience. Their expertise and resources are presented as part of the whole story about building capacity for safe and respectful approaches to sexual relationships. Like the actors and the play, they are seen as honest, respectful of audiences' ideas, real, approachable and relevant.

Sarah Flicker and co-researchers conducted a comprehensive study of teens called *Sexpress: The Toronto Teen Survey* (2009), which aimed to "enrich both the quantity and quality of sexual health information available to Toronto teens and improve the ways in which sexual health promotion and care are delivered" (Executive Summary sec. 1:4). They used a community-based research approach that included both quantitative and qualitative methods. In an overview of what teens identified as issues, the report found,

> *Canadian youth lack comprehensive knowledge of the risks associated with unprotected sexual activity and the necessary skills required to ensure the protection of their sexual health. At the same time, youth complain about their sexual health education claiming it focuses too much on biology, offers too little too late, provides few opportunities for discussion, is often non-existent, and is seldom sex positive in nature. Another concern is its relatively heavy focus on the risks and problems of adolescent sexuality to the exclusion of sexual desire and healthy sexual relationships.* (sec. 1:24)

The study examines what youth want to learn and the context in which they want to learn it:

> *According to youth, a good clinic is a place where: youth feel comfortable and welcome; all kinds of youth are accepted; they give you respect and understanding; youth feel supported, not judged; and where there is room for all teens to talk and let their feelings out.* (sec. 1:21)

Although the study focuses on clinics and the barriers that youth experience when accessing these resources, all of the elements teens identify for a good clinic are the foundational principles that underpin the AWTY theatre–health partnership.

Brian Parker, who was part of hundreds of *Are We There Yet?* performances and workshops, has this to say about what the health partner can expect on the road:

> *Health partners always make themselves available to the students, actors, and stage manager after the performance, in case a disclosure occurs or if an issue or concern*

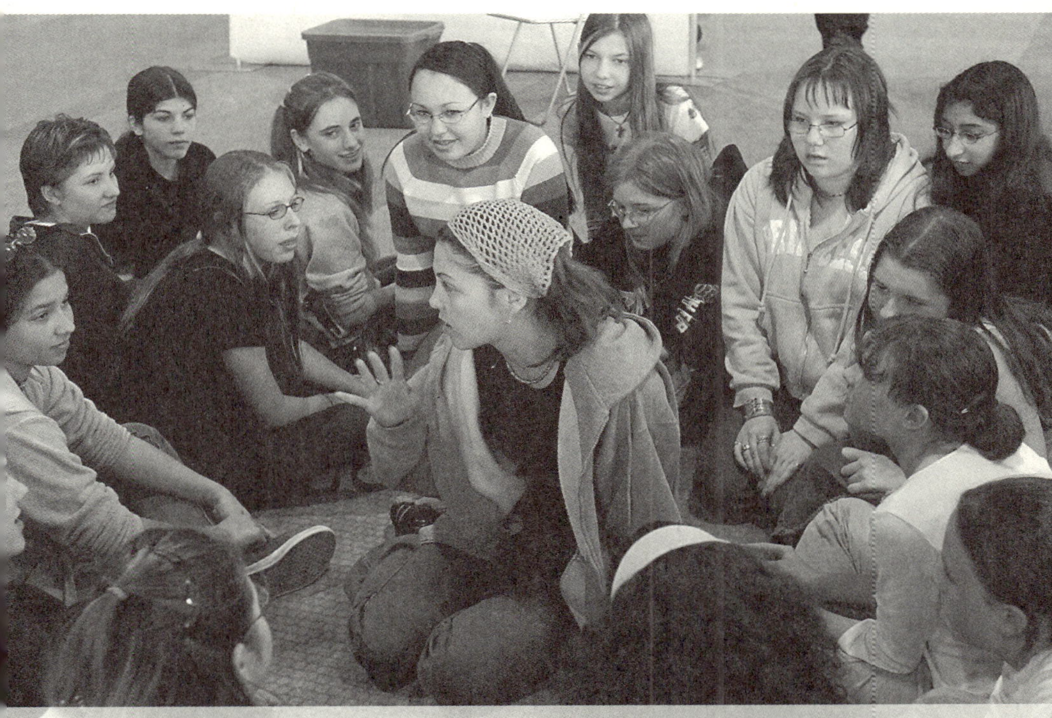

Character seeks advice
Shannon Larson, Concrete Theatre. Photograph courtesy of Epic Photography.

> *arises. To help make the health partner more approachable, we always stand up and mingle with the actors and the youth after each performance.*

Educators who were part of the adaptation and dissemination of the program during the research period agree that the play engages students through affect or the emotional part of themselves. In a common sex ed teaching model, the triad of information, motivation, and behaviours (IMB) includes both the affective and the cognitive, feeling, and thinking.

> *[The play] appeals to the affect [and] when we get to the affect then we can really deal with how people are interacting with each other, how this fits into relationships, what*

> *are the implications for relationships and what does that mean for you and the relationships you have.*
>
> —*Larry Brockman*[2]

The play breaks taboos and normalizes talking about sex. It gives the audience permission to speak up, publicly with peers at school, about sex. It clears some of the worst roadblocks and barriers and allows the more cognitive part of the program—the workshop—to not have to start cold.

> *You go in [to teach sexuality education] and everybody's embarrassed. Who wants to hear this? But now you have a play to follow that sets a tone that is upbeat. It's okay to talk about it, it's normal.*
>
> —*Leona Purcell*

The theatre engages the audience emotionally, through character, dilemma, story, and participation. The workshop links with and complements the play and the "sex educators can reflect back to scenes in the play to better explain certain aspects of relationships and/or sexuality" (Parker, interview). Brockman discusses this power: "The theatre reminds us of the power of the affect...it's delightful because so often when you're in front of a bunch of people it's so easy to get pushed to the cognitive" (Brockman, interview).

Because the play is powerful, students often seek out an actor or the sex educator after the show. It is important to be accessible. "To be approachable, actors and the sex educator can't go back stage at the end of the show. They kind of mock break down the set. And stay visible. That's the time you get the biggest stuff" (Parker, interview).

Disclosures

Although it is not the direct intention of the play to trigger a student's need to talk with someone about a situation that she or he has found her or himself in, this can happen. In these circumstances, the health partner is the expert and supports the student and the theatre company. Students approach the actors, stage manager, and health partner about all sorts of things after the play. It is important that the entire company expects this and is comfortable and prepared to engage in these conversations and knows when and how to refer a student to the expert, the health professional.

Although they are not a regular occurrence, performance-elicited disclosures of many types, from minor problems to disclosures of sexual assault, occurred over the course of the *AWTY* tours. In a northern Alberta town, a student disclosed being sexually assaulted at a party. She said that the Annabelle monologue in the play (Chapter 3, page 83) somewhat mirrored what had happened to her a few months prior. After a quick transfer from actor to health partner, we were able to determine that this was not a first-time disclosure and that this young woman had previously told their school counsellor and other adults. The health partner worked with the student for about an hour and ensured she had the support system in place to get the help she needed. The health partner also worked with the actors to make sure they could process their feelings about the disclosure.

In an Edmonton school, a student approached one of the actors after the play and revealed that she had been a victim of childhood sexual abuse. It was evident that the student was engaging in self-harm. After the hand-off from actor to health partner, the sexual health expert saw the student in a private office within the school for an hour. The discussion determined that the student had many supports in place, including the school counsellor, a youth worker, and foster parents who were helping her with this situation. Afterwards the health partner debriefed the actors.

Based on our experience, most students who disclose have many supports in place and want to connect with the character. In fact, in the Alberta region to date there has not been a first-time disclosure from a student after the play or workshop. Health partners should be aware that after a disclosure situation the actors generally request time to debrief. If the health partner has counselling skills, he or she will likely be able to deal with most of the situations that occur. If he or she is not trained in counselling, the health partner should know individuals or agencies to refer the youth (or adult) to for support. (See also "Rehearsing for Disclosures" later in this chapter.)

After the play sometimes someone might come up and talk about abortion or say, "I think I'm pregnant, I need an abortion, what do I do?" So youth obviously know they can talk to us about it, that underlying message is heard by them.

—*Brian Parker*

Leading the Follow-Up Sexual Health Workshop

The AWTY Program includes an important sexuality education workshop as well as the play. The workshop follows the play, normally by a week. It provides specific opportunities to reflect on the content of the play, address the play's content in other modes, apply some of the play's content to their own situations, and learn about options for birth control. Students' questions, provided anonymously, are also addressed. Sexual health and public health agencies who participated in *AWTY* each adapted the workshop somewhat to suit agency priorities and local school curricula. For a sample workshop outline, see Appendix 2.2, "The Teen Workshop."

The workshop allows students to see and handle different kinds of birth control methods, learn more of the facts about STI prevention and transmission, and to ask anonymous questions. Perhaps most important is the time the health partner/sexuality educator spends in the classroom making contact with students. As the actors move on to the next school, the educator standing in front of the class becomes the person who could help a young person make a healthy sexual choice.

At one level, the workshop provides another fifty minutes of much-needed sex education. In most cases, approximately sixty students see the play together and the students gather in the gym or library for the performance. The workshop is done with classroom groups of about thirty, so the smaller group allows for each student to have more opportunities to ask questions and participate. As Larry Brockman remarked, "You get a much higher level of participation and I think that's part of the learning...people having an opportunity to do something with their experience" (interview).

The play and workshop work in tandem. A workshop leader can use the play to extend the learning and combine the affective with the cognitive.

Brian Parker, the sexual health educator with the longest and most extensive experience with the play, uses scenes from the play in his workshop. He finds that the play "creates scenarios that are impossible for a sex educator to recreate in a classroom" (interview). Further, "two chances to cover the material is always better than one, better for filling gaps and better for retention. The play creates such an awesome memory and experience for students, the more it can be built on the more learning can come out of it in terms of long-term retention" (Brockman, interview). Given that students don't all learn in the same way, the workshop offers a learning mode that is different from the play: "If we just use one method we're only speaking to a part of the group. Often when it's just one method you're missing out on some very important people" (Brockman, interview).

As with the play, adapting this portion of the program to specific community conditions is important. For example,

> *In one school that has a high Muslim population, for the workshop we split the genders so all the girls were with a female sex educator and all the boys are with a male. It didn't seem to be an issue for the play but it was an issue in the workshop; the boys were overpowering the girls. We found splitting the genders solved the problem.*
>
> —*Brian Parker*

The play and workshop together are a potent mix that neither alone can match.

> *This was really exciting to me because we're trying to help educators become more comfortable with the topic. So for them to see the play and get the sense that there are lots of ways to get messages across to young people, that's great.*
>
> —*Leona Purcell*

The Teen Workshop

One of the key elements that links the play and the workshop very closely, and makes the most of both, is the exercise entitled Drawing the Line.[3] Brian Parker points out that one reinforces the other, and describes this important exercise in detail:

We put a line on a continuum and when they have seen the play I'll talk about Marcel and Delphi, the characters who talk about personal boundaries in the play. In every single part of the workshop we relate back to the play. So I'll say, "Remember the part of the play with Marcel and Delphi where they're talking about personal boundaries—what are personal boundaries again?" And they'll say: "where you draw your line, your bubble, your comfort zone." "Just like Marcel and Delphi, they were talking about personal boundaries, and they were talking about doing different things and that guy in the lab coat was talking about some different things they could do. Well, we're going to do that now. So let's say this is Marcel and Delphi or another couple, you guys are going to come up with some ideas or suggestions for what a couple could do, from no contact all the way to protected sex and maybe a little further. It's going to go from least intimate to most intimate. So it might be hugging and kissing around here on the line, getting naked around here, and they're going to do some more sexual things."

So like the play, I ask them for everything and they say: hugging, kissing, peck on the cheek, and they might say going to movies and I say, "just physical things," because we could be there for hours. So they say: hand jobs, fingering, oral, all this stuff. There are things that go off the line as well. Someone will almost always say anal sex. So I say, "Okay, where do you guys want to put anal sex on this line?" With anal sex they put it in so many different places. Some will say before intercourse, some will say it's the same, it should be in the same spot, and some will say off the line, it's gross. And there are some things I put off the line. If they want anal sex off the line that's what I do; it's their line. They will also say sex toys, whips and chains, threesomes, handcuffs, whatever, and those are things I put off the line. I don't put them off the line and say, "that's too kinky for this class." I say, "some people are into that, some people aren't, so we put it off this list." I don't make it a bad thing; I don't make it a good thing. They say all kinds of things but if they go crazy with it I say, "Okay, that's enough stuff off the line because we have limited time."

So then what we do is, just like the characters in the play, close their eyes to find their personal boundary. I read through everything they've put on the line and just like in the play I ask them to use an imaginary marker or just a yes or no in your head. "It's anonymous, don't tell anyone." I read the list, then I get them to open their eyes and ask them if everyone found where their line was. Usually, they say yes. Then I ask them if they knew where their line was before this or before the play and a lot of them will say yes. Then I ask them why is it important to know where your line is, and they'll say so you don't get in trouble and so you can tell a partner. And I ask them, "Do you think most people tell a partner before or after they've crossed a line?" They will usually say after—which is good 'cause it's true.

So we talk about that and I say where your line is today, six months ago it could have been in a different place and six months or two years from now it could different again. Then I say, "If your line is here today, could it go backward in six months or two years?" They say, "yeah, yeah," and I say, "It could move forward, it could move backward, it's totally cool." Then I talk about Marcel and Delphi having lines in different places, then I ask them what they told the couple in the play to do. And usually you hear compromise again. So I go over it again and because I have the lines on the board and the list written down it's a really good visual. And I can show them all the steps they would have to go through to compromise and explain compromise is great for some situations but not this one.

We show how the person with the highest line should move to down to the person with the lowest line. I then ask the students, "Would this couple just stay at this point?" The students generally say that they can slowly work their way up the line as a couple at a comfortable pace.

Then I talk about abstinence, using this line. I say, "Remember when we talked about abstinence in the play and what was the definition we gave of abstinence?" Usually they remember but sometimes they come back to "no sex." So we explore all those definitions. We talk about the main health one, and the one called "pure" abstinence—no contact whatsoever. Then I show it on the line as well, so if anal sex is on the line, I explain that the health definition is everything below that, so if on their line oral is before anal, they can do everything from oral down.

Now we're ready to move on to condoms and safer sex. I say, "Remember Mac and Carol Ann talking about needing to get condoms?" It's nice to bring it back to the play again so I say, "Where on this line should they be talking about using condoms?" So I use the line again and they might say, protected sex or oral or clothes off. Often people will say way down the line like holding hands! So we go back to the play and remind them of the guys who got introduced and one asks about condom use and that's too early. So then I talk about which are too late, dry sex is usually a really good answer because that can move to sex really quickly or clothes off is great, because if you're comfortable enough getting naked you should be comfortable enough to talk about condoms, even if it's going to be a year down the road before you need them.

I do a condom demo and I do a birth control demonstration. With youth, we do abstinence, condoms, and hormonal, we don't do diaphragms and sponges.

While I'm doing the condom demonstration I ask a lot of questions like: "How old do you have to be to buy condoms?" which is a trick question because you can be any age but lots of people don't know that. "Where should you store condoms? Where should you store them on your body? Where should you store them in your room? What two things do you need to do before you open a condom pack?"

So just like the play is participatory, so is the workshop. I talk and ask questions all the way through, like how do you open the package? Can condoms roll down one way or both ways? If you put it on wrong do you flip it over? (No, you don't flip it over.) I show them how to roll the condom down, give them the effectiveness rate. I show them another way to use condoms, using them with the withdrawal method because condoms are most likely to break at the point of orgasm. I ask them is there is any kind of lube not to use with condoms, like Vaseline and I do that demonstration, rub Vaseline on the condom and it busts right away.

Usually for the youth workshop we like to have a novelty condom like an elephant condom or a French tickler, because there's a lot of novelty condoms out there. I say, "if you have a glow in the dark condom, with a big dragon head on the end that sings happy birthday while you're doing it, you have a big problem." I use a lot of jokes. Humour with sex is great.

Then I show the plastic male condom, the female condom, dental dams, and ask, "If you don't have a dental dam what would you use instead?"

—Brian Parker

Contributing to Rehearsals

In addition to being part of the play and leading the post-play workshop, sexual health partner educators are called upon to prepare actors for the topic and for the possible consequences and issues they may have to deal with. There are three main goals for theatre company/health educator(s) meetings during rehearsals: first, to prepare the company for a sensitive topic; second, to rehearse the sexual health educator's roles in the production; and finally, to develop and practice protocols for dealing with disclosures by audience members.

The sexuality workshop for actors is most usefully placed after the actors have rehearsed for some time so they know the basic core of each scene. Rehearsing the sexual health educator into the play is often done toward the end of the rehearsal period. The final theatre company/health expert session, preparation for disclosures, is best held at the end of the rehearsal period, just prior to performing in schools. The sample rehearsal outline in Appendix 1.2 ("Rehearsing the Play: A Template Schedule") suggests the time the sexual health educator may spend in rehearsal for most productions. However, this will be adjusted to suit each partnership. For example, in the Vancouver adaptation, where the sex educator was in rehearsal full time, his role in the performance was somewhat increased and further integrated into the performance.

> *Being in the rehearsal process gets me excited and allows me to speak about the project a lot better and more articulately. If I were to come in and just watch a run through every week then it becomes harder to change because it's kind of embedded. If that were the case, I would share my thoughts with the director who could then pass it on to the actors. Protocol is important. Otherwise, it would seem like an authority figure saying, "You can't do that, this is critical and important," rather than that conversation of, "Hey you guys, it's been working great so far, how can we make it better? This is my suggestion." It's the process and having an understanding of that process.*
>
> —*Kenji Maeda*

Preparing the Theatre Company

In the original iteration in Edmonton, Options personnel worked with Concrete Theatre's actors, stage manager, and director to identify company members' own beliefs and values in topics related to sexuality. When this work is addressed early in rehearsal, an ease with open discussion of the play's messages and various beliefs in the company becomes possible.

> *The most important thing from a sexual health perspective in training actors is to get them comfortable with sexuality. A lot of time youth are yelling out things that actors might have issues with. They have to learn how to respond appropriately to that. They*

might be yelling out things that actors have never heard of. We can never give them all the information that an actor might need, but we try to arm them with enough information and skills to be able to deal with those situations.

—*Brian Parker*

This work sets the tone for clarity and openness regarding the goals of the play, responses from audience members, and dealing with sensitive topics among the company members. As actors are often the first people the audience contacts, they need training about how to be approachable and sex positive, and they have much to learn from a sexuality educator.

When we do training with the actors it is to work on their comfort levels with sexuality. Being sex positive and approachable is key. That means that inherently sexuality is a beautiful thing, it's a wonderful thing, and we don't want to be judgemental, we want to be respectful. What's really important for the actors is just to make themselves available. If you're approachable, a student will come up to you and if there's something they need to tell you or the stage manager, they will. So I think that's the key: be approachable with whatever topic that's out there. Through the entire performance, be approachable.

—*Brian Parker*

In addition to being open and approachable, actors need preparation for the ways students challenge the actors around this sensitive subject matter.

Because the play is participatory, some students will test the situation. Occasionally they will say very rude and inappropriate things, like "rape her." Not so common, but it happens and that can be a trigger. It can bring up a lot of emotions for somebody, so they need ways to appropriately deal with it without bringing the play down or making it like "Oh, the kids feel like now they can't talk or respond to anything," so there are ways we can work through things in the rehearsal workshop so actors are better equipped to deal with whatever situations come up later during performance.

—*Brian Parker*

While each sex educator and theatre company may approach this encounter differently, Options offers a rich sexuality workshop for the

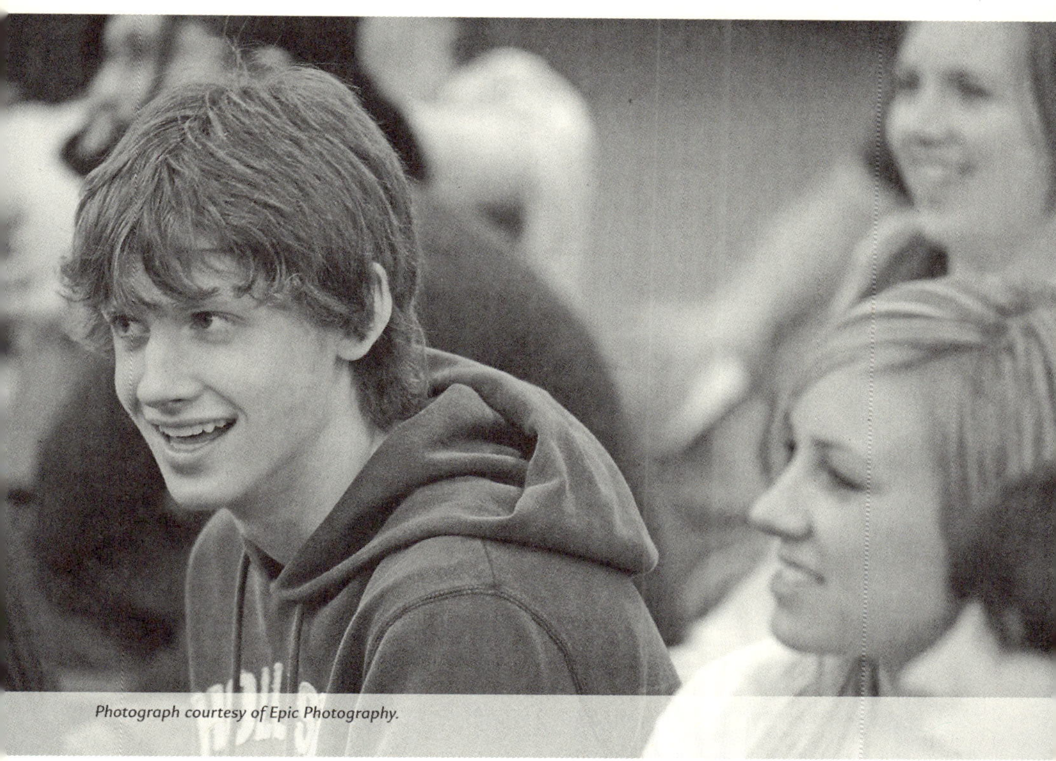
Photograph courtesy of Epic Photography.

theatre company. Brian Parker developed and refined a complete multi-step series of activities and exercises to prepare actors, stage management, and other theatre workers for a full, healthy, and positive engagement with the topic, the play, and the teen audience. The workshop begins with an examination of one's own understanding of sexuality, includes an excavation of personal attitudes and beliefs about sex and sexuality and moves participants toward the sex-positive stance required of actors. During the workshop, Brian both explains and demonstrates by example the supportive collaborations between theatre practitioners and sexuality educators required for the success of the program.

What follows is Brian's description of what he does in the workshop and why each activity, from introducing the project to reading teens' anonymous questions, is crucial. Throughout, he articulates the desired educational outcomes and emphasizes building an open and non-judgemental relationship with teen audiences.

Introduction

> *We do [an introduction] around the play itself, and our role in it...We let them know that we want to be as much a part of the play as possible. We started standing up when we speak as opposed to sitting on our little chair and being aside from everyone. We want to be like one of the actors so we're approachable as well because, ultimately, if there is a concern or an issue or a question that needs to be answered by the health professional, the youth [should] feel comfortable coming up to us. So the more we're involved, the better. So we explain that role—that we want to be with them and work as a unit with them.*
>
> *That's the first thing we do. Then we do training with them around sexuality. I would say half of the training with actors is about their stuff and half is training for what they might hear in the play.*

Where Did You Learn about Sexuality?

> *We ask questions like, what kind of messages did you hear about sexuality? Sometimes people, even adults, have never thought about some of these things. So it's a really good opportunity to share things and do some team building as well. For actors and for us too, we get involved in a lot of these activities and we'll share things as well; we're not just standoffish in the training. Everyone has a different story and we start from there.*
>
> *It's really important because what we're doing is sex ed. It's important to know where they came from, what kind of messages their parents told them, were they good or bad messages? Did their mom put a pamphlet on their bed after their first period? We hear that kind of thing quite often so we want to understand where they're coming from and that gives us a good idea. So we do that to get a foundation of where to start and that may lead off into little side conversations about stuff as well. Like maybe around religion or guilt and shame, masturbation. We hear all types of stories, which is awesome. People disclose a bit and you get to know them a bit more and you feel closer to them, which I think, in a play like, this is really important. I think it happens naturally too.*

"Triggers": Small Group Activity

This is something I developed because I think there are so many hot button issues when it comes to sex and relationships and adults, and parents and teens. We all get so many messages about sex and we all have hang-ups and issues and that's fine! That's great! Everyone is entitled to his or her opinion or what happened to him or her. My big thing about this is, it's not about you, it's about those kids. So that's really what a lot of this training is about: you are just the vehicle that's sending the message, and it's about those kids. So if there is something there you don't agree with, who cares? We can deal with that on our own time, but your job is to send the message without harming those youth. One thing I always talk about is that there are going to be things that come up in the play that affect you in different ways. This activity is around working out how to deal with those and I call it a Triggers Activity.

I write out ten (usually ten) different topic areas that could come up in the play. So some of them are quite general. I will put on a flip chart: teen sexuality, teen pregnancy, teen abortion, adoption, LGBT, and I do some more hard core ones, just to really work them, like bestiality. I do sexual assault, and sometimes BDSM.[4] *These are things they probably won't hear from this audience, but somebody might yell out "whips and chains," and if they don't really understand that, we want them to understand and not be thrown. So I'll pick two or three that are mild, some that are mid-range, and some that are extreme. Obviously there are thousands of things I could put up but I try to pick ones that might come up. So I post them around the room (one word per sheet).*

And I talk to them about the difference between wearing a personal hat and wearing a professional hat. And that it's very, very different. So I can believe whatever I want personally—I could be homophobic or anti-abortion—whatever I want to be and that's totally cool, but when I am a professional (sexual health educator) and especially when I am dealing with youth, people that I could really shape, or form, or hurt, then I have to be really careful with my personal beliefs and I have to take off my personal hat, hard as that may be, I tell them, and put on my professional hat.

But for the purpose of this Trigger Activity I get them to wear their personal hat, because that's what this is about—it's about their personal stuff. So each actor goes to each of those papers and they write what they feel personally about it...a word, a phrase a sentence, a novella, I tell them, if they feel inspired! Then they write whatever it is for each specific one. They do this individually and I ask them to read what other people have written but don't just write what everyone else wrote.

Then we go as a group from topic to topic and I ask for a volunteer to read what it says. We explore each one of those. And I give them more information. In the case of abortion, I'll give them the stats for Canada, pregnancy options, and in the case of a teenager, if it's an unplanned pregnancy, what would they be more likely to do. I explore each one deeper; give them stats to back things up. There are always times with the extreme ones that people may have problems with it. Even in some situations, someone might have a problem with the gay and lesbian stuff. Or there could be really extreme reactions to sexual assault (in the play) and that might be really important to explore. We do a separate training on disclosure where I really focus on that stuff.

It really shows where people are at. We don't really know who wrote what and we work through that and I reiterate, "it's totally fine to believe whatever you believe personally. And that it's totally fine to have a hot button or a trigger." So if abortion is someone's trigger, what I really want the actors to know, and I do the same thing with health professionals, is that it's okay. What's really important is how you deal with the situations within the context of the play. How harmful it could be to someone if we don't react properly. It might just be body language, or rolling of the eyes, and I talk about all this stuff. I give them some tips. Like if they were against abortion or they had some triggers around it, I tell them, "First stand in front of a mirror and say abortion ten times and see how you respond. Sometimes we think we're okay with things but we really aren't." We might say abortion and our body tightens up so I want them to kind of own those things and figure it out. And the more they deal with it, the better they'll respond in situations where it might come up.

That's how we do the Trigger Activity, and I say to them most of the things on the wall that we just talked about are going to come up in the course of touring the play, some of them daily. Every single performance they will be there...I think this is one of the most important pieces of the training that I do.

The Social Barometer Exercise

You've probably seen social barometers or social spectrums before. It's an activity around morals and values and beliefs. So we have three signs: agree, disagree, and unsure.

It works really well along with Triggers. This is more about what our beliefs are. I always say, "You are entitled to your beliefs—there are no right or wrong answers." But again we can tell a lot about where people are with stuff like this. The questions start off simply but get more complicated. With groups of actors they usually start off all agreeing or all disagreeing. They usually have several areas of agreement, for example, on gay marriage or GLBT *people having kids, so everyone is agreeing. But when you move along to paedophilia, that's when people are splitting and there is quite heated debate. So it's interesting what you hear. Again this is to get the company thinking about where they stand, where they come from. And a lot of this stuff comes up in the play, one way or another, so just hearing other opinions from their peers helps them to understand where people are coming from.*

So to wrap up "Barometer," I say, "It's cool to believe whatever you want, but in the play changing those hats (from personal to professional) is important." This is another step from the Triggers activity. That's the first part, a little tough; it might bring up some stuff for people. And we've had situations where actors come to us and they need to talk or disclose and that's part of our job too. Many of us who have been involved in the play, we're counsellors too.

Sharing Knowledge with the Theatre Company

The health educator can also update the performers' knowledge. From time to time new birth control options are developed and actors need to know what students may ask about or suggest to characters in the play. I tell them to keep informed of current sexuality information and resources because you need to be able to respond to the youth. Then I explain the cards [which are handed out to the audience and which list a wide range of resources for teens]. In almost all cases, the referrals kids need are on the cards.

It's really important if you can't handle a particular topic to find someone who can. Because emotion is always part of it. I tell the cast, talk amongst yourselves and figure out who's the best person to talk to if it's a gay question, if it's an emotion question, if it's a pregnancy question. If you know that this topic makes you uncomfortable and some else is better at it, refer the youth to another cast member or the health person.

I remind [the actors] it's totally cool, you don't have to know everything, actors are scared sometimes to be approached...I remind them that it's not about them; it's okay to say I don't know and refer them to someone else. They will be the first people the kids approach. And we do the hand-off, which has worked great. We're the experts and it's why we're there.

After that I explain why it's important to be sex positive and what that means. Often it's the first time they've ever heard that term so it's great to explore it. I say, "Sex is beautiful and powerful. And because it's so powerful there are a lot of negative things attached to it. Guilt and shame are huge. And as an expert, guilt and shame are big predictors for dysfunction, occurring later in life. If we can be part of movement to get rid of some of that guilt and shame and make sex a positive thing, that would be fantastic."

Obviously there are negative things that can happen too but I don't want to just focus on those things.

The Importance of a Sex-Positive Approach

Another thing I'm really passionate about is how to be sex positive and approachable, so I created a section about it, for actors and others. Obviously this play is sex positive so what I do aligns with that.

[It is important] to explain the difference between sex negative and sex positive... sex negative is saying, "If you have sex you're going to get pregnant, if you have sex you're going to die of AIDS." Unfortunately, a lot of sex education has focused in on the negative or harm reduction, which is good, but it just focuses on the negatives that can happen, and there needs to be positives in there too because sex is such a wonderful thing.

Sex negative just brings out so much guilt and all we feel is bad feelings when actually there's all these good feelings. Everything that I do at work is based around sex positive.

I talk to educators and to actors about being approachable and askable. Leave your baggage at the door. It's not about you; it's about the youth. It's totally cool if you have baggage, but leave it at the door. That's the number one rule about being a good educator around this stuff. Scare tactics don't work, I tell them.

Sharing the Teen Workshop Plan

I go over the workshop outline with them so actors have a good idea of that. I usually talk about...the workshop and do the Drawing the Line activity with them. That's the part of it that really relates to them in the play so I want them to know how I use that line in the workshop.[5] *After that I often take them through the part of the workshop on condoms and safer sex. They need to be up-to-date and know what may come up with the kids. I do a full condom demo and get the actors to role-play youth and I do a birth control demonstration. With youth, we do abstinence, condoms and hormonal, we don't do diaphragms and sponges but with the actors we do the entire kit, because someone might yell out: sponge or IUD and actors need to know what the kids are talking about. When we go through the hormonal stuff with actors, I tell them kids want to know about all the methods. They want to know: How does it work? Are there any side effects? Where can I get it? And, how much does it cost? So actors need to know these things even if they mostly send the kids to us for this information.*

Anonymous Questions

Then comes the favourite part of the training. We bring out the bag of anonymous questions. At the end of the workshop we get the youth to write down any question they would like to have answered about sex. So the last part of the training we do with actors is to show them the questions youth have given us. Each actor will take a pile and when they come to an interesting one or a funny one they'll read it out.

Actors want to know how I answer some of these questions and we talk about that. And I always say to the youth, "I'd love for you to ask a question but if you don't have one just write 'hi' or 'the play was great' or 'the workshop was great or it sucked or whatever.'" And I pass those along to actors particularly if it's the first time they are doing the show. Sometimes the kids will talk about a character like "when Delphi did this" and it's powerful for those actors.

Over the years of this program, teens have written myriads of anonymous questions, including:

- Why are men usually more sexually active?

- When you take birth control it makes your boobs bigger? Right?
- How long can sperm survive on hands, fingers, etc.?
- What's the point of oral sex, when you can just have sex?
- What kind of improvised birth control could you use?
- Do women have sperm?
- How to tell your man you want him to fondle your clit?
- Say if you partner is completely faithful doesn't cheat and if have unprotected sex, and they have only been with each other what STDs can you get beside herpes?
- Does taking birth control reduce the chance of a person being able to get pregnant in the future?

For more examples of youth questions, see Appendix 2.3.

Rehearsing the Play

> *Many health partners I trained felt they had to become an actor to participate in the show. In actuality, the health partner's role in the play is similar to how they would speak about the topic of sexuality in the classroom.*
>
> —*Brian Parker*

While the health educator has only a few small moments in the performance of the play, his or her presence throughout is key. Students see the sex educator's responses to the play and to student comments, and they build an impression of him or her. While the educator's active participation is brief, rehearsal is important so everyone is on the same page and so the educator has an opportunity to become confident within the play structure. It is useful to recognize the protocol of the theatre: a director shapes the play for rhythm and clarity and places the performers, including the health educator, to best suit the particular production. The educator should expect to receive some feedback and requests from the director as well as assistance with any questions about the text or staging.

Brian Parker shared with us how important it is to be part of the play, not just stand up when it's your cue, and then how much more the kids connect with the health partner and how they are more likely to really connect with the follow-up workshop.

—*Leona Purcell*

See Appendix 1.2 for suggested rehearsal schedules, which outline effective timing of health partner's participation in rehearsals. See also "Unpacking the Play" following the play script in Chapter 3, which addresses the purpose of each scene, including the sex educator's role.

Rehearsing for Disclosures

Management of potential disclosures is discussed and practiced. Receiving a disclosure can be difficult for the untrained and actors need to know what to do if it happens. The health partner, as the trained expert in the room, also trains the actors in rehearsal. Most often, youth will approach the actor they feel a connection with, after the performance. Since we don't expect the actors to be counsellors, a "hand-off" was developed, where the actor acknowledges the youth, but eventually directs the student to the health partner. In our experience, this has worked extremely well. Explicit and practical rehearsal for this eventuality is vital. In essence, a protocol for supporting the student and for taking the student to the health educator is articulated, practiced, and rehearsed.

In some cases, the partner health educator is not a sexual health educator/expert. The role of educator can be well-filled by those for whom public health is the focus, even where sexuality education is only a very small piece of the job. In this case, it will be important to arrange appropriate preparation for the health educator(s) as well as for the theatre company.

About a week after the sexuality workshop, when the company is well into rehearsals and has a feel for the play as a whole, the sexual health educator and theatre company work on how they will handle any disclosures that may be triggered by the topic and play. Brian Parker describes this work, which he developed with Concrete Theatre over the years they worked together on *AWTY*.

With disclosures it brings up so much for the actors, again the triggers. The most important things we try to stress with them is it's not about you and you should feel so wonderful that a youth approached you to tell you something like this, like [about] an assault or a rape or cutting or whatever it is, (sometimes it's non-sexually related) but really it's a gift. And that's what this play is about. I know it seems really scary but we really try and get across that a disclosure is a gift. If we can help that one kid get over whatever it is, like they're gay and they have questions about that or they are suicidal, this play came in and now they feel, "Oh my God, there are other people like me," then we did our job.

—*Brian Parker*

The Hand-Off

It's really important that there is a pass off between the actor and the sexual health educator because as actors we can listen and we can sympathize, but we can't really offer any help. It's the sexual health educator that is going to be the one that they need to speak to.

—*Kristi Hansen,* AWTY *actor,*
Concrete Theatre, August 27, 2010

If a student discloses to an actor or stage manager, the student is handed off to the health educator. There are three stages of the initial contact that actors must follow:

1. Acknowledgement or affirmation: "Thank you for telling me, you did the right thing"
2. Support and belief: "I'm sorry that happened (is happening) to you"
3. Action: "We're going to talk to (health educator's name) for more information or to get you some help"

Actors and stage managers are trained to ask a few questions if necessary but to not try to get all the details. The models for the hand-off in AWTY were based on *Feeling Yes, Feeling No,* a sexual abuse prevention program created by Green Thumb Theatre.

When we talk about disclosure we also talk about the law and the obligation that adults have to report abuse. We talk about how the hand-off works and then we do a lot of role-playing. Every single person (including the stage manager) plays both roles: the youth disclosing and the person being disclosed to. We always [place the role play] during the break down of the set, because almost always that's when it's going to happen, when the show is over and a youth can approach an actor more privately. We make up scenarios like "I'm gay," "I was assaulted," "I'm pregnant," and people role-play the youth. We try a simple hand-off and a more difficult hand-off and all the ways for an actor to get [a teen who approaches them] to us.

We make some of them difficult by asking the person role-playing the youth to not give much information or say, "I don't want to talk to Brian."

They practice bringing the youth to us, introduce us, and tell us a little about their story. We take the actors through what to say, like "I really suggest you talk to Brian, he's with Options and he really knows a lot about this stuff."

And the youth have seen us, we get off our chair, we've been with the audience, part of the play, so we don't have problems with hand-offs. The youth will come to us because we're part of the performance.

It's important to note that there has never been a first-time disclosure in all the years that this show has been running in the Alberta region. The show does not set out to solicit disclosures, so you don't need to freak out, you need to be ready but you don't need to worry that every day in every school you're going to have disclosures.

—Brian Parker

On the Road

[On tour] you need a sense of humour. Not all shows go as well as you want them to, [but] we all can talk about the previous show that just happened and how we can make it better. You're always going to miss things in a show [especially with participation], but then maybe you'll find some new stuff.

—Evelyn Chu, AWTY *actor,*
Neworld Theatre

In cases where the health partner as well as the theatre company are on tour for any length of time (tours to date have lasted from two to eleven weeks), the health partner plays an important role in sustaining the quality and effective growth of the production. While giving notes to actors is the purview of the stage manager and the director, with a play like this (its sensitive topic and participatory form) the health partner can be very useful as a company debriefs how it handled certain interactive moments and student comments. The health partner can also note how a group responds to the play or a section of the play and may have a role to play in bringing issues to the table. Certainly where any disclosure has occurred, the group is likely to look for some debriefing and reflection. Concrete Theatre builds in a weekly company meeting where any issues can be addressed. This is a vital part of letting the project grow well and supporting each other on the road. The health partner can be a major support in sharing information and sustaining healthy dialogue within this partnership.

> *A good health partner would have bravery for sure, fearlessness, the ability to talk to a teenager and recognize them for the questions that they have, but also be confident in the skills that you have, that you have something to share with them. An openness and understanding, patience, and an excitement and a passion for what you're doing. And friendly—please be friendly—otherwise, you know, nobody'll want to come talk to you.*
>
> —*Gina Puntil,* AWTY *stage manager,*
> *Concrete Theatre*

NOTES

1. For those in public health who decide to take on this project and who want to explore the workshop and health partner training in more detail, please see "A Guide to Facilitating the Are We There Yet? Follow-up Workshop." See Appendix 2.1 for additional information.
2. See Chapter 2 for more discussion of the value of this kind of approach to sexuality education.
3. See how this exercise, Drawing the Line, is used in the play (Chapter 3, page 75).
4. BDSM: Bondage, domination, sadism, and masochism.
5. Refer to the script for the Drawing the Line exercise (Chapter 3, page 75).

7

CUSTOMIZED

Adapting Are We There Yet? *for Community Specificity*

CONTENTS

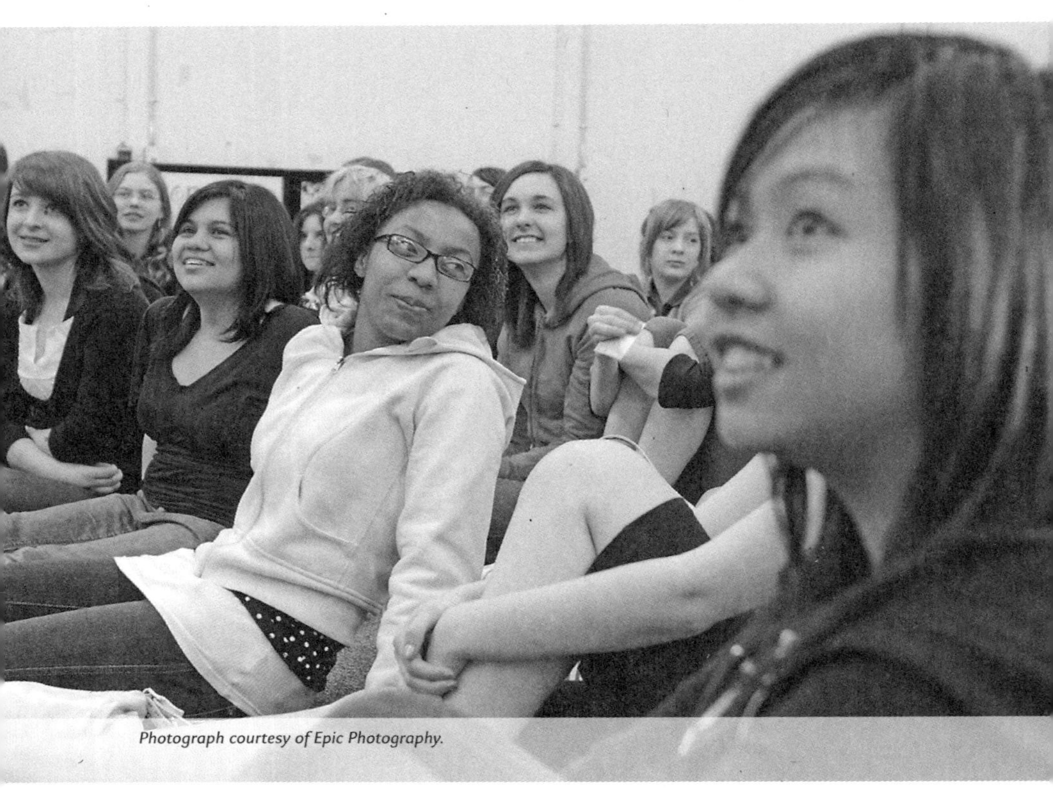

Photograph courtesy of Epic Photography.

The project was adapted in several different geographic and cultural settings. We discuss some of the highlights and discoveries that emerged as the project moved from rural Nova Scotia to downtown Toronto to boys' schools in Vancouver to small reserves in northern Saskatchewan.

> *You've never experienced La Ronge have you?*
>
> —AUDIENCE MEMBER

THEATRE THAT IS CREATED IN RESPONSE to a particular community's experiences, cultural expression, and expressed needs is not always repeatable, or it may have a different and often less potent meaning when transferred to a different setting. The community specificity may be understandable by others but it does not evoke the same level of recognition in every context. Thus, while we would set out to sustain the core intentions of *Are We There Yet?*, given that effective sexuality education is urgently needed in most areas of our country, we would adapt the play and workshop as much as needed, within and with each new cultural setting. Over the course of the Are We There Yet? research program, quantitative and qualitative program evaluations determined that the degree of positive change for participants was similar from region to region (see Chapter 9). These findings suggested that the adaptations met one of the challenges we set for ourselves; we wanted to discover how the piece should change in order to connect with our audiences and sustain high levels of recognition and identification in each setting. However, the adaptation process and outcomes were not always predictable.

Adapting Theatre for Varying Cultural Contexts[1]

Adaptation that embraces cultural and community conditions is vital if education and theatre projects are committed to transformation. In addition to finding the partnerships that are most viable in each setting, the program itself—the play and sometimes the workshop—needs reconsideration within each context.

There are many layers of adaptation in the AWTY project. To begin with, the play is regularly reviewed to update small details. Teen culture, its slang, jargon, and references change quite quickly, and specificity pays off in terms of humour, recognition, and, as a result, identification. While complications and pitfalls exist in this updating process, there are benefits when the company is very much in touch with and reflects their community's teens, language, and interests. Building up-to-date knowledge of the specific audience is an important part of the rehearsal process; even when actors are just a few years older than the audience, there are many tells if current community research is short-changed. At worst, authenticity is at risk. Teen audiences can easily become suspicious that the company (and play) is out of touch, or at best, sincere and well-meaning but not relevant. Small things enhance the audience's pleasure in the event, and choosing recognizable music, language, and physicality all make a difference.[2]

The play text may be altered in some details, but because the performance is so participatory, with actors improvising as they interact with the audience then returning to the script, research in the community may lead to adaptations that, while minor or even seemingly inconsequential in terms of alterations to the formal text, contribute significantly to the audience's perception of authenticity and local relevance. As the play is adapted, it must continue to represent audience diversity and range of circumstances. For example, as not every teen has access to a cell phone, some characters will and some will not have an option to use one, in order to be inclusive and build recognition among as many audience members as possible.

Beyond ensuring that current slang and popular references are in place, references to a particular audience's world are important. For example, the basic script, developed for urban audiences, has a character meeting her boyfriend for a serious encounter:

Carol Ann: ...I was so scared I just...ran out of there. (*She sets up the question for the* AUDIENCE.) Now I don't know what to do. I'm meeting Mac in a few minutes at the mall. What should I tell him? (*She* GATHERS *suggestions from* AUDIENCE *about her embarrassment and fears.*) Okay, I'll try. (*She goes into the scene.* MAC *is waiting for her at the mall. He's mad.*)

When the play was adapted in a rural county in Nova Scotia, the meeting place in most towns became at the bridge because there was no mall. While such details may seem minor, connecting the details in the play with the specific audience builds pleasure, identification, and trust. This relationship pays off as the performance continues. For example, later in the play, Mac asks audiences to give him ideas for where he can get a condom (Chapter 3, page 82). By this point, given strategic adaptation and effective community-based research, the play and actors' performances have established that this is not a generic sex ed lesson but one that is embedded in the audience's world.

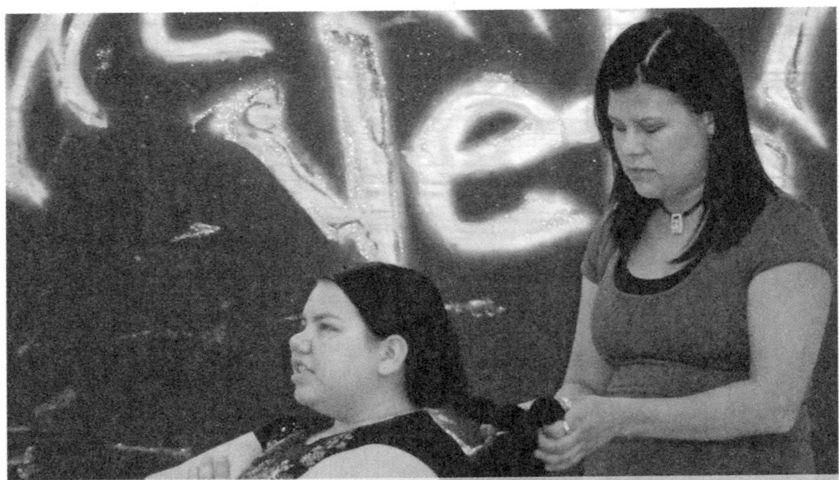

When can I learn to drive? Adaptation
Jennifer Dawn Bishop and Krystle Pederson, Saskatchewan Native Theatre Company.
Photograph courtesy of Jane Heather.

Mac: ...I've been thinking about it. Like how to get them. So I went to look, just check it out, a few weeks ago. I was just casually going up and down the aisles. I started to sweat, my mouth was all dry and it was really embarrassing. I passed the condom rack three times and I couldn't do it. The pharmacist was staring at me, the other customers, the lady at the till. I can't buy them, I'm too nervous. (GATHERS *ideas from* AUDIENCE.) Where else can I get protection? (GATHERS *ideas then* BLOCKS, *taking into account specific audience circumstances, such as cost, distance, quality, etc.*)

Community research during adaptation processes in Saskatchewan and Nova Scotia led to understanding that in small towns (or on reserves) there is often only one outlet with condoms, and usually teens know the person who runs it quite well. The character's particular difficulty in dealing with discomfort about going and getting a condom must change substantially. In this case the core script (quoted above) changes and the actor/character animates the discussion from a different set of given circumstances.

In addition to script adjustments, small but significant changes were made in staging specific scenes. A director, designer, and cast always make

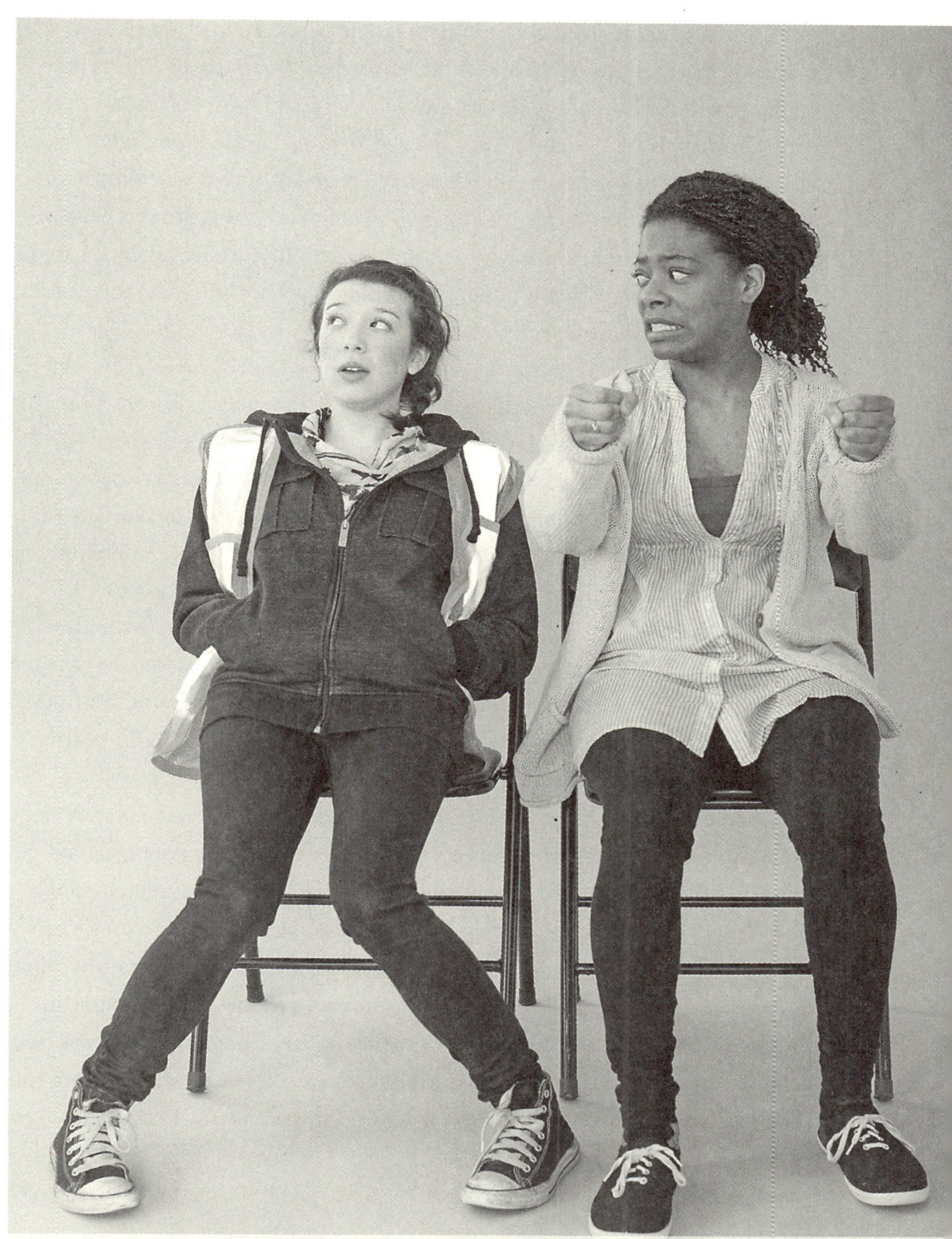

When can I learn to drive? Original
Ming Hudson and Monice Peter, Concrete Theatre. *Photograph courtesy of Epic Photography.*

interpretive choices, and each production held unique flourishes connected to the visions of these artists and their sense about how to reach out to their audiences. In the case of the Aboriginal version, adaptation for the cultural community was very evident. For example, in other productions, when we first see Alex and her mother (Chapter 3, page 69), they are driving. In Saskatchewan Native Theatre Company's production, the mother is brushing Alex's hair. Mom in this case is not taking her daughter to skating or the mall; they are having an intimate, personal moment together when the topic of sex arises.

Props also changed. In some versions of "Know Your Vehicle" (Chapter 3, page 70), the instructor uses two hand-drawn pictures of the human body (male and female) to demonstrate the body parts; in Saskatchewan, two drawings were used as well but the figures were fully clothed in simple, some would say cartoon, versions of traditional Aboriginal dress. The face of each drawing was cut out and actors' faces, one male and one female, appeared through the holes. This was a wonderful and very humorous choice as it recalled cheesy tourist activities where you can stick your head through pictures of various people or animals and have your picture taken. But the image also encircled audience and actors in a common culture and tradition. Only an Aboriginal company with an Aboriginal audience could make this simple image both a joke and something very serious.

A huge benefit of live theatre is that these adjustments can be made easily, as long as the playwright permits script changes and the producing company is truly in touch with the specifics of each community in which they play. Respect for teens' real issues, particular contexts, and world views can be expressed; all of these apparently minor elements add up to an authentic and respectful aesthetic and educational encounter. Our research into the importance of recognition and identification in this kind of theatre work (see Chapter 13) suggests these considerations are essential to making the most of theatrical interventions.

Adaptation Processes

This research program enabled an intensive and multifaceted approach to adaptation for Aboriginal audiences. The Saskatchewan Native Theatre Company (SNTC) worked closely with the original AWTY Program group to pursue a participatory research process. As this was *AWTY*'s first substantial adaptation, we imagined that the script revisions could be quite major; we knew that we must create conditions where this was feasible. Aboriginal co-playwright Kenneth T. Williams was engaged to work with the original playwright, Jane Heather. During the adaptation period, the creative team was in residence with SNTC for four weeks over four months. There were some important changes to the script; however, the process led to insights into other kinds of adaptation, changes that ultimately meant more to the success of the project.

In addition to ongoing consultation among the playwrights, SNTC's artistic director, and the *AWTY* principal investigator, the major methodology consisted of workshopping material, first with SNTC's Youth Ensemble and then with a wide variety of Aboriginal youth in urban and reserve communities. The Youth Ensemble had participated in Circle of Voices, SNTC's culturally-based theatre creation program, and was selected to continue training as they performed and created for the company. They explored the themes of the project using drama exercises such as snapshot stories, sculpturing, and improvisation, and worked on the participatory scenes from the play. These young adults participated in and gradually took on leading workshops, script testing, and exploration of participatory sequences with teenagers and community groups. This long-term engagement and evolving leadership approach was invaluable and challenging for everyone. Co-writer Kenneth T. Williams assesses these challenges:

> *Many of the problems we faced were historical, in the sense that Aboriginal communities have a history of someone coming in, identifying a problem then proffering a solution and leaving. Many Aboriginal people, especially youth, have been on the receiving end of the process. Now [in* AWTY*] we asked [the youth actors] to be on the giving end, the leadership position, so to speak. This was new and frightening, and I think we got a lot of resistance because of this. For all we knew, this was the very first group of*

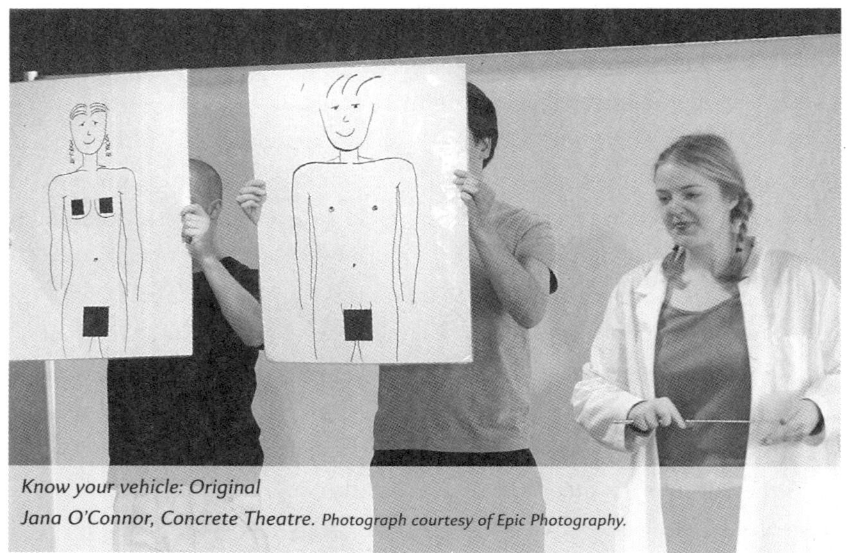

Know your vehicle: Original
Jana O'Connor, Concrete Theatre. *Photograph courtesy of Epic Photography.*

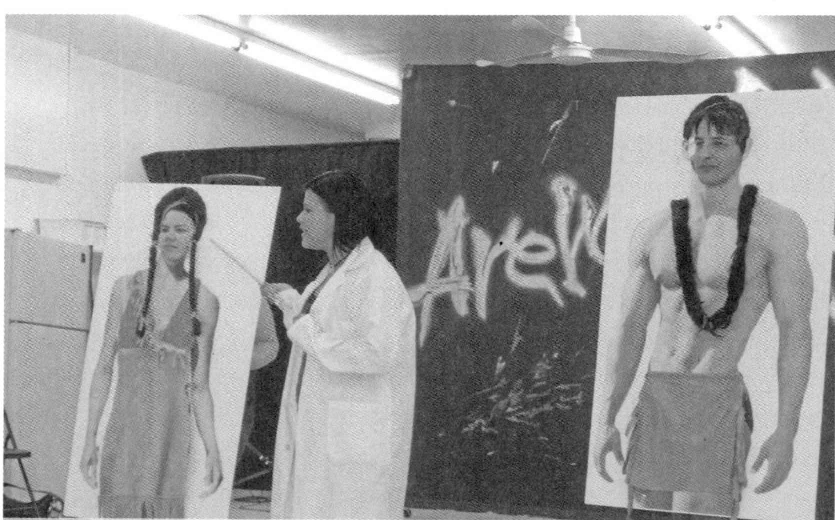

Know your vehicle: Adaptation
Jennifer Dawn Bishop, Krystle Pederson, and Clifford Cardinal, Saskatchewan Native Theatre Company. *Photograph courtesy of Jane Heather.*

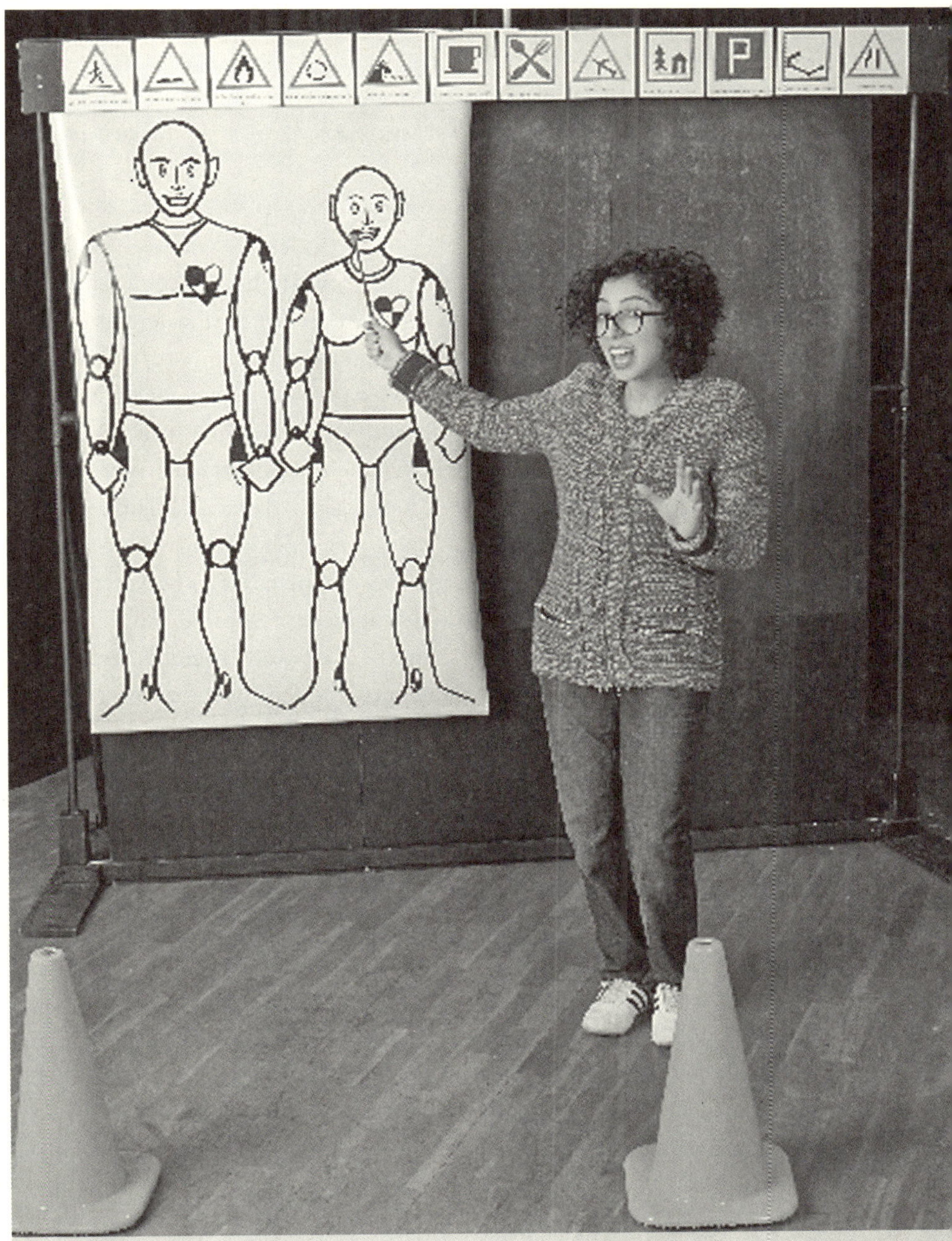

Know your vehicle: Adaptation
Azin Sadr, Neworld Theatre. Photograph courtesy of Tim Matheson.

Aboriginal youth who were leading this kind of theatre in their own communities. It's frightening. Resistance waned when they realized how they were empowering the youth in front of them. I think it's worth mentioning that when approaching this kind of theatre creation in communities that have been historically on the receiving end, there may be some resistance.

—*Kenneth T. Williams, November 16, 2010*

The form of theatre was new for the company, and public consultation events followed skill-building workshops for the young adult performers, as well as interactive events with a wide cross-section of rural- and urban-based teenagers. These community encounters led to many important insights. Discussions grappled with community acceptance, community silence on this difficult topic, youth safety, babies having babies, and much more.

In addition to the script considerations discussed earlier, a significant script adjustment came out of one of many participatory research events. The event involved SNTC's cultural advisors plus members of Saskatoon and northern Saskatchewan education and health sectors, hosted and led by SNTC's artistic director, Kennetch Charlette. The Youth Ensemble performed presentational and participatory elements of the play for and with a group of teenagers, as the community consultants looked on. An extended discussion about the content, community needs and varying sectors' priorities followed, involving the some thirty invited consultants. Discussion topics included advice, priorities, cultural issues, themes, cautions, and urgency of health issues (HIV and other sexually transmitted diseases, early pregnancies, and others). There was a debate about the values of abstinence messages versus recognition of teens' range of sexual activity. Discussions included varying views on the wisdom of using a theatre project such as *AWTY* to provide skills and tools for teens, on their terms. Several related topics were also put on the table, including sexual abuse, the impact of residential schools, gender, and culture. This stage was key in the adaptation process and building community commitment as well as providing opportunity for insights into how to adapt the play. The in-community and public statements of support for the project, while acknowledging the sensitivity and complexity of the topic for the community, were vital to building sustainability and acceptance.

However, as often is the case in community-based and participatory research, informal conversations around the edges of this event led to the most substantial adjustment of the script. During the course of the day, over lunch, coffee, and after the more formal consultation, an elder spoke with several of us one-on-one. She supported the initiative strongly and told us part of her story. This gift led to an important rewrite within one of play's monologues that focus on characters' difficult sex-related experiences and how they find ways to move on. Audiences commonly comment on the power of these stories, and many who were interviewed about their responses to the play chose to discuss their impact. This elder's personal response led to the following script adaptation. The original text, near the end of Hal's story, was:

Hal: ...My sister is a school counsellor and I looked at this pamphlet she had about date rape. I guess I knew before but I didn't really put it all together. Finally I did. I sexually assaulted my girlfriend in grade eleven. I wish I hadn't. (Chapter 3, page 84.)

The adaptation process changed this sequence to:

Hal: ...One day, they have this workshop at school about sexual assault. They made all of us go. I didn't want to. I never assaulted anyone, why did I have to go? And then I see my Kohkum and I wonder what she's doing here. Well, she gets up in front of everyone and she starts telling a story about something that happened to her when she was in school. About a boy she liked...and about what happened when he wanted to and she didn't. And how it had changed her. Man, I hated that guy. I wanted to kill him for doing that to my Kohkum. Then it hit me. I was no different than that guy. I sexually assaulted my girlfriend in grade eleven. I wish I hadn't. (Heather and Williams 2006, 30)

The elder's generous participation influenced how an Aboriginal teen character came to better understand his actions and make a change in his life.

Another substantial script adaptation came about through a combination of addressing community priorities and the overall change in climate and community acceptance of acknowledging same-sex relationships. As the project entered into the adaptation in Vancouver with Neworld Theatre and Vancouver Coastal Health, artistic director Marcus Youssef and sexual health educator Kenji Maeda felt the time was ripe for the inclusion of more LGBTQ material. Times change, and they felt that in their community, in 2009, a LGBTQ character would be accepted and not trigger school or parental backlash. This was an important opportunity to test new content and address (to some degree) a gap in the play.

The playwright and Vancouver team discussed many possible ways to include a LGBTQ character and Youssef and Maeda decided on a new monologue. They selected a male coming out story as the topic of the monologue as the best way to acknowledge these teens and communicate to them that the play and players were aware and attuned to their issues. Several versions of the monologue were written based upon the research and feedback from Youssef and Maeda; it was performed in the Vancouver adaptation and was subsequently incorporated into the Edmonton production as well.

While these kinds of script adjustments were extremely important to the project's success in disparate cultural conditions, ultimately the play script changed less than we had expected. On reflection, we believe that the relative stability of the original script is largely related to the participatory nature of the play. Other texts might change much more drastically when community specificity is sought. However, while this script changed only a little, the performance text changed a great deal.

Adapting Performance and Participation

The interactive sections of the play are planned but ever adjusting (see Chapter 4). These participatory sequences hold the text that is most affected by the culture of the audience and the capacity of the actors to encompass, react to, and inhabit that culture. While each interaction is initiated by the script, actors adjust and improvise extensively as the audience explores issues and advises characters. Recognition and communication at many levels (verbal, physical, emotional) are vital to the play's impact. To some

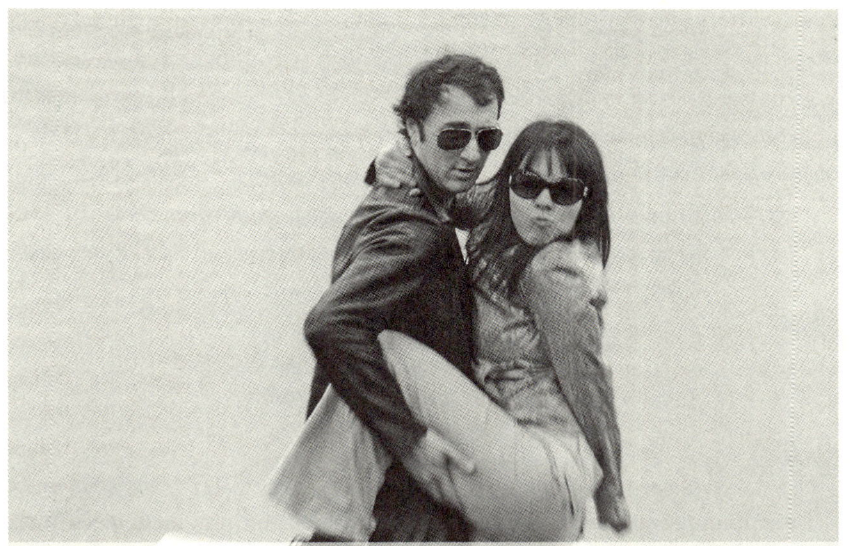

Fantasy date: Original
Jeremy Baumung and Nadien Chu, Concrete Theatre. Photograph courtesy of Epic Photography

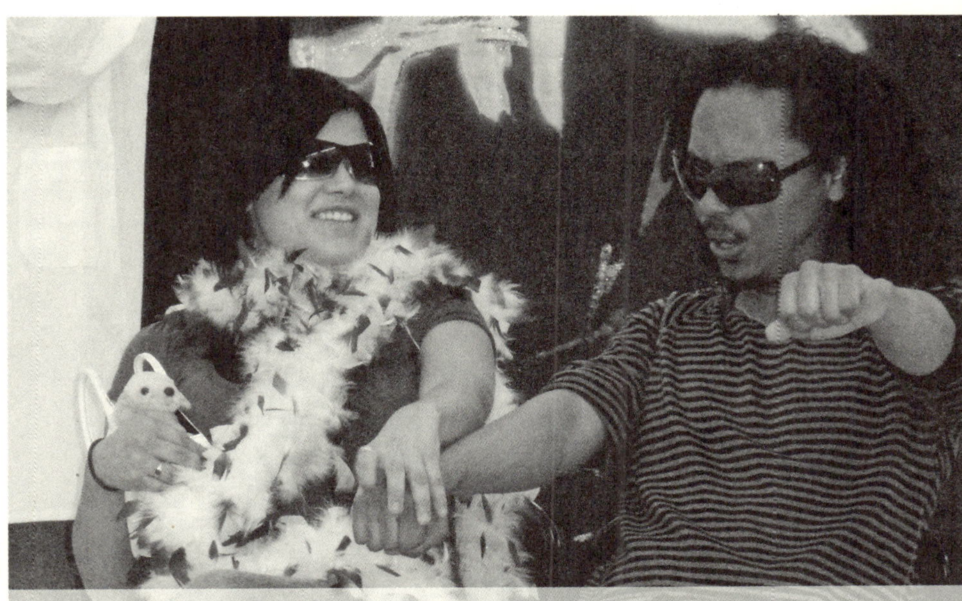

Fantasy date: Adaptation
Krystle Pederson and Arron Naytowhow, Saskatchewan Native Theatre Company. Photograph courtesy of Jane Heather.

degree, this level of engagement suggests adaptation for every single school and class:

> *Each time I do the show in a different school, there are different responses...just the demeanour of this certain class...they have a different idea of how to deal with a certain relationship and so suddenly that changes the way I'm behaving in the scene and as long as I allow myself to really just go there and not try to keep coming up with cookie cutter responses, then it's...more accessible to everyone and we get to open a better discussion with the kids.*
>
> —*Sheldon Elter,* AWTY *actor,*
> *Concrete Theatre*

This kind of adaptation is only possible in a live situation. Live theatre offers a tremendous opportunity to meet learners where they live and to flex a program's content and delivery to suit the specific situation. This approach relates closely with a model of education that links student need, students' starting points, and relevance to students' lived experience with educators' methods and content.

> *When I went to the all-boys school I felt like I needed to assert myself a little more. Maybe I played a little bit high status just so they'd go, "Oh, there is a female who can hold her ground." I think the general feeling sometimes in all-boys groups is that, "Oh, there's a girl, just do whatever you want." That's the feeling I got...Or in an all-girls school maybe I'll do something that's the easier choice for a girl...I'll go, "Oh, maybe I'll just hold his arm and he'll understand everything." Then it plays out wrong because the male Clay will go, "C'mon,"—he'll be more realistic with it. So it's interesting to push them that way. Say they're a pushy audience, well then take the pushy response and see what happens and then it goes wrong, not as they expected or it's not as easy as they think. Find the other extreme, find what they don't expect. That's what I do.*
>
> —*Evelyn Chu,* AWTY *actor,*
> *Neworld Theatre*

However, cultural differences involve both overt and subtle adaptation. In each setting (urban, suburban, rural, on and off reserve), the more deeply the actors knew the specifics of a situation, the more nuanced the participatory elements could be. We found that the overt details can be quickly researched and embedded once a theatre company identifies and prepares adequately for these adjustments. However, the deepest adaptation in a participatory play such as this comes from the carefully selected cultural makeup of the cast. Because so much of the play is about in-the-moment communications between actor and audience member, it is of paramount importance that the cast deeply knows, understands, and has lived the audience's cultural reality. Jennifer Bishop, an AWTY actor with the Saskatchewan Native Theatre Company, stated the following:

> *For me it's just...I can really...relate with the audience, like they see me as like I would hang out with them or go to school with them, so they don't see me as this big huge authority figure. They see me as just like a regular person I met so that they're more comfortable with us, you know.*

This view is put in another way by one of the northern Saskatchewan health partners:

> *The opportunity for youth on the reserve to see Aboriginal actors in their communities talking about issues that are relevant to them is such a positive experience. Some of those kids never leave the reserve...we say to them all the time, "You can do whatever you want...you can be whoever you want," but how many times do they get a chance to actually see that? Just the idea that they can see someone like them doing something like that [acting] is worth so much.*
>
> —*Leslie Brooks, communicable disease control nurse, Northern Inter-Tribal Health Authority, Prince Albert, SK, July 13, 2008*

Some of the variations from one cultural milieu to another are quite explicit, while others are very subtle. In watching the project adaptations in four quite different cultural settings, we observed that a key to the adaptation of this play is corporeal, most significantly held in the body and voice and way of being of each actor. Actors consistently looked for ways to incorporate cultural references gestures and language into the improvised participatory sections. A great deal of adaptation comes from the bodies, memories, and experiences of the actors. These can then resonate and, particularly in participatory sequences, are amplified by the audience through the actors. In participation, actors learn to play what they hear but also what they see. Cultural specificity is expressed in many ways. It is held in the nature of the jokes and humour. In the length of a silence. In all the ways each actor related to their audiences.

> *Like up North, just from being up North I notice like we talk different, we experience things different. Like from like an urban school, when you go to a reserve school, the kids, they learn things different and culture's really important to them, like everything's just a little bit different. It's the same but it's different at the same time.*
>
> —*Krystle Pederson,* AWTY *actor,*
> *Saskatchewan Native Theatre Company*

While challenging, adapting this play for specific audiences was accomplished most richly by investing fully in the training and rehearsal of a company most culturally connected to the intended audiences. Each context encountered different challenges in doing so. In the rural adaptation created by Mulgrave Road Theatre, one challenge was to find actors with sufficient current experience in rural settings. Generally, to get enough work, actors locate in cities. In this and in the Aboriginal adaptation, investing in training for the participatory elements of the play and particularly in creating opportunities to identify variations necessary in the non-urban settings were important. Early rehearsal opportunities to research with local teens and encounter their worlds were important, and workshop rehearsals (or test audiences, as this project calls them) assisted in this aspect of adaptation. In every version, the actors who found ways to make the most in-depth use of community knowledge and audience research as they built characters also most flexibly shifted gears from setting to setting.

> *When we were up North it was so easy to bring that Aboriginal flavour out, you know, because we had to change the show for them because if we presented it as it was [in the city], they wouldn't talk to us...My understanding of the Cree language and culture...*

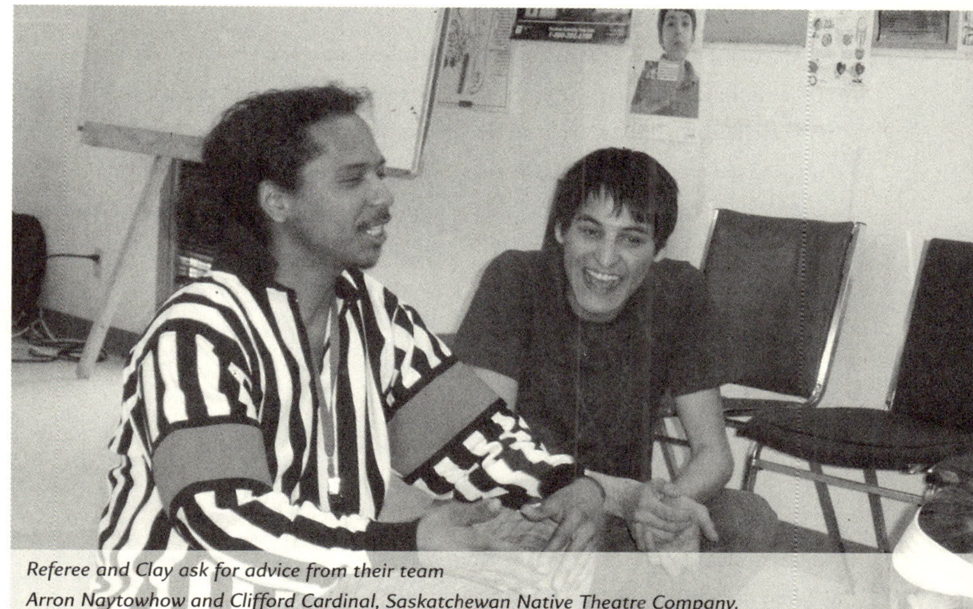
Referee and Clay ask for advice from their team
Arron Naytowhow and Clifford Cardinal, Saskatchewan Native Theatre Company.
Photograph courtesy of Jane Heather.

helped me out on stage...and they heard their own words. That does something for the kids when they hear, you know, they hear themselves—like okay then, we can talk to these guys.

—*Arron Naytowhow,* AWTY *actor,*
Saskatchewan Native Theatre Company

The urban projects have slightly different challenges. Performances can have an extremely wide range of teens from school to school and within each audience. Both the original company, Edmonton's Concrete Theatre, and the other urban production by Neworld Theatre in Vancouver, attempt to cast the play with a highly diverse cast. As the program evaluation research is proving audience recognition and identification to be so important, this strategy, long employed by both companies in a variety of their theatre productions, is vital.

A number of the artists found cultural affinity to be a very important factor:

I saw Are We There Yet? *when I was fourteen at my junior high, and then ten years later...I got cast for the show. Yeah, the role modelling effect, I mean...you just go up there and you be who you are and I think in terms of race there's sort of a quick access point for visible minorities...I saw the show when Jared [Matsunaga-Turnbull] was in it and that was the first time I'd ever seen an Asian actor onstage and that planted a little thing in my head that, "Oh, I exist up there too." And that was a neat thing for me [at fourteen] and I think I could see that [as an actor] in audience members too...if there's like one or two Asian kids and they see the one Asian guy up there, "Oh, I exist somewhere else." You know? There's just a little subtle thing that happens right there and it's not about playing any sort of race, but there's recognition in that you exist somewhere else.*

—*Richard Lee,* AWTY *actor,*
Concrete Theatre

It's so important, that sense of equality, that sense of "we're all in the same struggle," that sense of "we are," there is no separation.

—*Nadien Chu,* AWTY *actor,*
Concrete Theatre

So, deeply considered casting, which leads to cultural identification and supports the richest levels of authenticity and communication is vital to this work. Further, opportunities for rich, participatory research with the range of groups that will attend the play (considering age, culture, urban/rural, economics, class, etc.) and in-depth training and rehearsal opportunities, particularly for the interactive sequences of the play, are required to achieve the fullest productions with the highest impacts. In this work, the guiding principles must include a commitment to and search for both specificity and inclusivity.

Adapting the Program for Varying Community and Cultural Contexts

In addition to underlining the significance and power to be gained by casting the play with cultural specificity and providing rich opportunities for community-based and age-specific participatory research, the adaptation of the full AWTY Program to other settings taught the team a great deal about partnering the arts with other organizations.[3]

The original partners, Concrete Theatre and Options Sexual Health Association, created a particular partnership model, and initially we imagined that adaptations would follow that organizational structure. In the original model, a sexual health educator from Options attends every performance and returns to the school to lead a workshop with the students, usually about a week after the show; Options becomes a long-term resource for these teens. However, in Saskatchewan, another kind of partnership was required. While Saskatchewan Native Theatre Company was experienced in creating theatre around specific agency agendas or conference themes, they warned the research team that there would be jurisdictional issues as the project travelled to the theatre company's constituencies in northern Saskatchewan. Aboriginal health is both a federal and a provincial responsibility, and jurisdictional issues were indeed complex. As the company intended to tour to rural communities, reserves, and urban centres, finding a health partner that could serve many community circumstances called for a different partnership model. Ultimately, in most rural and reserve areas, local public health nurses and other health professionals provided the workshop component. Training was offered in a pre-pilot tour workshop by Brian Parker from Options. For the second, more extensive tour, training was provided by several of the original Saskatchewan health partners, Erin Schoenfeld and Brett Dow of the Saskatoon Health Region, and Wendy McPhail, a sexual wellness co-ordinator for the Mamawetan Churchill Health Region, who also supported the tour as jurisdictional issues allowed by travelling to several northern centres. It was patchwork at best, and this situation offered a lesson in some of the barriers to consistent and culturally sensitive health provision for Aboriginal communities. Tracy L. Bear, a PHD student and AWTY Community-University Research Alliance member, who conducted much of the evaluation processes for the Aboriginal adaptation, points out,

> *Every Aboriginal health conference I attend, I hear pleas and demands from Aboriginal communities for proven, sustainable programs on sexual health and wellness.*

> *Analysis of the qualitative and quantitative research proves undeniably that the AWTY project provides an innovative alternative from which to improve our approaches to teaching sex education within our Aboriginal teen population. I have seen it, I have experienced it. Government agencies and health officials can't say there aren't effective programs any longer. However, implementing programs like this one over the long-term will take dedicated financial support.*

Another important feature was implemented in the Aboriginal pilot tour, but unfortunately not repeated during the fuller tour the following year. An elder accompanied the actors to each performance; the importance of this choice cannot be overstated. Actors benefited from support and cultural consultation around this tough and sensitive topic. Teen audience members witnessed and felt this support, as did other members of each community. Liaison with the individual communities was invaluable, as was the demonstrated support for the project by a cultural leader.

Sharing Insights

Over the course of this combination evaluation and practice-based research program, findings in one community suggested ways forward for another, often quite different community. As each adaptation established a different partnership model, one area's model, born out of the specific conditions, helped another team address a problem. For example, the Nova Scotia production had a separate health partner embedded in each community, while providing central and collective leadership and training in sexuality education and in the health partners' role. This model helped members of the national alliance think about solutions to the jurisdictional problems in Saskatchewan and offered a way forward as Edmonton's Concrete Theatre started touring beyond Options Edmonton's mandated territory. Additionally, as a result of the national research program, several groups are considering whether or how to integrate Vancouver's model, where an independent sexual health worker is attached to their production. In this case, the health expert has historic ties to a sexual health organization, Vancouver Coastal Health, but is working on this project for the theatre company. The considerations of this rather attractive and efficient approach include looking for ways to connect the teens with an accessible and ongoing sexuality education community agency or resource after the theatre company moves on. Meanwhile, Options Edmonton has developed a training workshop with a DVD and workbook for new sexual health partners, which includes adjustments for those with sexual health backgrounds and for those with public health but not sexual health education backgrounds.[4]

Inventing a New Program Element

The most substantial adaptation to the overall AWTY Program was the addition of a community meeting in Saskatchewan. The theatre company suggested that, in the isolated reserves, the entire community needed to be involved in the project. In SNTC's experience, everyone in the community attended their performances, no matter the content or target age group. As the original *AWTY* is intended for teens, and seeks to create a space where teens talk openly with teens, we had to keep listening and keep talking with SNTC about how to negotiate this potential impasse. We all wanted to incorporate and honour the company's long-standing relationships with their communities, without losing what we thought was a core element of *AWTY*—teens talking with teens. The company felt that *AWTY* would generate interest for all community members, and that there needed be a way for all to be involved. Further, during the participatory research, community consultation, and adaptation process, adults and teens expressed that adults needed this kind of show as well as youth. Many expressed that their own sexual education had been rather poor, or absent, that they had learned a lot from watching pieces of the play, and they wished that they and their parents had had such a thing when they were young. Some of the elders at a community gathering spoke of the multigenerational impact of residential schools that left a legacy of silence and dysfunction in many families and communities. "Residential school affects my children," one said, and another offered, "Parents and communities don't heal. It's better now, they didn't talk about it twenty years ago." "It's hard," said one elder, "for some generations to look at [sex] but parents, elders are ready to do something about teenagers."

These were important discussions and ultimately the team determined that there was value to a show that allowed teens to discuss sexual choices and health among themselves, but that parents and other adults needed to be involved as well. Adults needed to learn about what their kids were experiencing. An interactive community meeting was devised, aimed at parents, elders, health workers, teachers, and other adults who engage with youth. At this meeting, the project and play were introduced, and some new participatory scenes especially for adults were presented. These were created by the playwrights, based on the youth company and SNTC's artistic director improvising from scenarios. Because the scenes were meant for adult participation, the situations place an adult character (parent, elder, relative) in a dilemma about a teen: the adult needs help from an audience of adults to work through an issue related to sexuality and the teens in their lives.[5]

The community meeting allowed us to ask, what is the participation for Aboriginal adults around this topic and play? We had a great ready resource at our fingertips to develop scenes. We had a rehearsal space, some time, and twelve young actors (aged eighteen to twenty-eight) from the Ensemble Theatre Arts Program (ETAP), SNTC's culturally-based training program, who were all well-versed in improvisation. We had Kennetch Charlette, artistic director, gifted improviser, elder, cultural advisor, and leader, as well as participation expert Jan Selman, and the playwrights. These were the perfect ingredients for a fun and productive day using theatre tools and participation skills to find the most potent scenes for this important issue: How do I (an adult) talk about sexuality to this teen?

To develop the adult scenes, we set up a series of improvisations. In each, a teen approaches an adult with a question or dilemma about sexuality and the adult asks for advice from other adults in the audience. Selman and Heather developed about fifteen possible presenting problems. These included:

- My vagina hurts
- I was having sex and the condom broke
- There's stuff coming out of my penis
- I think I'm pregnant
- I found this porno magazine, is it real?
- I think my girl friend is pregnant
- What's a blow job?

- Can you masturbate too much?
- I think I'm gay

We wrote each problem on a slip of paper. Just before the scene a youth actor would blind-choose one. The relationship between the teen and adult was decided, (father–daughter, uncle–nephew, etc.) and the scene would begin. Charlette offered many wonderful, rich characters for the young actors to play off. In one, he was a dad busy measuring the living room, preparing for the arrival of a new couch. In another, he was an older man, quietly and calmly repairing a fishing net. We saw truthful, urgent, complex, and compelling theatre. Each young actor took the exercise very seriously. This was a chance to show their chops and challenge their mentor/director/teacher/elder. After many days of learning a text, learning participation, and trying to learn how to be leaders, they got to shine and make tangible, significant contributions to exploring the topic further and creating new scene material. The scenes were fun and also dead serious but the participation was incredible. Charlette took to this form as if he were born to it. In one scene his daughter told him the condom broke:

K: You're having sex?
D: Well, yeah.
K: Does your mother know?
D: No, I don't think so.
K: Tell her, Tell her!
D: She's not here and I'm telling *you.*
K: (*Turning to audience*) Ahhhhh! What do I do now?

This is a perfect example of blocking through character and also through culture. This dad was uncomfortable discussing sex with his daughter and he wanted a female to take over for him, as is traditional. On the other hand, he wanted to support his daughter and respond to her need, not just duck out, delay, and hand it to his wife. It became clear that this kind of scene could evoke a complex discussion among adult audience members. We began to imagine, with great excitement, all the things a community meeting could open up for communities.

But there was more. For many days and weeks, the young actors had been working with the participation in AWTY while their peers, the playwrights, the project facilitator, director, and other adults and played teen audience members for them. Now they got a chance to play out how they believed adults would respond, and they were brilliant. One young man got up to perform the problem: "There's stuff coming out of the end of my penis." The young actors playing audience/adults were right on it, feeding Charlette the key questions such as, "Ask him if it hurts when he pees?" They also picked up on subtle visual cues the actor was projecting. Charlette got to a finish point in the participation, and he was able to promise the teen character that they would go to the clinic so the youth could be tested. The youth character had come into the scene in a frozen monosyllabic state, almost hidden in his hoodie. When the uncle character told the youth they would go to the clinic tomorrow, the youth said, "I don't know if I'll be here tomorrow." The audience jumped on this. "He's thinking about suicide," one person yelled out. The actor (Charlette) had thought the participation was over but it was not. His job as the adult in the scene suddenly became much bigger, as did the participation.

Slowly, it emerged that the audience was right. The teen character thought he had HIV/AIDS and felt suicide was a better choice than testing and finding out he had the virus. As the scene progressed, less and less acting took place and more and more we saw an elder—anxious, unsure, afraid—going on (with help from others) to get this precious boy back from the brink.

Ultimately, the AWTY Program is strengthened through flexible problem solving along with availability of effective resources and support as it is adapted to suit each community condition and each cultural milieu. Adaptation came to mean more than we first imagined. It refers to deep community engagement, and to how all elements of the program—script, participation, casting, evaluation, orientation, training, connections with prospective audiences, the workshop, the theatre–health partnership, booking the program in schools and communities, community-based research, involvement of the wider community, and more—are devised and delivered.

NOTES

1. Parts of this chapter draw on ideas first presented in Jan Selman et al., "Participatory Theatre for Change: Road Testing Cultural Adaptations," in *Creative Arts in Research for Community and Cultural Change*, vol. 2 of the Creative Arts in Interdisciplinary Practice Research Series, edited by Cheryl McLean, (Calgary, AB: Detselig Enterprises, 2011): 16–38.
2. See Chapter 9 for program assessment findings and Chapter 10 for a discussion of the role of pleasure in theatre's impact on audiences.
3. See Chapter 5 for a description of four varying theatre–health agency partnerships.
4. This resource can be accessed by contacting Options Sexual Health, Edmonton.
5. See Appendix 3.2 for an example of a participatory scene created for adults.

part III

RESEARCHING THEATRE FOR CHANGE

Interdisciplinary Research in Theatre for Change

THE FIELD OF THEATRE FOR SOCIAL CHANGE needs a more legitimate space to stand in and more capacity to demonstrate its powers. We are pressed to prove that it works. There are two pressure points, internal and external. Internal to the field, artists and organizations want to ensure that their efforts in using art for change has impact. Artists want to investigate questions about form, content, and context in order to make the most of their work: they seek meaningful impact. What works for participants and audiences? When? In what context? We want to ensure that our creative efforts are about more than our pleasure in creating and performing theatre. Organizations that partner with theatre practitioners to provide education and initiate change also want to know that the resources, time, and energy they commit will forward their mandates.

These committed artists and social organizations experience pressure from funders and other education and development partners to prove that theatre indeed works, that it produces the changes and growth they seek, that it is worth the cost and effort. Communities too want to know which agents and processes for change most deeply recognize their experience and support their goals. There are implications for many sectors. All players look for clearer articulation of how, when, and why theatre works and for more understanding and insights into ways forward. We all want to deepen and sustain the influence for positive change that theatre can have on participants and our communities.

While informal and anecdotal evaluations have been conducted, we need empirical and research-based information to back up our beliefs and to improve upon an already successful project.

—*Mieko Ouchi, artistic co-director, Concrete Theatre, quoted in* SSHRC CURA *research proposal, "Are We There Yet? Using Theatre in Teen Sexuality Education"*

Extant literatures on theatre and transformation, popular theatre, theatre and education, and theatre for development include a wide variety of case studies, and these sometimes report on some level of evaluation and analysis. Most of these are focused on one-off projects.[1] If we are to satisfy ourselves, our partners, and funders, and build the field's impact, there is a need to move beyond short-term, funding-related, and too often simplistic evaluation approaches and toward a deeper understanding of what is going on when communities participate at varying levels in theatre. There is a need to look at theatre's effects more broadly and to build a case for how and why theatre has an important role to play in creating change. It is a strong tool, as it reaches people holistically. It synthesizes issues, facts, information, and analysis with individuals' and communities' lives. But does it work? How? When? For what aspects of movements for change? The field needs these answers so that using theatre is most strategic. Michael Etherton and Tim Prentki (2006) see some unity in the group of players that do this work, and they challenge the field to extend its goals:

Common denominators have emerged. Perhaps the clearest of these has been the shared experience of the size of the gap between project evaluation, proving what was claimed to be done was actually done, and real impact in terms of changes of attitudes and transformed lives. But severally and collectively it is still not proven that applied theatre can today work towards those more substantial changes that many of its practitioners seek to make. (154)

While there is an increasing body of discursive consideration of this branch of theatre,[2] few are making much headway with this specific and tricky problem: Does it actually work? How? How not? How do we know?

The literature that assesses the more general fields of drama and theatre problematizes attempts at assessment and evaluation of theatre's impact. Theories of audience response, performance, and cultural studies are widely used to discuss and dismantle absolutes. Discussions that interrogate theatre of provocation, a kind of theatre that approaches aspects of the activist theatre discussed in this book, absorb some of these theoretic approaches and offer useful insights into the limitations of establishing a fixed view of theatre's impact.[3] Eschewing social science-based approaches, some argue that quantitative and many qualitative approaches to this problem are misguided, that only analysis through performance theories and cultural studies can adequately get at the complexity of what goes on in theatre and drama processes.

Those who argue the need to demonstrate impact more systematically and concretely than do postcolonial or philosophic discourses also point to the inadequacies of all of our tools. Nevertheless, there is a need to discover how to move on from these important insights about assessment limitations, not only for serving the funding systems' and arts-in-development's cyclical need for demonstrating impact but also for growth in the quality and depth of the practice of theatre for education and development. Thin evaluation tools and methods can lead to thin theatre. The theatre for social action field needs to better articulate and share expertise, not from a recipe book perspective, but from an understanding of foundations that are inherent to ensuring theatre's impact. This articulation will build theatre's success in contributing to deep education and change.

Answers may lie in a more interdisciplinary investigation than is often possible, using and integrating a wider variety of critical tools. The conditions of the Are We There Yet? research project led to significant opportunities to grapple with these matters, to respond to practitioners' interests in proving the value of their work, as well as to open up further questions. The extended term of this research project, its interdisciplinary academic team, and the partnership with many theatre artists and health educators from varying cultural centres created excellent conditions. What are the tools needed to conceptualize, unpack, and assess this kind of theatre? This project employed the tactic of comparing, integrating, and synthesizing a variety of disciplinary methodologies and perspectives. Beyond the case study on *Are We There Yet?*, this research program offered an opportunity to work on and develop a conceptual framework that could be useful to all stakeholders.

Over the course of the research program, researchers and practitioners moved beyond the initial thinking. We had proposed that university-based social science could develop appropriate methods and assess community-based projects that use theatre as a tool for change. We had suggested that this interdisciplinary alliance could improve overly simplistic quantitative approaches that are often employed in theatre project assessment and shift the theatre for change field from a largely anecdotal expression of theatre's impact. Insights, progress, and innovation were created by the social scientists' quantitative and qualitative approaches, and some of these are reported on in following chapters. However, over time we realized we had other powerful potentials latent in this five-year research opportunity. As we struggled with translation and mutual knowledge and acceptance across sectoral (community/university, artist/social scientist, and theatre/health) and disciplinary (social science/expressive arts) divides, we came to believe that greater insight lay in interaction and intersection. In many ways, the project became one of finding intersections that could challenge and lead to deeper interactions. Theatre theory, theatre processes, sexual health education practice, teen participants' experience, and actors' and stage managers' observation of audiences and the stories that emerge from many weeks of performances and workshops in many situations needed validation, not substitution.

Working the "inter" in interdisciplinary research and the "co" in co-researchers is where rich and layered understandings lie. As with pursuing transformative theatre's goals (social justice, equality), in this kind of research the most powerful answers lie in hearing every voice, every perspective, and not privileging one over others.

I think, as you go on through the run or through the years, if you do this a few times, when you start to see the kids more and more, it changes how you react to them, and how you see them. You come in and you could see someone with their arms crossed, looking down at the floor the entire time, and you can just assume that they're not getting anything from it. You can even try to engage them at times and say, "What do you think?" And they could possibly not say a word to you or maybe mumble something under their breath and you think, "Oh, I didn't reach that youth at all and oh, that's too bad," but then perhaps afterwards they'll be the one that comes up to you and says that was a really good show. Or possibly tell you something about themselves 'cause that could be an indication that they're going through something. So I think it's just really important to always keep trying to reach those the youth that you think, "Oh, they're not into it so I'm just gonna leave them alone," but I think it's important that you learn how to read them and learn how much they can handle, like if they don't want to talk, that's fine, but, you know, even eye contact is good. If they need to be left alone, fine but I think as you go throughout the years, you really learn how to reach your audience and to not assume that they're not getting anything out of it.

—*Kristi Hansen,* AWTY *actor,*
Concrete Theatre, August 25, 2010

Rather than being relegated to a position of mere anecdotes, these kinds of insights into how the piece (and pieces like AWTY) works for varying kinds of audience members must be absorbed into more formal analysis of how and whether and for whom the project has impact. While quick answers, encased in statistics, may be attractive to end users, a complex, hybrid approach to assessment and evaluation teaches us more. Quantitative assessment (based in tested, content-based instruments, learning theory, family studies, and demographic considerations) and formal qualitative investigations (based in current sexuality education theory) can intersect with stories and observations to provide richer analysis and insights.

The following chapters draw on some of the ways this research-educator-artist team integrated approaches and came to deeper and more nuanced understandings of the work we do and the impact we seek. Social science-based quantitative and qualitative assessments delve deeper when infused with theatre theories of engagement and distancing, as well as with understandings of the tools actors use to dig deeper during participatory parts of the play. Research based in theatrical criticism is enhanced by insights gleaned from various approaches to quantitative analysis. The importance and goals of participatory research are situated within the spectrum of essential tools for creating, adapting, and assessing theatre for change. The immeasurable powers of theatre can start to be captured in linking formalized interviews and questionnaires with insights into a particular audience's culture and traditional ways of learning and knowing. This section delineates some of these insights, methods, and findings.

> *I can see when they're resisting, I can see when they want to be rebellious. I can see when we win them over. I can see when they're having fun and they're listening. I have to work to be on their side and I think it happens in this show.*
>
> —*Evelyn Chu,* AWTY *actor,*
> *Neworld Theatre*

> *Before I was scared to just say what I was feeling...but the play really helped you to understand that...it is okay if you're not feeling the same as the other person or it is okay if you're at a different level and it is okay to tell other people your feelings...I think a lot of people are scared to actually say what they're thinking or show who they really are. And it's such a relief to people, like when you're like, oh wow, that's a really big burden off my back because now I know that I'm not the only one thinking it and I'm not the only one with these feelings.*
>
> *—Audience member, Nova Scotia*

NOTES

1. Notable exceptions are Dalrymple's (2006) discussion in "Has it Made a Difference? Understanding and Measuring the Impact of Applied Theatre with Young People in the South African Context" and Ross Kidd's (1983b, 1984) evolving analysis of puppet-based adult education work in Botswana. This work, called *Laedza Batanani*, as well as Kidd's assessment and critiques of varying forms of popular theatre practice worldwide both promoted and challenged the field to be more self-critical and accountable. See also Kidd and Byram (1983).
2. See the Bibliography for a variety of recent and useful books that add to our understanding of the range and approaches to community-based theatre and theatre for change.
3. See, for example, Piet Defraeye's insightful article, "The Romans in Britain and the Effect of Male/Male Sexual Iconography at London's National Theatre" (1999).

8

BRIDGE CONSTRUCTION—SLOW AHEAD

Creating a Play from Community Research

CONTENTS

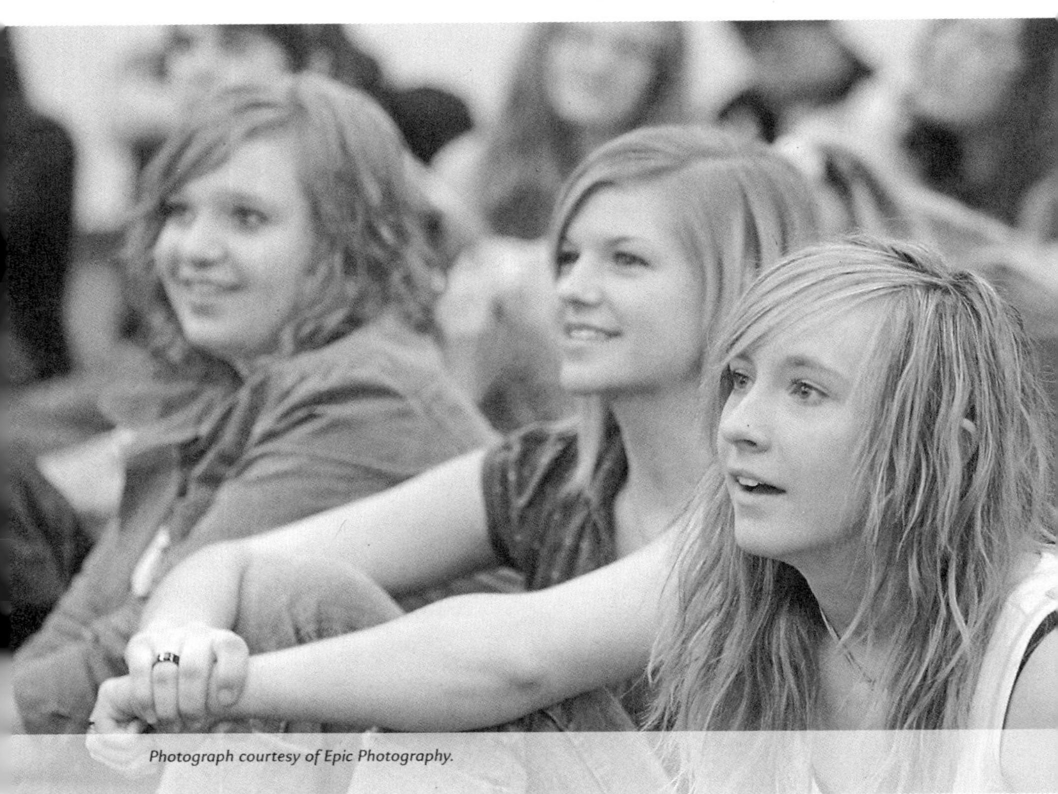

Photograph courtesy of Epic Photography.

Playwright Jane Heather discusses research processes and ethics involved in creating plays for and with communities.

> *The play sorta gave me the chance to have fun with sex, like, enjoy talking about it. It's, like, so serious in sex education and you're, like, okay AIDS, STD, crabs, okay, we know this stuff. Go away, please. It's, like, now you can have fun with it, you can ask the questions that you're not really sure to ask in sex ed. The play gave you a chance to shout out.*
>
> —AUDIENCE MEMBER

ARE WE THERE YET? IS A PLAY WRITTEN from community research. The development of the play, the choices of scenes, characters, participatory forms and style were informed by participatory research with teens. The research was gathered over time and in many different ways. The nature and intention of this kind of work and this play dictates that the audience/community be deeply involved in all the choices the playwright (and other artists) make. Some of the intentions of the play, as determined by Options, Concrete Theatre, and myself, as the playwright, were to engage youth in a conversation about how to make healthier sexual choices and to ensure that the expertise teens have about themselves and their world was acknowledged and incorporated into the play. The choice to use participatory theatre comes out of these intentions and is the foundation of all the other choices in the play. To write a play that intends to develop the trust and truth required to have deep, reciprocal interactions with audiences, community research is mandatory.

In 1997, when I first began to work on the play, sex ed in schools was much as it had been when I was an adolescent, but the world had changed considerably. At that time, HIV was not a chronic condition containable by drugs; it was a killer. No longer confined to specific groups, HIV was everybody's infection. AZT and the cocktail were promising but there was still a lot we didn't know. Internet porn and date rape, although not necessarily connected, were ubiquitous. It was a postfeminist world and women rejected sexual exploitation by others, empowered themselves and took over their own exploitation. It seemed the progress that we had made in the 1970s around gender and sexuality had failed, that adults were responsible for that failure, and the least we could do was improve the sex ed youth gets in school. The topic was urgent and the age group, never boring. Going into rooms to research sexuality with teens isn't everyone's idea of fun but it is surely one of mine.

Options had already done a lot of research with teens. The organization had developed a sexuality workshop for junior high school settings and was occasionally invited into schools to give this workshop for students. To create a play that would mesh with the workshop, and to begin thinking about how the workshop could incorporate and complement the play, several artists from Concrete Theatre and I participated in the Options teen workshop. One of the things that particularly struck me was the Drawing the Line exercise (described in Chapter 6 and as it appears in the play in Chapter 3, page 75). I loved the private, visual image each student could use to decide where to draw his or her line. It was so simple but also non-prescriptive, it acknowledged a wide range of sexual activity in a non-judgemental way, it could include any sexual activity, from making eye contact to full intercourse. Another function of the exercise was to cool down sex and begin to ask youth to consider sex as a choice not just a sensation or experience. Because the exercise is private and individual, it gave agency to each person to explore what he or she felt about each activity. It invited each one to think about what he or she really wanted and reinforced the personal choice aspect of sexuality. Knowing your personal boundaries may seem to be a natural and obvious part of being a human. However, it would be an error to assume youth, or even some adults, have considered this before. Moreover, the exercise places responsibility for determining one's sexual boundaries in the hands of the person engaging in the sexual activity. Parents, religious authorities and texts, the state, and other adults have tried to regulate sexual activity by fiat, across time and cultures, with limited success. The cognitive act of examining and choosing a personal boundary is a step toward making healthier sexual choices, in part because the idea of choice is introduced and reinforced. This was powerfully articulated by a male teen audience member in Saskatchewan:

> *The play helped me, umm...think more about if I want to have sex or not. Like, I already did have sex a couple of times but it was kind of not a specific decision but now I'm thinking if I should have or not.*

So, as I considered what the workshop could do and what the play could do, it seemed to me that because one's personal boundary often changes, that was a good reason to do it both in the play and the workshop. It then became clear that setting the line was the private, cognitive setup, and what the play could do is take the next step, helping teens to be able to communicate their decision to a partner. The play could move from the cognitive and safe (what workshops can do well) to the emotional and risky (what plays can do well). The Delphi and Marcel scene (Chapter 3, page 72) includes both of these stages. The characters get in communication trouble and an instructor intervenes; they draw the line for themselves and then communicate it to each other. This produces another obstacle that the characters need help to work through: their personal boundaries are in different places on the continuum. When the audience attends the workshop (usually about a week after the performance) the educator repeats the exercise, refers to the scene in the play, and expands the discussion. (See Chapter 6 for a full description of the teen workshop.)

Another part of the workshop is anonymous questions. At the end of the workshop the educator invites all students to write a question they have about sex on a small slip of paper. Everyone is encouraged to write something, even if they don't have a question. Students can write a comment about the show or the workshop, even a simple "hi" or drawing is encouraged. This helps the ones with real and urgent questions to not feel singled out or obvious. (See Appendix 2.3 for a sample of anonymous questions.) While researching the play, I read many of these questions and incorporated the most common ones into the play. Each time the play is rehearsed, actors also read comments that educators have collected from teens during workshops to learn about their audiences. There are thousands and thousands of them, more produced each tour, and they are a remarkably clear, intimate, and safe way for teens to speak and for theatre workers to find out what teens are thinking and what they want to know. The questions and comments teens make are also incredibly revealing about what they don't know, what they worry about, and what they find puzzling, or odd, or hilarious, about sex. Reading anonymous questions was an early form of community research for this play.

Options also made available to me as part of the research some anonymous survey work with teens, which asked them to identify questions they had about condoms. The survey, not very big or formal, indicated that young people most wanted to know how to raise condom use with a partner. This research also became part of the play. I also read reports about teens and sexuality produced by various provincial and federal bodies. Each of these research activities helped me build the dense, intimate knowledge of the audience required for participatory theatre.

Because of extensive previous work with this age group, I knew the play had to be engaging, entertaining, daring, honest, challenging, and, most of all, funny. In other words, my intention was to write a good play. To do that, talking to knowledgeable adults, reading reports and anonymous questions was invaluable, but I needed to talk to teens, lots of teens, and for that I turned to participatory research.

I first became aware of this kind of research and its application to theatre in the 1970s. At that time, creating plays collectively, based on interviews with community members, was a popular technique for theatre companies across the country. Early examples of plays created by this kind of research include *The Farm Show* (Theatre Passe Muraille, 1972) and *Two Miles Off* (Theatre Network, 1975). In most cases, a company of actors lived for a period of time in a community, established relationships with community members, and collectively created a play with the stories they discovered. In some cases, the resulting play was a verbatim piece; in others, stories and characters were blended together, text was imagined or some was verbatim and some not. Some of this work was broadly or specifically political, some claimed to have no particular political intentions. Politics, overt or otherwise, were always a factor in decisions such as where the theatre company located its project and what was revealed or discarded in the final script.

Participatory research with the community using theatre processes (and other techniques such as focus groups) is, in my opinion, the research that tells you what of all other research is valuable. Although I began writing AWTY in 1997, I began the participatory community research many years before. All of the plays I have written or co-created with other performer/creators were built from community research. I learned how to write participatory theatre first by being an actor doing participation and making a lot of mistakes. AWTY contains an accumulation of ideas, stories, participatory experiences, work with many teens on many topics, work with many artists, and a great deal of participatory community research. It took many years to get to AWTY These are some of the plays I wrote and experiences I had that impacted the writing of the play.

Stand up for Your Rights

Stand up for Your Rights was a participatory play for and with adults with mental disabilities. As a performer/creator, I researched to discover what issues were important to this community and to find a character. During one research session, I met with a woman with mental impairments in her apartment to interview her and get an idea of her life and world. She was incredibly energetic and full of joy but difficult to understand. Part way into the interview she pulled out a *Playgirl* magazine full of pictures of hunky men in provocative poses. She pointed out her favourites and laughed and laughed. I learned what is now obvious: you can't tell by looking if someone is interested in sex, and it's funny to everybody.

High Stakes

I was commissioned by the Alberta Alcohol and Drug Abuse Commission (AADAC) to write a play for and with high school students about risk, with a focus on HIV prevention. I travelled to a small, northern town every few weeks to work with teens in school. I did focus groups, interviews, and many drama sessions. The group I worked with role-played, improvised, and created images and sculptures that I used as the foundation of the play. One young woman was pregnant but staying in school, despite the censure she felt from some of her classmates and the mean gossip she endured. There was a lot of fear there and both underground and blatant homophobia coming from some of the students, the boys particularly. In an early improvisation, one boy spoke what many felt: "Fags deserve to die of AIDS." The young, pregnant woman said what became one of the key lines of the play: "I don't think people deserve to die just because they weren't careful about sex." Everyone looked at her belly and the wind shifted.

A group of teens from the school that had been involved in the creation of the play subsequently performed it for their classmates. The performance showed me some of the problems with this configuration. They were not equipped to deal with the material; the sexuality was too much for them, as was the topic of HIV/AIDS. In their school, in front of their peers, the risk of exposure was overwhelming. Everyone in the audience knew them, and although they did their very best, they had to stand away from the material. Too many people in the audience could only see them, not their characters, and the performers' level of anxiety prevented them from committing to what they were doing or saying. I saw a group of courageous, frightened teens, praying to get off the stage as soon as possible. I had written the play to be participatory, and again the students did not have the maturity or the skill to pull it off.

Teens can and do create and perform plays about healthy sexual decision making. Insight Theatre in Ottawa is a Planned Parenthood program that has been operating for twenty-six years and is very successful. The work is sketch comedy, fast, funny, and informative. Both performers and audience seem to enjoy themselves very much, and this work is to be commended. In this case, older teens create theatre for younger teens. That bit of distance seems to work very well and might have solved some of the problems with *High Stakes*. Participation is another matter, however.

Talk is Cheap and *Rap it Up*

These two plays, also participatory, were about teen–parent communication. To research the plays, I did workshops with groups of young people in urban areas and travelled around to a number of small rural communities. I had asked for teens but, as is common, the teens were a little too cool to come, and I often got rambunctious groups of ten to thirteen year olds. The topic was the difficulties teens and parents have communicating with each other, and I was looking for the stories and the issues. In most cases, they identified overscheduling, money, school, household chores, hair, curfews, and the like as contentious issues between them and their parents. We laughed a lot and jumped around, being goofy. In one town, as I neared the end of the workshop I asked (as usual) what were the most difficult subjects, the hardest things, for teens and their parents to talk about. One very young person told a story, in a small and hesitant way, about finding out his uncle had died. He wished that his parents had told him and grieved that they hid this, and the funeral, from him. Everyone knew we were getting down to the ground here, to the bones, and a dignified hush full of yearning fell on us all. In the quiet, another little voice said, "And sex, it's hard to talk about sex." So sex and death, things that young people wanted to talk about but felt unable to discuss with parents. The story about the uncle became an important scene in the play.

I could not have conjured this in my own brain and imagination. I could only set the conditions where the story could be told and heard. I'm always seeking this moment in the research, listening for the inhale that signals the exhale that will open up territory unknown to me. I follow the path marked by great listeners such as Studs Terkel and Anna Deavere Smith. Deavere Smith's book *Talk to Me: Listening Between the Lines* (2000), describes this moment: "Over time I would learn to listen for those wonderful moments when people speak a kind of personal music" (36).

Wabasca Native Youth Theatre

I worked with several groups of Aboriginal teens in a remote northern community, facilitating several projects created and performed by the teens about their concerns. I lived and worked in this community periodically for three years. For the first two years, I was part of a team of theatre workers, Aboriginal and non-Aboriginal. The youth created and performed stories from their lives and lives of people in their communities. I was not the playwright but I facilitated and shaped their words and scenes. Each time I returned I re-established old relationships and built new ones. Many of the youth I worked with came back again and again to do more drama. They often visited me at my home when they came to the city. I got to know parents, siblings, aunties, teachers, social service workers, elders, the waitress at the café. And they of course got to know me. Many of those youth (now in their forties) are still part of my life, and I have continued to do theatre projects with two of them. It is rare to be given an opportunity to work over such a long period of time in a community not your own. I learned countless things, everyday, many of which I cannot name. I only know that when I went to Saskatchewan to work with SNTC, I could access a language, a way of being, a kind of humour, and a sense of spoken/not spoken that I learned in Wabasca. This is not to say all Aboriginal people are alike, but that if you are Cree from northern Saskatchewan, you share some things with the Cree from northern Alberta.

> *When you leave that house of what is familiar to you—your family, your race, your social class, your nation, your professional area of expertise...you will end up standing someplace in the road...On the one hand, they are not comfortable places; on the other hand, in them one acquires the freedom to move...In my work I have moved across many cultural boundaries...I've developed a lot of stamina for being where I don't "belong."* (Deavere Smith 2000, 24)

The theatre work I did and the ways that I was gradually invited into people's lives cannot be transferred from one community to another, even if they are similar. One's history is never evident on the outside, but you never start exactly from zero again. Perhaps the most important thing that I was able to take from the Wabasca projects to working with the Aboriginal community in Saskatchewan was a reduction in the paralyzing anxiety that plagues well-intentioned white people. What if I inadvertently insult someone? What do people want to be called? The world seems filled with invisible and unknowable potential gaffes and disasters. This feeling diminishes over time, thankfully; my errors were pointed out to me and I learned. This process is ongoing in my life, and I hope I continue to have opportunities to learn.

Appropriation of Voice

I think it would be reasonable to say that no one ever writes a play without researching. Even if the research is into their own memory and the hidden pathways of their heart, the process of creating a play requires interrogation, ordering, and making choices about what to emphasize and what to leave buried. If a playwright chooses to step away from their own lived experience, the research they do into how others live, think, talk, and what actions they take requires at least curiosity about others and perhaps some specific kinds of reading and conversations. The further the playwright steps outside his or her own skull, the more research is required. Playwrights who go into the lives and actions of those completely outside their own experience can flounder into deep water and drown.

There is a case to be made that there are experiences and situations that are universal and human, but a play (usually) requires someone to speak and embody a character, so some things cannot be disguised as they might be in a novel. The author of a novel can remain somewhat hidden behind their book, (although currently, any reader who is curious can go to the Internet and find out if an author is writing from their own identity and culture). However, as novelists quickly point out, if they are only able to write their own culture, identity, and community, what a dull, narrow, airless form the novel would be. A novelist might also say they aren't trying to be someone they are not; they are trying to imagine someone they are not, and surely imagination is their job and their gift.

This becomes a more difficult problem in the theatre because of representation. Who can represent whom on stage is a complex question. Because an actor is already performing someone they are not, it is a short step to asserting that everybody can play everybody, women can play men, white/black, old/young, gay/straight, disabled/abled, and so on. However, the appropriation of voice in text becomes the appropriation of body, culture, history, and memory as well in the theatre. In a novel, the character is imaginary. On stage, the character may be imaginary but the person, the actor, is real. Things can get ugly, awkward, and it turns out not everybody can play everybody in all cases.

Can a playwright write anybody? Well sure, there's no law against it but if you want, as a playwright, to tell stories and create characters from and with a community not your own, and have that community recognize their own voice, stories, and truth (or some of it), if you want shared ownership, you have to work on inhabiting other people's reality.

David Foster Wallace, in a commencement address at Kenyon College in 2005, spoke about truth and freedom as being rooted in our efforts to get out of our own lonely, self-referential skulls. We need, he stated, to force ourselves to consider other people's reality and to use our educated brains to disrupt our "automatic, unconscious belief that I am the centre of the world, and that my immediate needs and feelings are what should determine the world's priorities" (2008, 14). Not because it is moral or nicer but because it is the true freedom:

> *The kind [of freedom] that is most precious you will not hear much talk about in the great outside world of wanting and achieving...The really important kind of freedom involves attention and awareness and discipline, and being able truly to care about other people and to sacrifice for them over and over in myriad petty, unsexy ways every day. (Wallace 2008, 14)*

This is hard, Wallace reminds us, "because the so-called real world of men and money and power hums merrily along in a pool of fear and anger and frustration and craving and worship of self. Our own present culture has harnessed these forces in ways that have yielded extraordinary wealth and comfort and personal freedom" (14). In this case, Wallace is speaking to university graduates in America, perhaps some of the most privileged people in the world. Recognizing how difficult it is to challenge our present culture and what it has created, Wallace calls on the students at the commencement, and all of us, to stay conscious and alive to something other than ourselves, to pay attention. I cannot claim any extraordinary skill in this endeavour. I too stew in my own ego juices, but I know that I need to try to get out of my own skull in order to do the work I want to do.

I know if I can pay attention even for a short time, people will tell me their reality and it will be different from mine. A play can then be written and performed that carries that reality back to the community and to others outside the community.

The playwright is compelled to cross the border to see another's reality and try with all her heart and mind to hear what she is listening to and see what she is watching. Some borders are much more difficult to cross than others and relative power is always a factor. Margaret Atwood, in her essay "Writing the Male Character," says that, because of the power imbalance between the genders, it is easier for women to write male characters than it is for men to write female characters. This is in part, she explains, because

> *Women...have a relatively large pool of experiences [with men] from which to draw... their own experiences with men, also their friends', since, yes, girls do discuss men*

> *more than men...discuss women...If men are going to talk about their problems with women to anybody it's usually...to another women...women are likely to know more about how men actually behave with women than men are.* (Atwood 1982, 424)

Women understand men in a way men do not understand women, partly Atwood suggests, "because it was necessary for survival. If the other fellow has the heavy artillery, it is best to be able to anticipate his probable moves" (429). Those with less power, be it social, economic, historical, or political, closely study those with power over them, in order to stay alive.

Most theatre for change (including my own) begins with entering a community as a representative of the powerful. Often, the community researcher/play maker, by his or her race, age, gender, class, education, health, or other status marker, has the heavy artillery and has not been forced to study the other in order to survive. Perhaps that is changing, and the survival of the human race will turn on our ability to learn from marginalized people, but generally, the survival of the powerful has entailed ignoring, vilifying, and silencing those on the other side of the wall. Those who cross the border or jump the wall (and there are many) do so as an act of will, a choice that rejects the current structures of power as a system that threatens everyone's survival. Individual and global self-interest play a part in taking on this work, as do guilt, curiosity, and other more venal desires. Encumbered with history and unearned privilege, projecting the shape of an abhorrent system, the playwright staggers into someone else's community, culture, and world asking for something. Trust me, talk to me, for one is virtually impossible without the other. That community researchers and community members do come to trust one another and talk to one another is remarkable. The power imbalance, historical and contemporary, never goes away but some things can, if not erase the barriers, at least allow for some trust and some exchange to occur. Time to listen, honouring difference, and looking for things in common, genuine curiosity, complete transparency in the process, and in the plans for the research, can help to go beyond tourism, appropriation, and re-colonization and move toward a reciprocal alliance.

Participatory, community-based research and theatre for change is always welded to reciprocity. While researching, the researcher is also being researched. Sooner or later, usually sooner, people can see who you are. The

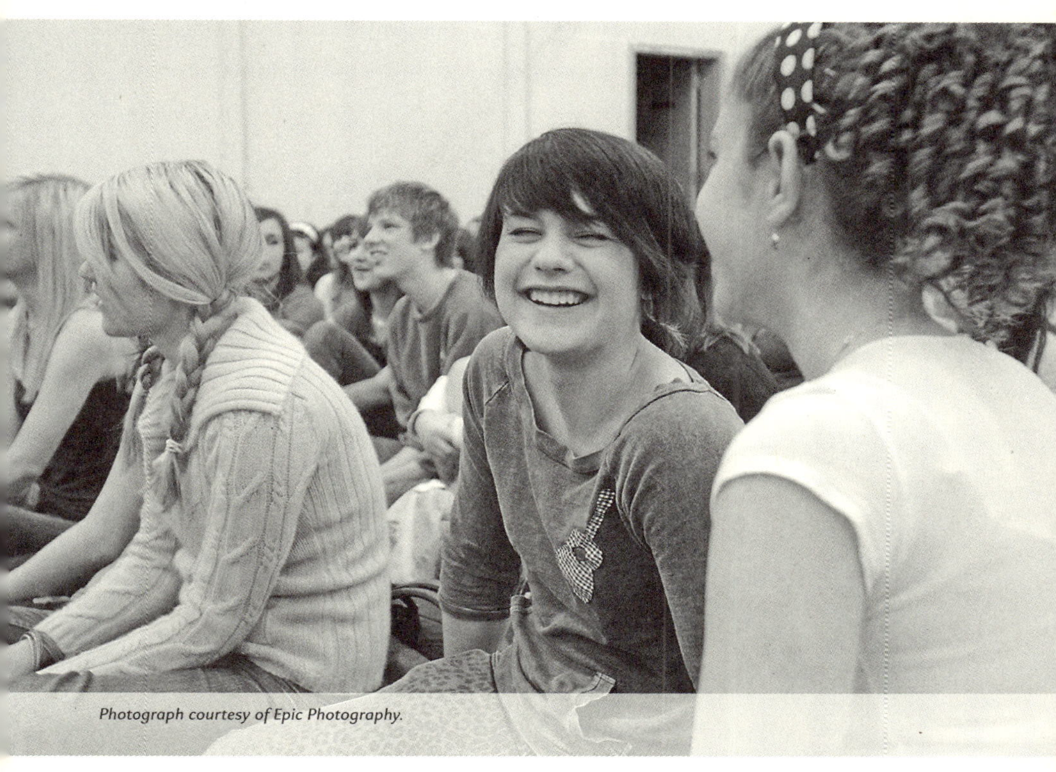
Photograph courtesy of Epic Photography.

biggest error would be to imagine that the researcher is hidden, a neutral receptacle for a story or a gesture or an exchange between participants. You are seen; all public behaviour is measured as your request to be trusted with stories is considered. People are really smart; they are very astute and attuned to your intentions. Waste no time performing, they can see who you are.

Once you have passed inspection, the hard part begins, the listening. One's assumptions and prejudices surface in alarming and unexpected ways. As the naïf, you can and will be played. You may not hear what you expect, you may not hear what you want to hear, and you listen to what is not being said as hard as to what is. You may never understand a lot of what you hear and see. As you ask a community to see you, not the privilege you carry around, they ask you to see them, not whatever cliché of oppressed people you might have in your head. And because no race, class, gender, age, sexual orientation, or other group has a monopoly on mendacity or honour, you will begin be able to sort the creators from the destroyers. Often this is common knowledge and when you begin to see what others in the community know, a deeper level of trust and talking ensues. There is reciprocity in more complex seeing and knowing. Most of who you are is seen by community members through what you do, during the research and with the research.

All of the theatre projects described here (and many others of this kind of theatre) built community involvement and reciprocity throughout the entire process of research, creation, and performance. As with social science research with human subjects, the intention of the research, the writing and consultation process, and the disposition of the research are carefully explained and informed consent is sought. Open rehearsals are held, and community members, especially those who have shared a story, are invited to contribute to a play in process. Scenes are tested with groups and/or individuals. Comments, complaints, and suggestions are solicited. The research continues throughout the creation and production process. No community is homogeneous and it is not possible to represent all community views of an issue in one play. One play can, however, spark fruitful debate about a contentious issue, or identify an omission or misrepresentation. Out of that discussion, another play that corrects or adds to how a community is represented, or how an issue is examined, could be created.

The processes, contradictions, conundrums described here come from the experience of having written many plays created from community research. I have entered communities as an outsider and conducted drama workshops, interviews, focus groups, and story circles with groups of teens, prison inmates, women survivors of domestic violence, Aboriginal women, union members and the labour movement, Black women, seniors, and urban homeless people. I have also performed a person with mental disabilities to rooms full of persons with mental disabilities. In some cases, the community is close to my own lived experiences (I was once an adolescent) but in most cases I am writing and creating a voice not my own. The prohibition against appropriation of voice is correct, and I would not attempt to claim that it is ever possible to have a relationship that is free from exploitation, or the possibility of appropriation of voice. Even with every possible ethical provision in place, a research process and researchers can make mistakes. I think it is possible, however, to move from a way of working that seems, to the community, like the most obscene and exploitative resource extraction for the benefit of the extractor, toward something that is more like a collective work bee to dismantle the Master's house.[1]

There are, as well, some advantages to being an outsider. Outsiders can talk about things that are too delicate for anyone in the community to name. In some cases, the community is grateful that the sore spot was touched or exposed and even more grateful that it wasn't them that had to do it. My co-playwright, Kenneth T. Williams, commented on this phenomena when reflecting on the Aboriginal adaptation process in northern Saskatchewan:

> *Yes, it is true, voices and stories have been stolen and we must be careful not to do that. But there is advantage to being an outsider, many times people cannot tell their stories, their secrets, what's truly in their heart to someone within the community and an outsider provides a safe way to reveal, get it off their chest or express a deep dark secret. The problem with a small, well-connected community is everyone knows your business and you're less likely to expose yourself, even to a professional, if you know you're going to see them in the coffee shop, the bingo hall, or the hallway of the school. Last thing you want is for people to know you're talking to a professional. An outsider is sometimes the safest option for revealing.*

Insider, outsider, or other, when someone tells you their story they place a precious gift in your hands. How you listen, the time that is spent, the process, and what is done with the story will determine, to a large extent, how a person or people in the community feel about the work and the possibility that the work can be part of making positive change.

> *I wanted to get people to talk to me, in a true way. Not true in the sense of spilling their guts. Not true in the sense of the difference between truth and lies. I wanted to hear—well—authentic speech, speech that you could dance to, speech that had the possibility of breaking through the walls of the listener, speech that could get to your heart and beyond someplace else in your consciousness.* (Deavere Smith 2000, 51)

NOTE

1. Audre Lorde (1984) taught that it is not possible to dismantle the Master's house using the Master's tools, but these tools (theatre) never belonged to any master, so we can steal or borrow them or build our own and use them for our own purposes.

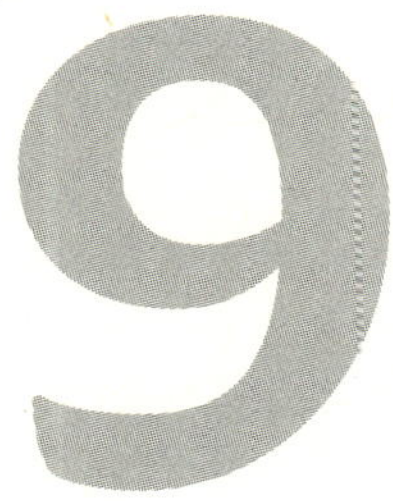

CONSUMER REPORT

Yes, But Does it Work? Program Assessment

Shaniff Esmail, Brenda Munro, and James McKinnon

CONTENTS

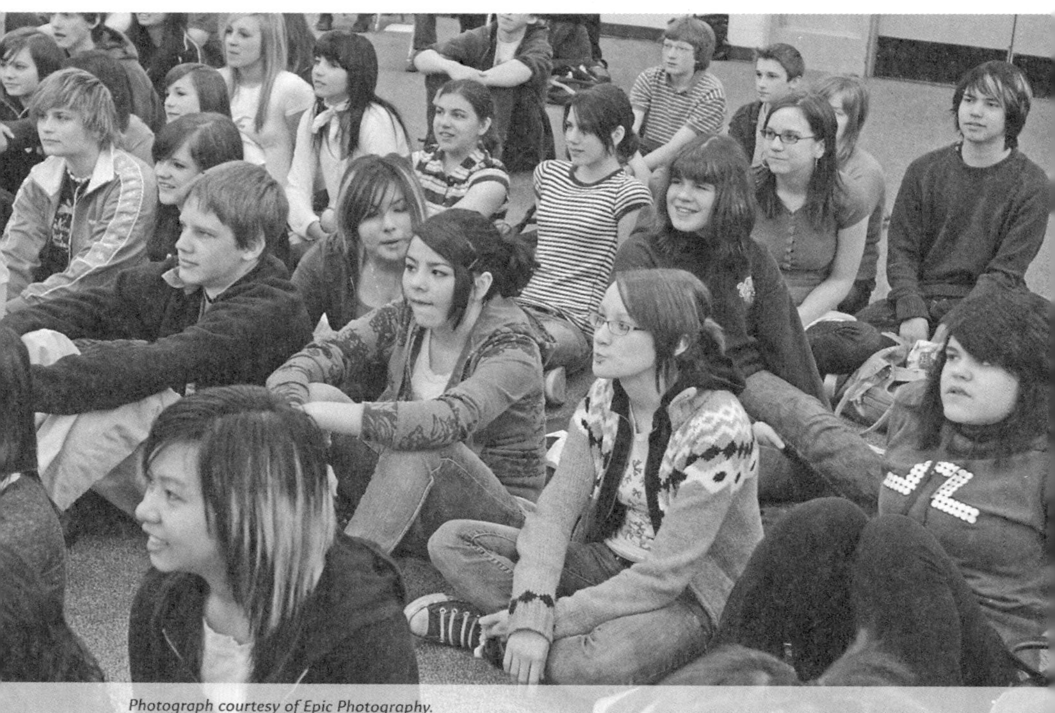
Photograph courtesy of Epic Photography.

Are We There Yet? was the subject of an extensive research and evaluation project. While there is a lot to report, this chapter provides a summary of the most significant findings from the quantitative and qualitative evaluation research and suggests implications for sexual health education.

> *[Health region administration] value the research. For public health, the evidence-based research is huge; the research component connected with this and the fact that it was an external research assessment, separate from who's doing the play. Then the research speaks for the project and theatre as a medium to do other kinds of education.*
>
> —LEONA PURCELL, PUBLIC HEALTH NURSE AND CO-ORDINATOR, GUYSBOROUGH YOUTH HEALTH AND SERVICES CENTRE, GUYSBOROUGH, NOVA SCOTIA

Why Do Research?

SEXUAL HEALTH EDUCATION STILL VARIES tremendously throughout the world, but generally speaking it has come a long way in the past four decades, shifting from a focus on abstinence and moral absolutist principles (McKay, Pietrusiak, and Holowaty 1998) to more comprehensive approaches that emphasize sex-positive messages and the importance of deliberate and informed decision making (Finklea, Gruendemann, and Harris 2004).[1] This growth reflects a desire to improve efficacy; new programming seeks to succeed where old ideas failed to bring about desired changes in unsafe sexual behaviour, STI transmission rates, and teen pregnancy rates. While this growth in programming is driven by concerns about efficacy, that efficacy remains difficult to measure: sexuality education is still difficult to research due to the sensitivity of the topic and the potential physical or psychological risk to the vulnerable populations involved. Talking about sex, which may include talking about sexuality, abuse, relationship, and/or family breakdown, can raise extreme emotions, provoke feelings of dread or fear, increase awareness and impact of violence, reveal or cause stigmatization, expose illegal behaviour, and result in controversy and/or conflict (McCosker, Barnard, and Gerber 2001). However, this range of risks and traumatic experiences associated with adolescent sexual behaviour only accentuates the importance of evaluating sexuality education, an effort that depends on the cooperation of many stakeholders.

Our study sought to measure both the extent to which the program brings about the targeted behavioural changes in its participants and the extent to which those results are tied to the unique form of the program: participatory theatre. Therefore, in addition to assessing degrees of change in the participants, we investigated how teen audiences experienced the program as theatre, measuring levels of enjoyment, involvement, and participation. This approach allowed us to evaluate the efficacy of the Are We There Yet? Program in particular while working toward insights about the efficacy of theatre-based sexuality education in general.

What Type of Research Was Done?

This research deployed both quantitative and qualitative methods. Using multiple methods allowed us both to quantify the general impact of the play on adolescents and to understand and describe unique experiences of individual spectators. We were able to look at how the play impacts a general population, how it works differently with three different identity styles within that population, and how it is experienced by individuals.

Quantitative Research

Quantitative research allows us to make general observations about the program and its efficacy, to measure the statistical significance of pre- and post-treatment changes, and to quantify objectively the impact of the AWTY Program. It also allows us to isolate important correlations between different variables so that we can ask whether the impact of the program is affected by a participant's gender, ethnic background, identity style, etc. The advantage of quantitative research is that a larger sample of students can be gathered, which allowed us to generalize findings to those who experienced the AWTY Program. However, quantitative data does not offer detailed insight into the participants' individual experiences or the range of experiences activated by the performance. Nor does it capture the unique and important consequences the program may have for individual participants—particularly given that the participatory, semi-improvised nature of *Are We There Yet?* means that every performance is different and that any spectator or audience can influence the tone and even the content of the show.

The quantitative evaluation for this study was designed to measure how participants' attitudes toward sexual decision making changed from pre- to post-treatment, and how AWTY affects different groups of students within the group as a whole. We also wanted to know how the program's efficacy is tied to its theatrical form and its participatory aspects. These objectives presented serious challenges. How would we distinguish groups of students within the general population? What kinds of questions would establish the participants' attitudes toward sexuality and sexual decision making, and how could we ensure that those questions matched the objectives of the play? As with all quantitative studies, we needed to be sure that our questions actually measured what we wanted to know and that they would produce reliable, consistent, valid results. This process forced us to think carefully about what AWTY actually tries to do. For example, since the play does not teach spectators how to use condoms, there was no point in asking the spectators whether they use condoms correctly or whether they learned such skills from the play. We needed to be sure that our questions reflected the play's true objectives, which are primarily communication and conflict-resolution skills.[2] In addition, we wanted to know how the program's theatrical form affects its effectiveness, which required us to develop a unique set of questions. Finally, we had to do all these things with maximum efficiency because we quickly discovered that students would become fatigued and frustrated by an overly long survey.

Developing the Quantitative Survey

A questionnaire was developed by an interdisciplinary team with backgrounds in sociology, family studies, occupational therapy, developmental psychology, and theatre. It requested participants' perceptions on topics previously identified in research on both theatre and adolescent sexuality. After it was pared down to suit this age group's attention span, the resulting survey took about twenty minutes to complete. It was administered both before and after a performance and workshop of AWTY at participants' schools.

The survey consists of several scales, that is, sets of questions (or items) that measure similar things. The scales address three broad categories, which are described in detail below. First, we wanted to know whether and to what extent AWTY is an effective sexuality education program, so we surveyed the students about their sexual communication skills before and after the program (and compared the pre- and post-treatment results to a control group that did not participate). We know that this age group includes some who are and are not sexually active, and we asked questions about sexual activity levels to assist researchers to determine whether the program assists both or only one of these groups in identifying and communicating sexual boundaries and making healthy decisions about sexual activity. Second, we wanted to know whether AWTY is more or less effective with certain kinds of adolescents, so we gathered data that would allow us to analyze the results based on gender, social or ethnic background, and in terms of three different categories of identity style orientations, as described below. Finally, in order to gain insight into how the program's efficacy is tied to its theatrical aspect, we asked questions about the specific effects of theatre.

Scales and Scale Development

Sexual Behaviours These questions assessed comfort in sexual communication and knowledge transfer of sexual health information. The AWTY Program emphasizes the importance of learning and practicing communication skills related to sexuality, so we wanted to know how participants performed these skills both before and after participating. In order to measure decision-making skills, we adapted the Mathtech questionnaire, a widely used inventory about adolescent sexuality, because its efficacy, reliability, and consistency have been well established in several studies (Kirby 1984; Kirby 1998; Mishel 1989). Kirby's Mathtech Adolescent Sexuality questionnaire has two objectives: first, to evaluate the most important knowledge areas, attitudes, values, skills, and behaviour that will either bring about a positive and fulfilling sexuality, or reduce unplanned pregnancy among adolescents; and second, to evaluate the effectiveness of sexuality education programs (Kirby 1984). Kirby's questionnaire consists of three separate inventories, which measure knowledge, attitudes and values, and behaviours. For the purposes of this research, which measures how theatre influences action, we used the sexual decision-making scale from the behaviour inventory, which assesses three aspects of behaviour: the skills one requires to perform the behaviour, one's comfort with performing it, and the frequency with which one performs that particular behaviour. This scale covers a range of behaviours, including frequency of sexual activities, numbers of partners, and contraceptive behaviours. Respondents use a Likert scale of 0 to 5 to indicate how often they perform the behaviour, ranging from 1 (almost never) to 5 (almost always), including a 0 item (corresponding to *does not apply*). We focused on learning about participants' awareness of and capacity to: (1) identify personal sexual boundaries, (2) communicate their sexual boundaries, (3) make decisions about sexual activity, and (4) identify the practice of safer sex.

We chose five outcome measures identified from previous research that matched the goals of the play (Kirby 1984). These measures included: (1) three items on general attitudes/beliefs about sexual relationships; (2) four items concerning embarrassment when talking about sexual issues; (3) four items pertaining to comfort in discussing sexual feelings; 4) five items on sexual self-efficacy (i.e., a sense of control or ability to manage sexual encounters); and (5) three items regarding an ability to identify and exercise sexual limits or boundaries. The outcome measures all exhibited adequate reliability.[3]

Identity Style and Attachment In addition to collecting basic demographic information (gender, age, sexual experience, etc.), we used questions about identity style (Serafini and Adams 2002) and attachment (West et al. 1998). The former enabled us to group the participants into three basic identity/decision-making styles—diffuse-avoidance, normative, and information-seeking—and determine whether different learning and decision-making styles lead to varying responses to the play and workshop. To measure identity style orientations, we selected items from previous work (Berzonsky 1989; Berzonsky and Sullivan 1992) to assess diffuse-avoidance, normative, and informational styles. All item responses were obtained using a 1 = "not at all like me" to 5 = "very much like me" Likert-type scale. The diffuse-avoidance orientation was measured by items reflecting uncertainty as to why the participant was in school, avoidance of worry about problems, and delay or procrastination in making self-relevant decisions. Normative identity style was assessed by items reflecting the adoption of parental values, behaviours that are expected by others, and a desire to know what is expected and to behave accordingly. Informational identity style was evaluated with items assessing the degree of information gathering before making a decision and time taken for thought and analysis about self-relevant choices.[4]

Measuring the Efficacy of Theatre Although there are many theories about how theatre affects spectators, we found no appropriate methods to measure spectators' responses to theatre. To this end, we drew on contemporary theatre theory to build our own scale composed of five subscales. Theatre-based variables were identified from a review of previous literature.[5] Subscales measured the degree to which the youth liked the play (i.e., pleasure, three items), identified with the play (three items), empathized with characters (three items), participated in the play (four items), and were impacted by the play (three items). We tested the questions for face validity by asking experts in this area to critique them, then administered them to 247 youth to test them for reliability, validity, and internal consistency. Both the scale and subscales proved to be extremely reliable, valid, and internally consistent.[6] These questions were included in the post-test questionnaire only.

Qualitative Research

Qualitative inquiry "explores the experiences of people in their everyday lives" (Mayan 2001, 5). Our goal was not only to quantify and measure the play's impact on the students but also to gather their perspective on what they got out of the play. By entering into a conversation with students, we wanted to gain insight into the personal impact the AWTY Program had on the participants, particularly in regards to their attitudes about sexual decision making.

While the stories told by individual participants cannot be generalized to the larger population, they give the researchers insight into the play's impact on individuals. Individual responses also tell us about possible consequences and outcomes of the program that cannot easily be predicted or measured by quantitative methods. For example, after watching the play, one grade nine student decided to end an abusive relationship, and another realized that she was a victim of sexual assault and she needed to go for help. These types of personal stories add to the richness of our evaluation. While no single response should be taken as a general summary of what the audience thought, taken together they suggest a continuum of possible responses to the show. Moreover, once we heard many unique stories, some similar themes started to emerge. These themes were like pieces of a puzzle that, when pieced together, gave the researchers insight into the impact of the play, and thus of the potential of participatory theatre as a medium for sexual health education. These themes, like the individual responses, revealed important insights that might not have been revealed by quantitative methods alone.

Gathering information about individual experiences is also important because the participatory nature of the program means that no two performances are the same: each audience influences the content, direction, emphasis, and overall atmosphere. In addition, each student operates from his or her own perspective and each constructs meaning from the event within his or her own unique framework.

> *[The play] made me realize that everybody is not in the same place, like everybody is at different levels...Like just because you're ready for something doesn't mean that someone else is.*
>
> —*Audience member*

> *Participation gives the kids a sense of ownership and it makes them proud that they can give their input and the fact that they did it in a group takes away some pressure because they don't have to be shy.*
>
> —*Teacher*

Each student has a highly personal experience of the program because no one reality exists for students when it comes to sexuality and sexual health education: some are sexually active, while others are still quite inexperienced. In addition, whereas questionnaires constructed by researchers inevitably reflect what researchers think is important, we wanted to hear the students' perspectives on what was notable or important about the experience. To this end, our interviews were semi-structured: rather than asking participants to answer our questions, we used open-ended probes that encouraged them discuss whatever they thought was important. Our goal as researchers was to remain objective in our qualitative data collection and to give the students an opportunity to tell their story as it related to the play.

The objectives of the qualitative component of the research project evolved over the course of five years. In year one, our goal was to understand and describe students' experiences of the AWTY Program; we used one-on-one, semi-structured interviews. In year two, the research focus shifted to understanding the play's impact on student's sexual decision making and behaviours. In addition to individual interviews, we also convened focus groups, in each case directing questions toward the students' perceived impact of the AWTY Program on their knowledge, skills, and behaviours. During year three, we replicated the qualitative component in Saskatchewan and Nova Scotia. In addition, based on the quantitative findings, we conducted focus groups with students who were separated based on identity styles. Year four of the project focused on adults, with interviews to gain their perspectives on the AWTY Program. Year five of the project aimed to assess the longitudinal impact of the AWTY Program, again using both interviews and focus groups, this time with students one-year post AWTY Program.

Semi-structured Interviews

The popularity of interviewing as a method of data collection for phenomenological studies has been increasing (Lowes and Prowse 2001). Students who indicated on their consent form that they would be willing to participate in interviews or focus groups were randomly selected, usually by the school contact. An in-depth semi-structured interview, approximately thirty to forty minutes in duration, was conducted with each student in a private space. Each one-on-one interview began with the investigator reviewing various components of the AWTY Program to help the students remember and focus on the play. Although interviews were framed with a series of probes, participants had opportunities to discuss other issues they felt were relevant. The primary goal of the interview was to give students an opportunity to share their stories through conversation. The role taken by the interviewer was both one of a traveller and one of a miner (Kvale 1996). The traveller may explore a specific site or just roam freely discovering new and unique information (Kvale 1996). The miner digs or probes at specific locations, using more focused questions related to the research objective, to unearth details and nuggets of essential meaning.

Qualitative Focus Groups

In addition to individual interviews, we conducted focus groups to elicit discussion and build on data collected in both the interviews and the quantitative surveys. We used results from the other components of the research to develop probes, discussion items, and activities for the focus group. Two trained project members conducted the focus groups, which lasted ninety minutes to two hours, in a private space within the participants' school. The focus group leaders encouraged relatively open discussion, using a semi-structured approach to address specific areas of skills, attitudes, and behavioural changes as they relate to sexual decision making, boundary setting, and their experience of the play. Because the focus groups dealt with sensitive issues, and because participants in this age group are highly adept at saying what they think adults want to hear, we took measures to ensure that participant comments and discussion reflected their experiences rather than an effort to provide what they thought were socially desirable responses. For example, we had participants write their responses down before sharing them and provided them with scenarios that they worked through based on personal experiences. The participants were told at the start of the focus group that our goal was not to gain consensus but to facilitate discussion regarding their thoughts and perceptions around the AWTY Program. Our objective was to elicit main themes and priorities that ran throughout the discussion as well as to confirm, clarify, or refute various themes/ideas that emerge during the research process.

Qualitative Data Analysis

We subjected interview and focus group transcripts to a constant comparison content analysis method. This process was developed by adapting a fourteen-stage approach described by Burnard (1991), as well as a six-step guide to analysis as described by Kvale (1996), and a general approach described by Maykut and Morehouse (2001). Each transcript was read repeatedly using an iterative process in order to observe and record notes on frequently occurring themes. These data were then narrowed down using the process of condensation, categorization, and interpretation (Kvale 1996) to determine some consistent overriding themes.

Findings

Who Participated: A Breakdown of Participants by Location and Gender

We sampled youth response in an urban location in Alberta, a rural location in Nova Scotia, and in an Aboriginal community in Saskatchewan. A questionnaire was administered to youth prior to the AWTY Program, right after the AWTY Program, and one month after the AWTY Program. We also sampled a control group, which was given the questionnaire at two points, two weeks to one month apart. The sample included 154 students from Nova Scotia, 202 from Saskatchewan, and 496 from Edmonton. One hundred and fifty students were part of the control group.

Not all students filled out all of the questionnaires (i.e., pre, post, and follow-up) and thus the analysis numbers were smaller. The sample consisted of 45 per cent males and 54 per cent females. The age of students ranged from twelve to sixteen; however, most youth were fourteen or fifteen years old, and most were in grade nine. While most students described their gender orientation as heterosexual (90 per cent), a small percentage saw themselves as homosexual (1.2 per cent), bisexual (3.7 per cent), or were unsure about their gender orientation (5.2 per cent). Most youth lived with both parents or with mother only. However, a small percentage of youth lived in other situations.

We conducted interviews and focus groups in Edmonton, AB; La Ronge, SK; Vancouver, BC; and several cities in Nova Scotia. The majority of student participants were grade nine students ages fourteen or fifteen. Adult participants consisted of teachers, sexual health educators, sexual health service providers, and parents who had an opportunity to watch *AWTY*.

Impacts

Responses to the Theatrical Elements of AWTY

We found significant changes within the treatment group between pre- to post- and pre- to follow-up treatment (for actual tables of analysis, see Munro et al. 2009). Differences were small but statistically significant; while the lay reader may find the degree of change apparently small, when compared with other educational interventions and research, this change is actually quite significant (Willett 2007). Students who experienced the AWTY Program thought they were more able to make sexual decisions and communicate them to others. All significant changes indicated a positive change in attitudes and behaviour. The findings were in direct contrast to changes found among the students in the control group. In all cases but one, the pre- to post-change for control students did not significantly change, and if the change was significant it was in a negative direction; that is, control group students

YEAR ONE: In year one, twelve interviews were conducted with four boys and eight girls. In year two, this qualitative research component was expanded.

YEAR TWO: The participants were divided into four sets.

Group	Total number	Females	Males
SET 1: EDMONTON, ALBERTA SCHOOLS			
Teen interviews	16	8	8
Teen focus group (boys)	1	N/A	7
Teen focus group (girls)	1	7	N/A
Teen focus group (mixed)	1	4	4
SET 2: LA RONGE, SASKATCHEWAN TEENS			
Teen interviews	9	6	3
Teen focus group (mixed)	1	4	4
SET 3: LA RONGE, SASKATCHEWAN ADULTS			
Adult interviews	10	5	5
Adult focus group	1	4	4
SET 4: EDMONTON, ALBERTA TEACHERS			
Teacher interviews	5	3	2

YEAR THREE: Interviews and focus groups were conducted during year three.

Group	Total Number	Females	Males
SET 1: EDMONTON, ALBERTA SCHOOLS, TEENS			
Teen focus group information seeker	1	5	3
Teen focus group normative	1	6	0
Teen focus group diffuse	1	3	3
SET 2: NOVA SCOTIA, TEENS			
Teen interviews	6	3	3
Teen focus group (male)	1	N/A	8
Teen focus group (female)	1	8	N/A
Teen focus group (mixed)	1	4	4
SET 3: SASKATCHEWAN, TEENS			
Teen interviews	10	6	4
Teen focus group (male)	1	N/A	6
Teen focus group (female)	1	4	N/A
Teen focus group (mixed)	1	3	3
SET 4: SASKATCHEWAN, ADULTS			
Health partners	1	3	1
SNTC	1	3	1

YEAR FOUR: Sixteen (12 female and 4 male) interviews were conducted with adults in order to gain insights from parents and teachers. Both constituencies were impressed with the content and the theatrical delivery. They were particularly impressed with the level of participation from teens.

SUMMARY: Years one to five

Group	Total number	Females	Males
Teen interviews	53	31	22
Teen focus group (boys)	3	N/A	21
Ed. teen focus group (girls)	4*	25	N/A
Ed. teen focus group (mix)	6	23	21
Adult interviews	31	20	11
Adult focus group mixed	3	10	6
Total number of interviews student and adult	84	43	29
Total number of focus groups student and adult	16	58	48

*The normative focus group was all girls.

felt less able to make sexual decisions and felt less able to communicate their sexual limit post-treatment when compared to pre-treatment scores.

Participants responded strongly to all five of our scales that measured the theatrical elements of the play. Almost all students reported pleasure; only 3.2 per cent of students disagreed or strongly disagreed when asked if they liked the play. As a result, there was little variance: no substantial group found the play more pleasurable than any other groups. A large majority of participants identified with the play (62 per cent) and empathized with the characters (63 per cent), and 56 per cent said they participated in the interactive parts of the play. Moreover, these students thought that the experience would help them in the future, and many commented about the play's power and its ability to keep their interest as well as make a lasting impression. Sixty per cent of students agreed or strongly agreed that they will were highly impacted by the program, and 74 per cent of students agreed or strongly agreed that they will use the information from the play to make healthier choices for themselves.[7]

When asked directly about the play during interviews or focus groups, the students consistently reported that the AWTY Program was not what they expected. All participants reported enjoying the play, specifically mentioning the use of humour, the age-appropriate analogy between sex education and driver training, and the fact that audience participation was seen as important and relevant: "I like how it used humor to teach us that because it was better than just sitting there and listening to lectures"; "[we were] able to participate not just sit there passively while the teacher tells you stuff." They also described the open comfortable atmosphere created by the play: "I really liked how it was really open and it really talked like it wasn't really anything that was sort of hidden." They described how they were easily able relate to the characters and situations: "The actors in it...were young and they were open and stuff. We weren't like afraid to say stuff, like, 'if you get up.' They would go along with it." As well, the students could identify the scenarios with problems and issues that they themselves may face (or had already faced), and this seemed to have a lasting impact on the students and how they would deal with situations in the future.

Certain scenes and elements were particularly influential for the adolescents. The play's realistic scenes had a strong impact, and students emphasized the importance of the real-life scenarios:

> *It was really real. And I think that's the part that everyone liked about it. Because it was just so...like happens in everyday life and I think a lot of people in there could relate to different skits that they did because of maybe the things that they said or the actions they played.*

Since the scenes were perceived as things they might deal with in the future, students felt they left a more lasting impact. Some students even addressed current or former sexual and relationship situations through information they got from the play. On the other hand, the non-realistic, participatory elements also made a strong impression, particularly the body moulding, Clay scenes (Chapter 3, page 89) in which groups built an ideal male or female. This process allowed students to see that everyone has their own preferences, to reflect on their own conceptions of their own body and beauty, and to build confidence: "[It's] interesting to see the different things people thought were 'ideal,' everybody likes different stuff and brought out the importance of being yourself."

The Mac and Carol Ann sequence (Chapter 3, page 80) also left a strong impression on students. Both the male and female character feel they are ready, but neither knows what the other is talking about. The students often cited this scene as an example that demonstrates the importance of communication.

Students' Perceptions of AWTY *vs. Other Forms of Sexuality Education*

Students told us that they preferred *AWTY* to other forms of sexuality education, such as classroom-based lessons with their regular teachers or discussions with their parents. Parents were not considered the best people to go to for advice when it comes to sex or relationships because teens perceive their parents to be uncomfortable discussing sex with them and because they perceive parents as discouraging any sexual activity or thoughts of sex, rather than helping the teens deal with their questions or situations. Most students who talked to their parents about the play stated the conversations tended to be general and did not lead to deeper discussions regarding sexual choices or relationships. Interestingly, some females did have very open and deep conversations with their mothers following the play, whereas males said they did not communicate with their parents at all for fear of embarrassment. Also, students mentioned that addressing parental reactions within the play would be a beneficial addition to the program.

Students preferred *AWTY* to conventional classroom-based sex education partly because they perceived it as being more sex positive and partly because they were more comfortable discussing sexuality with a trusted neutral party than someone they see every day in the classroom. While students expected the program to be lecture style and to focus on negative aspects of sexuality, they were pleased to find this was not the case. Several key themes that they took away with them came up in interviews in focus groups. They heard and apparently heeded its message about the importance of communication and boundaries. They also agreed that the play sent a positive message and by this, they did not mean a message to go have sex, but a message that sex is a normal part of a healthy life. They felt the play focused on being safe, waiting until one is ready, and learning how to make good sexual decisions by thinking and communicating before acting. They also expressed an increased openness in communication and an awareness that everyone might be in a slightly different place when it comes to sex, and that no one should need to feel pressure to be sexually active. Some students expressed relief that they no longer worried their thoughts or feelings about sex would seem weird or strange if they voiced them to their partner. Many said they felt less alone in their feelings and decisions about sex. As a result, many stated they felt more confident around the opposite sex and more comfortable discussing sex as a result of the play. Interestingly, they mentioned the importance of openness both in relation to the atmosphere of the play and to their own lives.

How AWTY *Changed Sexual Behaviours*

Regarding communication about sexuality and communicating sexual boundaries, students typically said things like, "I never really realized how important it was to kinda talk about that kind of stuff."

The following data combines results from Edmonton, Nova Scotia, and Saskatchewan and compares it with the control group (students who did not receive the program). Results show a significant difference between the treatment group and the control.

Communication about Sexuality

Figure 9-1 and 9-2 show how the students' ability to communicate about sex increased after they received the AWTY Program. The items tested pertained to difficulty and embarrassment discussing sexual topics and sexual limits with a partner (example: *It is difficult to discuss your sexual limits when you first start dating*). The Communication about Sexuality Scale ranged from 5 to 25 with 5 being the lowest and 25 the highest level of communication about sexuality. While the treatment group started at a higher level of communication about sexuality than the control group (15), only the treatment group increased in perceived level of communication about sexuality while the control group did not.

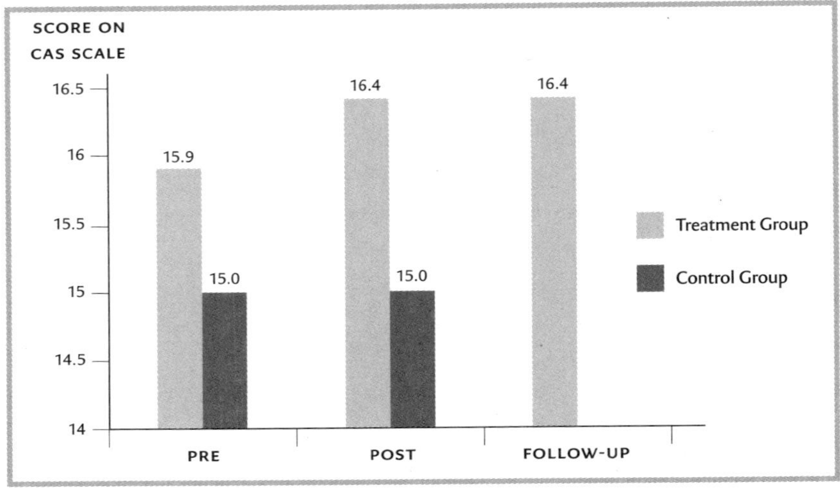

Figure 9-1 Communicating about Sexuality
Communicating about Sexuality (CAS) Scale ranges between 5 and 20 with 5 being the lowest and 20 the highest level of communication about sexuality.

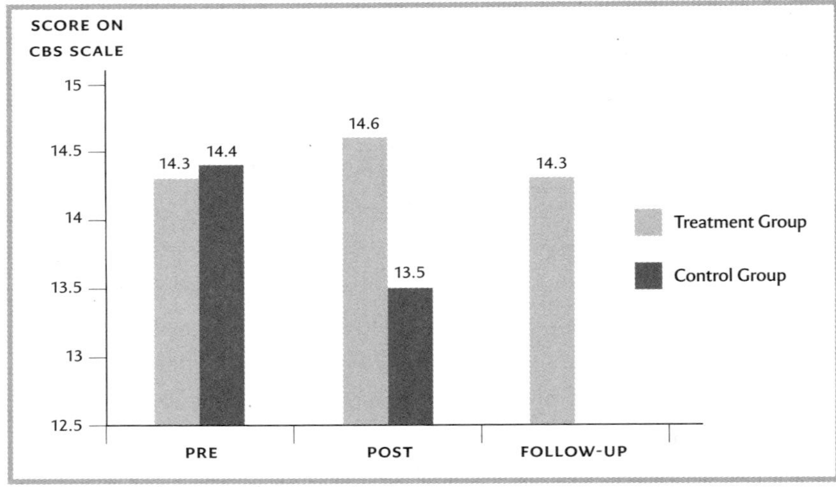

Figure 9-2 Communicating Sexual Boundaries
Communicating about Sexual Boundaries (CBS) Scale ranges between 5 and 20 with 5 being the lowest and 20 the highest level of communication about boundaries.

Communicating Sexual Boundaries

These items tested for the students' difficulty communicating sexual boundaries to a partner (example item: *It is really hard to bring up the issue of sexual boundaries with my boy/girlfriend*).

Interestingly, while the results remain the same from the pre-test to the follow-up for the treatment group, the control group actually saw a decrease in their ability to communicate sexual boundaries in their post-test without the AWTY Program. The program served to reinforce the age group's ability to continue communicating sexual boundaries.

Qualitative data supported the quantitative findings. Participants felt that communication about sexuality and communicating their sexual boundaries were important themes in the play. Many of the students used examples from the play to describe how a good relationship requires open communication between partners and being comfortable with the topic of sex: "All the scenes were about...well, obviously, one of the main things was communication and stuff like that. So, it's like, be real, don't like beat around the bush or whatever, just be open and stuff." Others related this topic to the concept of respecting and communicating personal boundaries:

> *For me it actually helped a lot because I was in this kind of relationship thing before the play. Well, I wasn't getting too active about sex, right; it had nothing to do with sex, right. But like, it showed me that you have to be able to communicate in your relationship in order for it to work out and it showed me I was having an unhealthy relationship, so it helped me just deal with it.*

A recurring theme emerged from the interviews: tell them no and then tell them why. That is, the students consistently said that if a partner pressured them into sexual activities that made them uncomfortable, they would assert their boundaries, or rather, say no. However, all students interviewed claimed that they would talk it through with their partner rather than make a hasty exit. The students emphasized communication and discussion as the preferred option and proposed breaking up only if the partner did not respect their wishes:

I would just tell him that I wasn't comfortable and at first I wouldn't really be mad at them. I'd just be like, "okay, I know you're really horny" or "calm down" (laughs,) but if they kept pressuring me more I'd be like, "you can't respect my boundaries then we're gonna break up because you obviously don't respect me as a person."

Honestly the only impact it had on me was just stressing out how much you need to communicate with your partner, that for the relationship to actually work and for you to feel comfortable in that relationship, and stressing out the use of protection.

Like you know in your head why you're leaving but they don't know, like they can't read your mind. You have to tell them why you don't want to do this.

In general, the evidence shows that the play equipped participants with a valuable skill set of strategies and decision-making skills surrounding sex.

How AWTY *Speaks to Different Genders*

Given that boys and girls often respond differently to different styles and media of teaching, we wanted to know if *AWTY* was equally effective for boys and girls; or, if it turned out to be more effective for one gender, what might be done to create or adapt a program that would be equally effective for both boys and girls. We discovered that *AWTY* is effective for both boys and girls but (not surprisingly) effective in different ways, which reflects the fact that boys and girls face different pressures and challenges in regards to sexuality.

Females were more likely to report that they enjoyed the play, empathized and/or identified with the characters and situations, and were impacted by the program. Males were slightly more likely to report that they participated in the program. Not all differences in outcomes were the same for men and women. Only the significant findings are discussed below.

Females changed more than males in regard to communication about sexuality. It is interesting that males went into the program feeling that they were more able to communicate about sexuality before experiencing the program. Thus, while females changed more than males as a result of the program, both males and females ended the program feeling equally confident in their ability to communicate about sexuality.

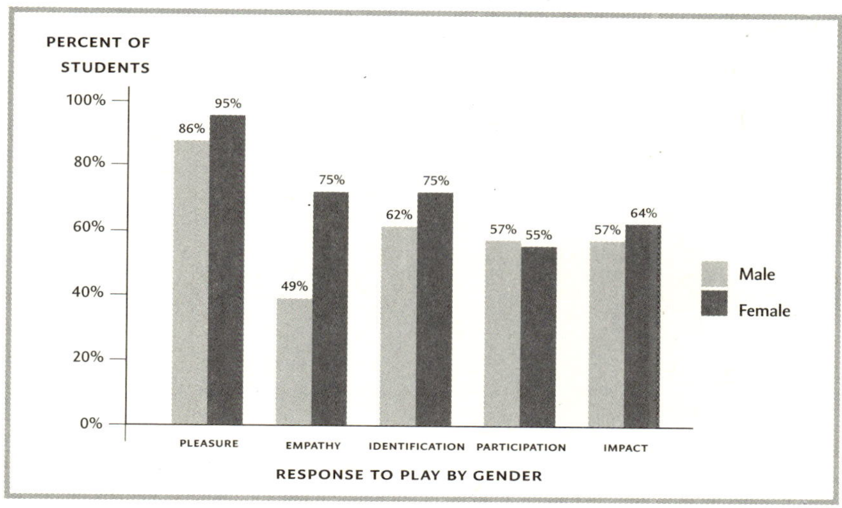

Figure 9-3 How Males and Females Experienced the Play

Figure 9-5 shows falling levels of discomfort with saying no or, rather, increased confidence in one's ability to resist pressure to engage in unwanted sexual activity.

As a result of the program, females felt less uncomfortable saying no to unwanted advances. Males did not feel that their comfort level had changed much and, at the time of the follow-up, felt less able to say no to unwanted sexual advances.

Females

In the qualitative findings, the main skills that girls claimed they learned from the play are communication, and the ability to conceive, set, and respect sexual boundaries. They felt that learning to think about and communicate their boundaries helped them to shape their beliefs and values in relation to sex. Several female participants said that if they felt pressured in a relationship, they would end it. Communication, both about what each person wants in the relationship and about the use of protection, was deemed to be important. One participant stated that as a result of the communication skills she learned in the play, she is more comfortable speaking

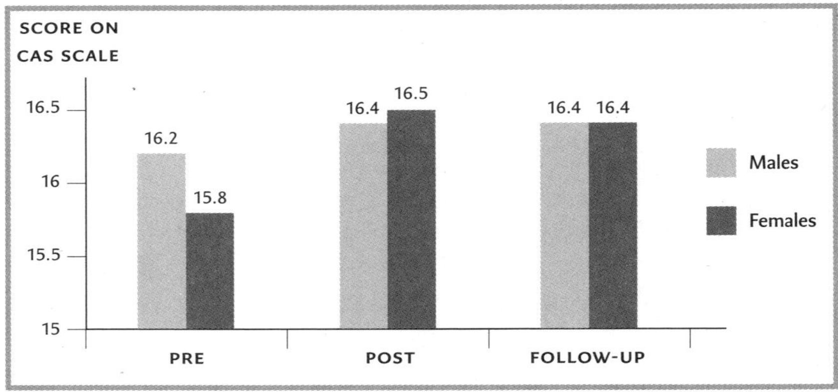

Figure 9-4 Male and Female Change in Communication about Sexuality
Communicating about Sexuality (CAS) Scale ranges between 5 and 20 with 5 being the lowest and 20 the highest level of communication about sexuality.

to her friends about sex and related issues: "Now that I saw examples...I think I will be more ready to handle situations. I feel like I could give candid advice to a friend now like you know because of the participation aspect of the play." All of the girls talked about being impacted by the play, especially the content on boundaries and the different scenarios represented in the play. The play increased the girls' level of comfort with communicating personal boundaries and with resisting pressure to engage in sexual activities that they are not comfortable with: "I talked about how we did set boundaries and I talked about...I'm gonna be honest, he doesn't have many boundaries but I talked about that I should really draw some strict ones if I don't want to do something, I should tell him and all that. Because I think he feels that he could kind of push me if he wanted so..."

Even though the participants had experience with the concept of boundaries, many students mentioned that they found it helpful to complete the exercise to determine where their line is, and how to communicate this to their partner:

> *Yeah, it made me think more like waiting, like abstinence and stuff like that, because sometimes sex can make you closer and sometimes it can drive you apart from the person.*

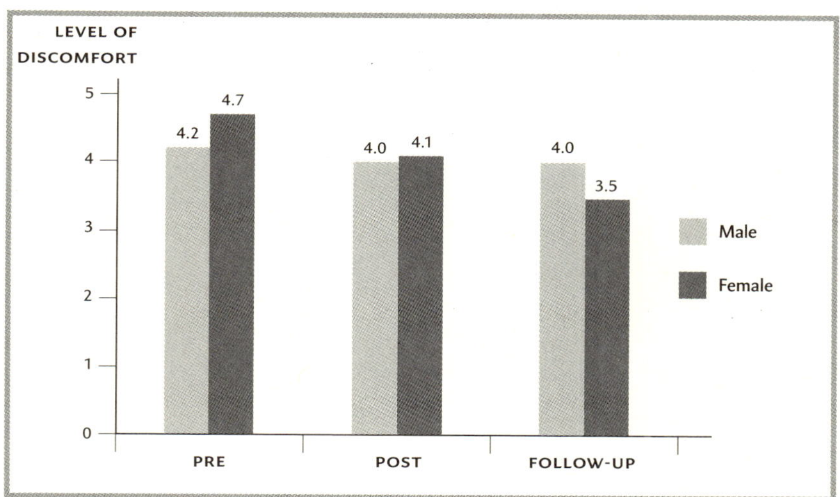

Figure 9-5 Level of Discomfort Saying "No"

Note: Level of discomfort saying "no" ranges on a scale from 1 (low level of discomfort in saying "no") to 5 (high level of discomfort in saying "no"). The level of discomfort dropped, i.e, after seeing the play, participants were more comfortable saying "no" to pressure.

> *I think personally it impacted me by making me happy to see that there are people out there with similar boundaries to mine and people out there who actually thought it was okay to say no.*

Males

When the boys were questioned about learning, there appeared to be a general consensus that they had already learned the information, and that this was simply an overview. However, the boys felt that some people would have acquired new information from the play, such as how to handle sexual situations. Many of the boys commented on the realism of the examples, and how these examples could be applied to future situations: "It was like shooting a dead duck. It was like going over the same stuff. It was like, 'no duh,' but I mean some people don't know as much about it I'm just...not saying anyway that I'm better than anyone else; I'm just saying like that it was—for me at least—just reiterating stuff that I've been told since I was a kid."

The boys felt they did acquire some skills from participating, including the importance of respecting their partner. They also felt that participating changed their behaviour in terms of establishing boundaries within the relationship, and communicating with their partner: "I found it didn't really get down to the nitty gritty of sex. It was more about like the, starting your car before you drive it, it was more about that, I found it didn't get down to the hardcore, not to do it, (laughter) you know what I mean."

Similarities and Differences between Female and Male Teen Focus Groups

Similarities between the female and male groups included belief that participation was beneficial; that the play was a better method of teaching sexual education than regular classroom approaches; and that the content was appropriate to their age, experience, and maturity level. However, both groups stated they already knew much of the information presented; the program focuses on using information and knowledge rather than the transmission of information. Neither group felt the play was explicit and both groups felt the play could be presented to a younger audience, although, as stated by the boys, this would be highly dependent on individual experience. Both groups also recognized the importance of establishing boundaries and communication within a relationship. Both felt that negotiating personal boundaries is not about meeting in the middle but actually understanding where the other person is. They felt the play made them feel confident that they could bring up the boundary conversation with their partner. Interestingly, the boys spoke of the importance of boundaries in terms of respecting one's partner's boundaries, while the girls spoke in terms of the importance of one's partner respecting one's own boundaries. Although both groups stated that open communication is important in relationships, the girls further developed this section to explain why, whereas the boys did not expand in this way. Finally, both groups stated that the play would be very beneficial to individuals who had less knowledge in the area of sexuality.

Differences between the two groups were more difficult to notice. However, an important difference was noted when participants were asked what other material they would like to see in the play. Overall, the boys requested further information on the how to and the consequences of having sex, while the girls requested more information on pregnancy, birth control, and Internet dating. In addition, boys found the boundaries theme more difficult to notice and identified free condoms as an area of information within the play. They also mentioned the play's humour more. Girls stressed the importance of having someone who is not your teacher provide sex education, and the importance of being comfortable with discussing sex. Girls also frequently reported discussing the play after watching it with other girls, while this was not apparent for the boys.

General observation and review of field notes revealed an interesting phenomenon: the gender composition of the focus groups significantly affected the level of involvement and types of responses given by both genders. The boys tended to be more open during the mixed focus groups and tended to give more socially acceptable (expected) responses during the males-only focus groups. The girls, on the other hand, were less open in the mixed focus group but very assertive and at times quite explicit during the female-only focus groups.

The participants' responses, when asked whether the play targets boys, girls, or both, also produced some intriguing gender differences, depending on whether the question was asked individually or in an all-male, all-female, or mixed groups. Female participants in one-on-one interviews and female-only focus groups said that the play was designed for them more than the boys. They perceived themselves to have taken the play more seriously. Females felt that the males had a more immature reaction to the play and that they made a joke out of it. Some girls got the impression that the guys thought they knew everything already. By contrast, when the same question was asked of males during individual interviews or male-only focus groups, they consistently felt the play was primarily targeted to them. However, when asked the same question in mixed focus groups, both boys and girls consistently responded that the play was designed for both male and females.

The Impact of Identity Type on Reception of AWTY

In addition to gender, we assessed the impact of *AWTY* on three identity types: diffuse-avoidance, normative, and informational decision-making styles. We asked, first, if there was a correlation between the level of each identity type and perceived response to the play and, second, whether changes in sexual communication and decision making, pre to post to follow-up, were related to identity types.[8]

After reviewing the quantitative data based on identity styles, we chose to conduct separate focus groups with students with each identity style. Probes for these focus groups were selected from probes used in previous one-on-one interviews and focus groups in order to compare students with specific identity styles to those from mixed groups. We also created probes targeting each identity style.

A majority of the students with all identity styles reported experiencing pleasure, empathy, and impact, and they participated and identified with characters from the play. Significantly, the youth's perceptions of the play and their experience were not always related to the play's actual, measurable impact. For example, diffuse youth perceived themselves as less empathetic and less impacted by the play than other groups; however, the change from pre- to post- and pre- to follow-up suggests that, in reality, diffuse youth were significantly impacted by the play and could relate to the situations. For the information seekers, perceptions matched outcomes. This group reported feeling empathy and being impacted by the play, a perception that was confirmed by the quantitative study results. The play had the smallest impact on normative youth, who neither perceived as much impact nor experienced actual behavioural changes to the same extent that other groups did.

Both diffuse and information-seeking groups showed significant positive change in sexual communication and sexual decision making and greater comfort with saying no to unwanted sexual advances after participating in the play. We anticipated that information-seeking identity style would be associated with higher levels of outcomes, as their locus of control is based on their personal experience supported by information they have gathered (Berzonsky 1990). However, we would not have predicted a high association of diffusion with change in major outcome variables.

This disconnect between what diffuse teens say about their experience and what is revealed through analysis of the outcomes yields an important insight. Qualitative and quantitative findings suggest that diffuse-avoidance adolescents, who may be most at risk, claim less empathy, less engagement, and less impact when they talk about the play. Yet when surveyed about future behaviour, they report increased self-efficacy and ability to communicate sexual boundaries. The play has significant impact, even though they are either not conscious of this, or loathe to admit it, or both. We wonder whether the theatrical medium and or the participatory style reaches this group, perhaps in spite of themselves, with all of its powerful but unstated messages, messages held in the emotional responses of characters and audiences.

By contrast, adolescents with a normative identity style, who rely on social convention and norms rather than experience to regulate their behaviours, did not change as much as the other groups. It appears that these youth took more of an observer role during the play, as many of their comments were observations of their classmates. They did not appear to relate to or identify with the play's situations as much as the other groups. They agreed that the situations presented in the play were realistic; however, they gave the impression that these were more relevant for their classmates than themselves. Self-control, in this perspective, is to be found in the norms or conventions of one's social environment; normative types rely on the past generation and adult norms to guide their conduct. This was evident in many of their comments and attitudes, which can be described as socially expected responses (i.e., the play was too sex positive or the play was giving permission to students to have sex). In this case, self-control is not so much internalized into the self as it is constrained by the social conventions of adults.

This investigation is novel in an important aspect: it introduces the potential role of identity theory into research on sexuality and sexuality education using the concept of identity style. Much sexuality research has not incorporated human development perspectives as a common theoretical perspective. For example, the role of identity formation and individual differences among adolescents in their identity-based self-regulation systems has not been directly investigated. Our findings may be the first to look at the potential for identity theory in predicting adolescent sexual behaviour and limit setting. This analysis has significant implications: assessments of programs aimed at providing youth with skills to act more safely and respectfully in their sexual relationships may well need to account for the likelihood that different educational strategies have varying impacts on different kinds of youth. With this study, we open up one way to pursue this deeper analysis of sexuality education.

Causal Modelling and the Significance of AWTY'S *Theatrical Elements*

As our data suggests, and as we anticipated, different youth experience *AWTY* in different ways. Individual factors such as age, gender, sexual orientations, identity types, family types, and sexual activity backgrounds impact the efficacy of the program. We expected this, but we also predicted that the theatrical elements would outweigh all of these factors. Our theory was that theatre, by virtue of its power to influence individuals' thoughts, emotions, and future behaviour, would prove an effective medium for sexual health education, and that the biggest factor in the impact of this program on a given individual would be whether or not he or she enjoyed the play. That is, we expected that youth who found the play pleasurable, who participated, empathized and/or identified with characters, and those who felt impacted by the play would positively change their sexual communication, boundary setting, and future behaviour, and that these responses to the play would have more impact than the personal attributes of the individual experiencing the play. This is important because any method that only works on certain types of individuals, or works much better or worse on some groups than on others, is of limited utility in public education.

In order to verify this theory, we used a process called causal modelling,[9] and in particular we used a two-stage regression. First, we determined that different types of youth do indeed experience the play in different ways. Second, we determined that experiencing the play in different ways did in fact impact the target areas (sexual communication, boundary setting, and behaviour) more than other individual attributes (such as, age, gender, sexual orientation, identity, family type, sexual activity). As the theatre components are statistically more important than any individual difference, theatre can indeed be said to be a broadly effective medium for teaching sexuality education. We also analyzed the relative importance of the impact of theatre experience in comparison to other attributes of the individual using a process called stepwise regression.

Findings

The overall impact of the theatre components (pleasure, participation, identification, empathy, and impact) were tested separately. Only significant findings are presented here.

While almost all student participants found the play to be pleasurable, those who enjoyed the play most were female and from cohesive homes. The more pleasurable participants found the play, the greater they perceived their ability to communicate about sexuality, and the more able they thought they were at making sexual decisions.

Most students felt they participated in the play, but those who felt they participated the most were information seekers, while sexually active students felt they participated less. Those who felt they participated more had a greater change in perceived ability to communicate boundaries and felt that risk-taking behaviour would be reduced.

While most participants identified with the characters in the play, those who identified most strongly were female. The more strongly an individual identified with characters in the play, the more change there was in his or her perceived ability to make sexual decisions.

While most of the students empathized with the characters in the play, those who empathized the most were females and those from cohesive homes. Diffuse youth empathized the least with characters. Students who felt they empathized more with the characters also perceived a positive changed in ability to communicate boundaries and felt that risk-taking behaviour would be reduced.[10]

Most participants felt impacted by the play, but two groups felt most impacted: females and information seekers. Students who felt more impacted by the play experienced more change in perceived ability to make sexual decisions, felt more comfortable saying no to unwanted sexual advances, and perceived an increased ability to communicate boundaries.

Based on these findings, our theory was confirmed in most cases. Youth with different attributes did experience the play differently. In addition, and most importantly, in most cases the participants' experience of the play was more significant than any other individual factor in predicting how they changed in terms of sexual communication, boundary setting, and predicted future behaviour.

Adult Responses

As part of the qualitative component of the research project, we surveyed parents, educators, and sexual health educators and service providers, asking their opinions about sexual health education in Canada and about how the Are We There Yet? Program addresses the key topics considered necessary for adolescents to make healthy and informed sexual health decisions.

The adult participants focused on concerns about sexual education, skills parents hope students will gain, the role of adults in providing sexual education, and parents' opinions of how sexual education should be taught. We found that parents are concerned about the current state and content of sexual health education in Canada, especially in rural areas. Parents felt that sex education should be holistic, focusing on human biology as well as relationships. The skills adults hope students will gain include postponing sex, developing a friendship with their partner prior to initiating sex, and exposure to LGBTQ content to help with future challenges and experiences. Parents acknowledge that they should be engaged in what their children are learning in sexual education at school but are concerned that the potential for embarrassment prevents either themselves or their children from initiating the conversation.

Major themes that emerged concerning the AWTY Program dealt with how the adults experienced the play, knowledge gained by students, the effective method of delivery, and some overall impressions regarding this type of approach for sexual health education. The parents overwhelmingly felt that the play was presented in a manner that is conducive to learning about sexuality and sexual relationships. They commented on how the setting relaxed students and made them feel more comfortable with the topic:

> *It [participation] was fun. I think it made it easier for people to talk 'cause everyone was yelling things out and it was a lot more comfortable and people definitely got more comfortable with it by the end because they weren't putting people on the spot. I think when teens are in a position where they vocalize and verbalize their advice, they're more likely to stick to that advice.*

The adult participants felt that in general the play enhanced students' knowledge in the areas of sexuality and relationships. Areas that they felt would have the largest impact or lasting impression included information on open communication and creating and respecting boundaries. Participants felt that students picked up on communication strategies modelled by the actors. Students also had the opportunity to practice these skills by giving the actors advice. Personal boundaries were demonstrated in the boundary setting exercise, which was thought to be beneficial to students. As one participant remarked, "all the input that the kids had in the decision from the guy's view and the girl's view made them feel like they had part in the decision making. They [audience] think that if I can help them [actors] make a decision, maybe I can make a decision on my own."

Adults perceived that the use of outside educators, professional actors, and humour all helped to disarm the youth and encourage open discussion about sex in a non-threatening environment. They felt that the driving metaphor effectively held the students' attention because teens could relate to the topic. The play was designed to encourage participation, which the adults believed improved the atmosphere, empowered the students, and increased their attention. Adults thought that the play let youth work on important skills, such as communication and decision-making skills, and to build confidence in dealing with sex and relationship issues. The play was thought to function as a starting point for sexual health discussions at home and with peers by providing students with an opportunity for exploration and interaction while creating a sense of togetherness with their classmates. After watching the play, parents reported that it could help open the door for discussions at home as they have knowledge of what topics were covered. They felt the play also opened their eyes to how teenagers act and think in today's society.

Teachers' reactions unanimously emphasized the benefit of having alternate sexual health educators come in for the teens, particularly the importance of learning from people the adolescents perceive to be experts. They observed that having actors who are closer to the students' age conveying the information, however still perceived to be older, more experienced, and more knowledgeable, meant that teens found the material relatable and credible. Other adult participants also recognized the value of the sexual health educators who were part of the play because they have more freedom to discuss controversial topics, topics often excluded by teachers and parents.

The adults recognized that the youth feel greater comfort in discussing sexual health with outside educators because, unlike their parents or teachers, they do not interact with them on a daily basis. Overall, parents and educators considered *AWTY* a valuable and effective resource for teaching sexual health education to adolescents.

The adults had various opinions and debated the realism of the play in terms of the communication among characters as well as its scenarios. In terms of communication, the majority of adults believed it was true to life. However, in contrast to teen responses, some adults felt that the content presented was beyond the level and knowledge of many of the students; "they were not ready for it." Interestingly, the teachers and sexual health educators felt the play was pitched at the appropriate level and was not too explicit for the students, while parents were more likely to feel it was too explicit. This possibly speaks to the fact that teachers and sexual health educators see a very different side of youth than the idealized identity that all parents want to believe in (and which most children, even adult children, both consciously and unconsciously manufacture for their parents' benefit).

Conclusions

In general, the students who experienced *AWTY* enjoyed the program and felt theatre was an effective form of sex education. Students reported that they prefer learning about sexual health through a theatrical presentation to a classroom setting. Participants enjoyed the active role of providing suggestions to the actors and shaping the relationships and scenes of the play, and this enjoyment helped them maintain their attention throughout the presentation. Many students identified with characters in the play, which enhanced the relevance and impact of the information it presented, and resulted in more effective and enjoyable learning. Both students and educators emphasized the age-appropriateness of the approach and the benefits of humour, describing how the performance fostered a comfortable and relaxed setting that encouraged open discussion by the audience. Additionally, the fact that the material was presented by and through young actors who were open, relatable, non-judgemental, and who were neither their teachers nor parents, contributed to the students' comfort level and engagement in the program. This experience helped students realize they are not alone in their thoughts and feelings about sex.

Students noted that the play was presented in a sex-positive manner, specifically focusing on communicating and respecting personal boundaries, waiting until they feel ready to become sexually active, and being safe when sexually active. Despite feeling that the information presented was a repetition of their current knowledge, participants thought the information and skills conveyed were helpful for less-experienced students and a useful refresher for the more-experienced. In keeping with the goals of the play, the aspects of practice were emphasized over information. Students reported a significant change in their decision making as the play offered them a skill set of different strategies, allowing them to choose how to approach sexual situations and topics with their partners. As a result of the experience, students felt more comfortable talking about sex, more confident about knowing and communicating their personal boundaries, and more capable making sexual decisions.

What Areas AWTY *Impacted*

Knowledge

The more prominent themes in student feedback included increased knowledge of the importance of communication and an awareness of personal boundaries and safe sex. By developing an awareness of boundaries, students learned how to set them and how to implement or communicate them within a sexual relationship. They also developed an understanding of how to know when one is ready to change boundaries or take a physical relationship to the next level. Students gained insight into the other gender's perspective, aiding their ability to approach conversations with more openness, sensitivity, and understanding. The participants felt they acquired information about issues they may face in the future and skills for dealing with them. Based on the frequency with which communication is mentioned in the participants' responses, the AWTY Program meets its original goal of improving teens' capacity to communicate sexual boundaries. The program provided students with the words and understanding to express and discuss sex and boundaries, giving teens an opportunity to learn and practice these skills in a safe environment. Additionally, the participants gained an appreciation for the importance of communication in relationships.

Skills and Behaviours

The play appears to positively impact the students' skills and ability to make sexual decisions, communicate, and set sexual boundaries. Students involved in *AWTY* reported a marked increase in their ability to communicate about sex, anticipating less difficulty and embarrassment. Students reported that they felt they learned how to communicate, having acquired a skill set that includes strategies on how to broach topics with their partner and deal with sexual situations. Following the play, participants reported a greater ability to assert themselves and stay within their personal boundaries; they felt they could establish what they were and were not ready to do with a partner. Some students reported discussing the play with their partner and asking about their personal boundaries. Participants also stated they were more likely to use proper protection and think before acting when it came to sex. They also developed decision-making skills based on self-reflection of their own boundaries and their knowledge of safer sex. It is worth noting that some of the students were observed to behave with increasing maturity and less silliness toward the topic of sexuality as the play progressed.

Attitudes

The AWTY Program had a significant impact on participants' attitudes, changing how they felt about themselves, their boundaries, and their ability to communicate. Students reported feeling more comfortable with themselves and their personal boundaries after viewing the play. They developed a strong appreciation for the importance of respect within a relationship and gained an understanding that it was normal and acceptable for everyone to be at differing levels of comfort and experience with sex. The participants agreed that no one should feel pressured to have sex or avoid a conversation about it for fear that the other person might judge them. They also reported an increased appreciation of the value of communication and of the importance of discussing sexual activity and personal boundaries. They felt more confident in their decisions and more comfortable with their thoughts, feelings, and boundaries regarding sex. They also agreed that it was important to consider carefully the consequences of sexual activity beforehand.

Normalizing the Topic of Sex

Many students felt the theatrical medium served to neutralize a dangerous or uncomfortable topic. Instead of feeling embarrassed, students understood that discussing sex with a partner is not only important but is a healthy and normal conversation to have. Most students appreciated the sex-positive approach. Learning in a non-judgemental and safe atmosphere allowed them to normalize feelings about sex and gain confidence that may not have been possible if the messages were focused on the negative aspects of sexuality.

Insights Gained

The evaluation process gave us insight into various areas related to sexual health education. For example, AWTY as an educational tool has shown to affect boys and girls differently. The instructor/facilitator teaching sexual health education must understand that students will react differently when in a mixed gender group as opposed to being in company of their own gender or individually. In addition, male and female participants tend to learn (or perceive as important) significantly different knowledge and skills. Knowing this, sexual health educators can shape interactive sexual health education to accommodate the varying gendered concerns.

We also gained insight into how students with different identity styles vary in their reaction to sexual health education, in terms of both perceived/reported impact and actual impact. For example, normative students will tell the teacher they learned a lot and the session was great but in reality they were impacted minimally, while the diffuse students may state the session was ineffective but in reality were most impacted. What you see is not always what you get! These findings suggest that identity theory may play a role in adolescent sexual behaviour and decision making as well as how sexual health educators may choose to approach their class. Future research should look at both the predictive value of identity types and the need for a variety of education strategies to account for the varied reception of information. Moreover, this data sends clear messages to sexual health educators: first, while students have a lot to tell us about the efficacy of sexual health education, they aren't always able to perceive those effects accurately or objectively. Second, the same applies to educators: while it might be tempting to focus one's efforts on the students who appear to be most receptive, our study suggests that, in contrast to the appearance they may be trying to project to themselves and others, students with diffuse/avoidance identity styles have the greatest needs and benefit the most from the AWTY Program approach.

Implications

Implications for Sexual Health Educators

Based on these findings, sexual health educators can be assured that participatory theatre is an effective tool for adolescent education. Adolescents value participation and learn more effectively when they are directly involved in the performance, which allows them to practice the skills they are learning and to influence the outcome of realistic scenarios, which enhances their confidence and understanding. Many students enjoyed the sex-positive perspective, appreciating that the program does not use negative messaging or scare tactics. They also responded well to the presence of youthful actors and sexual health educators who were not their teachers or parents. The students are able to believe that the actors really can understand their perspectives and problems, partly because they do not wear the trappings of authority figures, and partly because their age gives them a sense of authenticity. Educators must also adapt the information conveyed and expect varied participation based on the presence or absence of the each gender. Separating the audience by gender for certain activities may allow for greater participation and allow for information that is more specific and applicable for each gender.

Implications for Parents

Involving parents in the experience may facilitate further sexual health education discussion outside the classroom. The few parents who had the opportunity to watch the play generally felt it was successful in enhancing the students' knowledge of sexuality and relationships and believed it could encourage more open communication about sexual health education at home. The community meeting model, reported in Chapter 7, offers a way forward for future projects. As parents felt the areas with the most impact were open communication and creating and respecting boundaries, it is likely these areas would continue to be reinforced if further discussion could be facilitated between parents and teens at home.

Implications for School and School Board

Our research shows the benefit of using outside educators who are not directly linked to the school or students to deliver sexuality and sexual health education. Students are more comfortable discussing sexuality with a trusted adult who is not their regular teacher, for a lot of good reasons. In addition, encouraging sex-positive messages in the sexual health curriculum is important. Many students learned how to broach the topic of sex and personal boundaries with a partner and that such conversations are not only not taboo but also an unavoidable, vital part of a normal, healthy sexual relationships. This finding could indicate a need for more focus on these areas in sexual health education. Participatory theatre stimulated involvement; the students enjoyed the role of directing what the characters do and exerting control over how the scene played out. Participatory theatre should be considered within the sexual health curriculum and in other sensitive curricular areas because it proves effective, enjoyable, and engaging for students and can open up areas of the topic that other approaches cannot.

Implications for Policy Change

In the wider social spectrum, our work points to the importance of a using sex-positive approach and emphasizing communication skills and an awareness of personal boundaries. This approach allows teens to address a wider variety of situations, not necessarily foreseeable in the scope of current sexual health education programs, which may equip children with a lot of information about the reproductive organs, STIs, and prophylaxis, but not with the attitudes and skills required to negotiate a fulfilling, healthy sexual life whenever they decide they're ready for it. Giving teens a skill set, including the ability to assert themselves, feel comfortable asking questions, and reflect on their own values, allows them to develop a healthy approach, both emotionally and physically, to relationships and sexuality. The facts of life are necessary, but no less so are the skills of life.

Summary

Sexual health is a sensitive and controversial topic, making it difficult to complete comprehensive research on the efficacy of sexual health education programs. However, the community partnership and multidisciplinary research team behind the AWTY Community-University Research Alliance research project allowed this project to hear the voices and meet the needs of the community of interest. The research presented in this chapter provides important evidence of the efficacy of the AWTY Program as a tool for sexual health education. Using participatory theatre, this program engages the students by giving them more control over the direction and content of the presentation, which leads to increased understanding and retention, and positive behavioural change. *AWTY* has been shown to have a considerable impact on adolescents' ability to make healthy sexual decisions. These findings demonstrate the growing need for research on the effectiveness of sexual health education strategies; our research on *AWTY* only scratches the surface and suggests there is value in future analysis elaborating on identity types, gender variations, and elements of theatre and participation that influence learning. With demonstrated efficacy, new sexual health education strategies (such as participatory theatre) can be used as a tool by educators to promote a more sex-positive attitude that better engages the students and provides them with the skills, knowledge, and attitudes needed to make healthy sexual decisions.

NOTES

1. See Chapter 2 for a full discussion of these developments.
2. For another perspective on determining the goals of the play, see the playwright's discussion of her process, Chapter 8. See Appendix 1.3 for the statement of the goals of the play, produced by the playwright for this interdisciplinary research program.
3. As assessed by Cronbach's alpha: 0.50, 0.74, 0.76, 0.55, and 0.77, respectively. Cronbach's alpha is a measure used to calculate the internal consistency and is used as a test of reliability (i.e., are all items testing for the same construct?) of a questionnaire. "Alpha was developed by Lee Cronbach in 1951 to provide a measure of the internal consistency of a test or scale; it is expressed as a number between 0 and 1. Internal consistency describes the extent to which

all the items in a test measure the same concept or construct and hence it is connected to the inter-relatedness of the items within" (Tavakol and Dennick 2011, 53) the test.

4. Each scale had three items and the alphas were 0.50 or better with each set of items positively correlated with the total score (ps < 0.05). Subjects assessed themselves on all three sets of items.
5. For a discussion of the theatre theories involved, see Chapter 13.
6. We used Cronbach's alpha to measure reliability, factor analysis to measure construct validity, Pearson r correlation to measure internal consistency. Alpha values ranged from 0.61 to 0.85, factor loadings ranged between 0.62 and 0.86, and Pearson r correlations ranged between 0.70 and 0.82.
7. For an explanation of the rationale for theatre-based scales, see Chapter 13.
8. We used Pearson's r correlation to determine correlations between identity type and perceived response, and Hotelling's trace analysis to look at the relationship between identity style and changes in sexual decision making and behaviour.
9. Causal modelling is a systematic representation for understanding one possible cause of a phenomenon in the context of other factors (Blalock 1985). Causes and causal processes can be inferred by observing patterns in data and constructing arrow diagrams connecting two or more variables (Asher 1983). The causal models developed can lead to the creation of clearer causal hypotheses between variables under investigation (Asher 1983). "Causal models incorporate the idea of multiple causality, that is, there can be more than one cause for any particular effect...even when there are only three variables under examination many different models of their relationship are possible. Thus, investigating all the different possible models is an important step in the analysis of data, and in linking sociological theory to empirical research" (Marshall 1998, 66). This process of causal modelling goes beyond predicting a phenomenon and provides greater insight into the topic being investigated, by understanding the direct and indirect effects of one variable on another (Asher 1983; Norris and Munro 1997).
10. Each kind of analysis needs careful consideration. For example, while this finding about diffuse participants provides important insights, so too does the finding that this group demonstrated significant change in a number of the sex education goals (see "The Impact of Identity Type on Reception of *AWTY*").

10

CAR TOONS

The Pedagogy of Laughter

James McKinnon

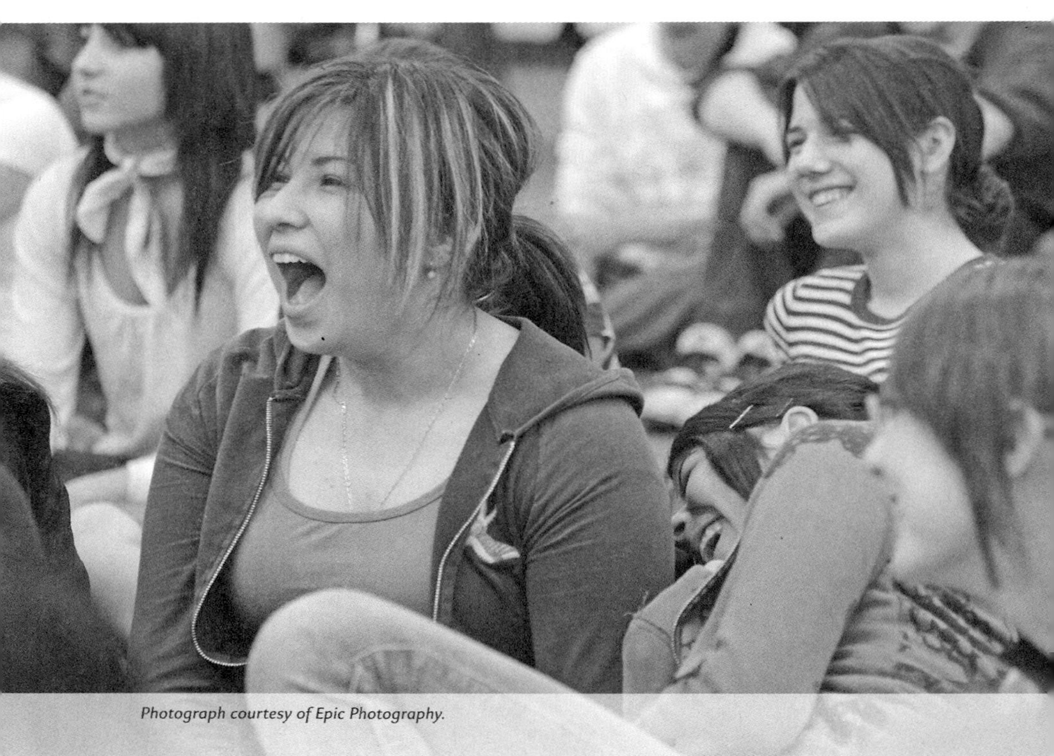

Photograph courtesy of Epic Photography.

Using cultural theory and insights from performance studies as well as the program assessment findings, James McKinnon investigates audience response and the role of humour within the play.

> *Like, it was funny, not just, like, you know, boring old adult saying, like, just giving you the facts and stuff...Yeah, it was, I liked it.*
>
> —AUDIENCE MEMBER

IN A SCENE IN THE 1980S FILM *War Games*, a biology teacher asks students to show they have done the assigned reading, asking, "Who was the first to propose asexual reproduction?" The question provokes a flurry of whispers and a localized eruption of laughter. The teacher detects the source of the laughter—a student played by Matthew Broderick—and tries to make an example of him, repeating the question: "Who was the first to propose asexual reproduction?" Broderick's character, David, replies: "Your wife!" Now the laughter explodes throughout the classroom, and the humiliated teacher punishes the student's ignorance with a trip to the principal's office.

In fact, as will become evident later, David's jest actually suggests evidence of learning, not ignorance, but for the moment I cite it as an example of why many teachers work to maintain a serious learning environment: because laughter is considered disruptive, antisocial, and mocking. As Michael Bristol (1989, 125) points out in *Carnival and Theatre*, serious writing about laughter throughout the Western critical tradition typically connects it to "what is socially and intellectually low and commonplace" and thus opposes it to learning; laughter privileges "logical contradiction and equivocation," and, as such, it "appears to be incompatible with philosophical statements," that is, "serious" thought. Where there is a strong cultural association between learning and seriousness, laughter signifies an absence of seriousness, and therefore implies the absence of learning. In addition, seriously inclined philosophers generally take a dim view of laughter because it is associated with emotions, passions, and thus the base, earthly, mortal, and degenerate aspect of humanity. From the perspective of Platonic, Christian neoplatonic, and rationalist discourses, laughter signifies an embarrassing loss of self-control or at best a regrettable symptom of the venting of dangerous passions (a sort of emotional flatulence, so to speak). Laughter represents a lapse into sensual pleasure, and thus the failure of both external and internal authority: a breakdown of discipline and the failure (both individual and collective) of rational order. Medieval theologians debated whether Jesus laughed, and whether, therefore, laughter should be considered godly and unique to humanity, or a base, animal impulse.[1] Finally, while authority (religious, moral, and otherwise) sometimes tolerates laughter insofar as it serves to point out the "aberrations of...sinners and the deformity of their sin" (Bristol 1989, 126), this kind of laughter is not often sanctioned in classrooms because of its negative, scornful character, which can be harmful and stigmatizing to its target.

Readers who have experienced such corrosive and disorderly laughter in the classroom may therefore be surprised by the consistently positive acknowledgements of laughter in accounts of *Are We There Yet?* cited in this book. No one expects sex ed to be funny, least of all when it happens in a junior high school. Sex ed classes are often viewed with dread and apprehension by students and teachers alike; a *Globe and Mail* article neatly evokes the collective mortification that prevails in such an environment: "Traditional sex education has long been a source of squirm-inducing torture for young people, who are forced to listen as their phys. ed. teacher explains the location of fallopian tubes and who rarely get up the nerve to pose any embarrassing personal questions" (Agrell 2008). If this description evokes personal memories, you may be doubtful that humour could facilitate adolescent sexual health education. In fact, the atmosphere of dread, embarrassment, shame, and fear is exactly why a humorous approach to sexual health education is not just possible but, I argue, absolutely necessary. In this chapter, I show why commonplace notions of laughter as a sound signifying the opposite of learning are wrong, and how laughter and humour are not corrosive to learning but indicative of it and conducive to it. Using Mikhail Bakhtin's theory of laughter, I show how conventional practices of sex ed work against learning, and by focusing Bakhtin's critical lens on AWTY I show how laughter is not merely a benign byproduct but a vital constituent element of the learning experience.[2] Moreover, I use the spectators' own responses to prove it!

The prevalence of laughter throughout performances of AWTY is not only observed by performers and health educators but also firmly established in the qualitative and quantitative data gathered by the team of social science researchers studying AWTY: both the students and their teachers frequently mention laughter in interviews, and 92 per cent of the participants agreed that they enjoyed the humour in the play. So we know that almost everyone finds the play humorous and enjoys the humour.[3] The more important question is whether the humour actually supports learning, and here, too, the findings are clear: while AWTY generally produces positive results in all the areas measured by the researchers (for example, improvements in communicating about sex, communicating sexual boundaries, confidence in one's ability to say no to sex, sexual behaviour and self-efficacy), its effects are strongest in participants who enjoyed the humour.[4] Participants who enjoyed the humour also felt more comfortable with the material. In other words, humour is not indicative of mockery, mischief, or a failure to pay attention, an assumption often made by teachers who act instinctively and aggressively (and to the chagrin of the actors) to surveil and discipline students who appear to be having fun, or cutting up. Rather, students who find the play funny are also more significantly affected by it.[5] In AWTY, comedy correlates with efficacy.

But how? After all, this finding flies in the face of traditional understandings of laughter, particularly in the classroom. The first-hand experience of students and teachers alike confirms the traditionally suspicious view of laughter described above: laughter in the classroom often does signify something other than attentive learning. Laughter may indicate harmful, negative mockery of a classmate, the subject, or the teacher; it can signify distraction and diversion from the lesson at hand; and in either case it reflects an antisocial, rebellious impulse, an attempt to subvert the learning environment. Therefore, in order to preserve the sanctity of the learning environment, to maintain their own authority over the classroom, and to protect themselves and students from scorn and mockery, teachers often discourage laughter, sometimes by stigmatizing students themselves. Most students shun the label of classroom clown. So how do laughter and humour work positively to stimulate learning in AWTY.

To be fair, not all serious thinkers view laughter as corrosive. Recent research demonstrates many positive impacts of humour on psychological, physiological, and social health, linking laughter to improved respiratory activity and oxygen uptake rates, lower blood pressure, and immunity (Mooney 2000). Humour is also known to lessen feelings of anxiety, fear, anger, frustration, and pain (Boyd and Hunsberger 1998), has been identified as a "means of enabling communication, fostering relationships, easing tension and managing emotions" (Dean, Kinsman, and Gregory 2005), and may even be an integral aspect of spirituality (Johnson 2002). However, none of these therapeutic constructions of laughter explains a positive correlation with learning.[6] For this we turn to the work of the influential Russian sociolinguist Mikhail Bakhtin (1981, 23), who associates laughter with freedom and discovery:

> *Laughter has the remarkable power of making an object come up close, of drawing it into a zone of crude contact where one can...examine it freely and experiment with it. Laughter demolishes fear and piety before an object, before a world, making of it an object of familiar contact and thus clearing the ground for an absolutely free investigation of it. Laughter is a vital factor in laying down that prerequisite for fearlessness without which it would be impossible to approach the world realistically.*

There is perhaps no context more suitable to illustrating how laughter dispels fear and enables free investigation than that of the conventional sex ed classroom: the mortifying effects of fear and piety are clearly evident in the (perhaps caricatured) lesson sketched out in the *Globe and Mail* article cited above.

The fear will probably be more evident to readers than the piety. We all know, because we can all remember, that the newly or not-quite-yet sexual body is a source of (literally) visceral fear and abjection for the adolescents who inhabit it. For some of our audience members, sex has already been a source of shame or trauma; for most, it is an aspect of life that is said to be universal (and that certainly saturates the culture in which they live), but from which they have thus far been excluded (or protected). Sex is unknown to most, but apparently inevitable. Ironically, among all the subjects taught in school, it may be the one that students have the greatest anxiety about failing: most fourteen-year-olds have figured out that one can succeed in life without mastering trigonometry, but no one wants to fail at sex! Yet few adolescents have a clear idea of how to succeed. Even those with direct knowledge, when they look back on adolescence as adults, will be very unlikely (and if so, very unlucky!) to wax nostalgic about having the best sex of their lives in grade nine.

Most adolescents are terrified of what they don't know about sex but also of asking questions that might reveal their ignorance, since sex-saturated popular culture makes it seem like everyone should know by now. Nor are teachers immune to such fear. Even after sexuality has been disarmed of some of its terrifying mystique by experience, for many adults the human body remains a site of shame, embarrassment, and mystery. Teachers are no more confident than the general population about their sexual expertise, nor are they likely to be comfortable sharing it with their students, whom they regard as children. For the teacher, as much as for the students, there is a terrifying risk of misspeaking, of revealing one's ignorance; pity the sex ed teacher who is corrected by a thirteen-year-old on a matter of sexual anatomy, and thus compromising one's status and authority in the classroom, which is after all based on the notion that teachers know what students need to know.

This is where the piety comes in. Not religious piety necessarily (although this is invoked in some abstinence-based sex education programs); there is a kind of piety at work in medical and scientific discourses about sexuality too.[7] Science and medicine, like religion, are privileged paths to knowledge that distinguish themselves from common-sense ways of understanding the world by their specialized, complicated (and typically Latinate) language. Most of us accept science and medicine, again, like religion, on faith, because while we accept the principles of empiricism and reason, most of us lack the resources to their lofty claims: very few of us can say that we know diseases are caused by invisible animals, or that the sudden alarming appearance of pubic hair is a result of certain changes in our internal chemistry. Because science and medicine are privileged fields, scientific language dignifies whatever it speaks of as worthy of rational inquiry, and mundane things are exalted by their grandiose, official Latin names; a common cold is no excuse to take a day off, but if you call in sick with a rhinovirus, your boss might beg you to stay at home.

This elevation of the mundane by official language is an integral part of most sexuality education; indeed, in some cases sex ed seemingly consists of nothing more than learning to explain how babies are made in Latin. As discussed elsewhere (see Chapter 2), the first generation approach to sex ed was based on the futile hope that transmitting clinical facts would stimulate behavioural changes that would result in fewer unwanted pregnancies and lower incidence of STIS (Hubbard, Giese, and Rainey 1998). By focusing on technical knowledge and using serious, official language, such programs attempt to mitigate the awkwardness and embarrassment of talking about the sexual body by conceptually dissecting it into anatomical segments and explaining it in abstract, Latinate language. Teachers and students alike embrace this scientific jargon because it neutralizes the unruly, messy potential of the adolescent sexual body by reconstituting it in sterile technical terminology, which (both because it signifies scientific authority and because it is essentially foreign) mitigates shame and embarrassment: to discuss sexuality in terms of progesterone, testosterone, gonads, and zygotes is to distance ourselves safely from it. But using scientific language to sterilize the bawdy body actually exacerbates students' fear and anxiety: explaining puberty, reproduction, and sex in abstract Latinate jargon does not address students' fears about real events in the material world; it directs their attention elsewhere. The sexual bodies we speak of in the discourse of sex ed are objects of piety, belonging to an exalted, abstract realm that has little to do with real bodies in the real world, least of all our own.

Later approaches, which included a firm (and equally serious) message (e.g., abstinence only or always use a condom) have proven no more effective, and to the extent that they attempt to sidestep embarrassing discussions about prophylaxis by instilling terror (of disease or the shame of unwanted pregnancy), these approaches, too, exaggerate rather than dispel the aura of fear and mystery around the subject of sexuality. Moreover, using scientific discourse only adds to students' anxieties by associating mastery of the body with the mastery of an arcane terminology. When I condescend to explain your own body to you, using privileged language and terms of my own choosing, and to evaluate your mastery of your body by testing whether you can master the vocabulary I have given you, I am essentially telling you that I know more about your body than you do: an act of appropriation, more or less. Thus, the explanation that sex ed offers to adolescents comes at a price, requiring that they submit their will and even their bodies to the discourse, agenda, and priorities of the curriculum. Ultimately, conventional sexual education programs, whether based on transmitting knowledge or moral dicta, attempt to control and contain the dangerous sexual body by constituting it in sterile, clinical, or moralistic language. By neutralizing the unruly teenaged body with clinical jargon, explaining sexual desire as the uncontrollable outcome of chemical imbalances (or original sin), and focusing on the myriad negative and stigmatizing outcomes of sex, conventional sex ed practices exacerbate the problem, which is not that teenagers do not know the location or function of fallopian tubes, but that they are too fearful, anxious, and embarrassed to talk about sex.

This is the fear and piety that laughter can dispel. Fortunately, the topic of sexuality lends itself well to laughter: as Bakhtin points out, the scatological and reproductive aspects of the human body, "the lower bodily stratum," to use his euphemism have always formed the very basis of comedy (Bakhtin 1984, 23). From the ancient Greeks and Romans, to Rabelais and Shakespeare, to Chris Rock and Tina Fey, comic language, imagery, and action have been rooted in the unruly, uncontrollable, messy aspects of the human body (if your familiarity with Australian slang is causing you to snicker, it only proves my point; if not, ask an Australian what root means). Indeed, the extreme liability of sex to comic appropriation is the very reason that conventional sex ed emphasizes abstract technical jargon. Both the characteristically dry, serious tone and the focus on abstract information and general knowledge about the human reproductive system, typically presented through set lectures, films, and abstracted diagrams and visual aids, reflect the general desire (of all parties) to prevent uncontrollable eruptions of laughter. After all, laughter is dangerous in this context, because everyone lives in fear of becoming its target. (I like to think repeated exposure to this kind of laughter throughout my teaching career has immunized me, but then again I have never had to teach grade nines how to use a condom.)

However, as we have seen, effective sexual health education (i.e., that which leads to safer behaviour) requires the ability to conquer this fear in order to discuss the topic freely and confront its material aspect, not merely to master the abstract discourse of general anatomy. During a performance of *AWTY* that I witnessed, the students demonstrated the extent to which fear and anxiety drive their sexual decision making. During the scene between Marcel and Delphi, the audience is asked for advice on how to resolve a conflict based on different comfort levels with sex. The students who spoke were unequivocal: break up!

A knee-jerk adult reaction to this response might be to punish the students for not taking it seriously.[8] But they were. For many people the mere prospect of discussing sex with a partner is so mortifying that they will go to great lengths to avoid it, even if it means breaking up, having unsafe sex, or oscillating wildly between extreme caution and utter recklessness.

Conventional sex education produces poor results because it has no answers for this fear: cross-section diagrams of the uterus, grainy films about hair down there, and relentless assurances that only condoms/abstinence will protect you from disfiguring diseases/shame/damnation are useless to someone who is being pressured into an experience he is not ready for, or who feels so terrified about botching the purchase (let alone application!) of a condom that she would rather just hazard unsafe sex, or who feels constant anxiety about how a decision to have or not have sex will arouse the derision of his or her peers. The teens' comic response is not trivial; it is a collective recognition that, absurd though it may be, Marcel and Delphi's dilemma is very common: many couples do break up because they cannot openly discuss sexual conflict, adult as well as adolescent.

The rarefied discourse and vocabulary of sex ed is useless here: abstract concepts and jargon do not help us grapple with the messy, material realities of sexuality. So instead of describing sex in abstract terms, *AWTY* brings the participants back into what Bakhtin (1981, 23) calls "crude contact" with sex, using the driving analogy to create an alternative vocabulary for discussing it. This vocabulary, no less than the official discourse it replaces, is euphemistic; but its euphemisms are rooted in the immediate, material world:

> *The engine* (points to heads)*: the control centre, everything is routed through here including the gas pedal and the brake pedal. Signal lights* (mouth)*: to signal to others when you want to slow down, stop or change direction. The windows and mirrors* (ears and eyes)*: must be kept clear to hear and see incoming messages and signals. Other standard equipment includes: headlights* (breasts)*, gearshift lever* (boy parts)*, glove compartment* (girl parts)*, and various other knobs, buttons, dials, gauges, etc., scattered through the vehicle* (whole body sweep). *(Chapter 3, page 70)*

In contrast with the opaque discourse of sex ed, which maps the sexual body with unfamiliar Latinate toponymy/taxonomy, this transparent analogy brings the body back down to earth, using common, familiar language to create "a zone of crude contact where one can finger it familiarly on all sides, turn it upside down, inside out, peer at it from above and below, break open its external shell, look into its centre, doubt it, take it apart, dismember it, lay it bare and expose it, examine it freely and experiment with it" (Bakhtin 1981, 23). Like conventional sex ed, AWTY offers participants a special language, but it is one that makes the subject more familiar, not less. In addition, whereas elite discourses are exclusive, the AWTY metaphor is inclusive: it invites the participants to appropriate and experiment with it. One student's response indicates how important this is:

> *Um, we, there was a lot of discussion after the play and a lot of it was kind of like, people joking around about the driving analogy, stuff like that. You could hear in the halls, everyone talking about driving, and stuff like that...which was pretty good, cause then you know that they were listening.*
>
> *—Audience member*

This student's comments suggest that she or he and other students continued to engage with the play's material long after it was over, investigating sex and sexuality on their own terms, in their own language. In contrast to scientific discourse, which controls them, they control it. They may even use it as a point of entry to initiate their own awkward conversations. Unlike conventional sex ed discourse, the vocabulary used in AWTY can be used to facilitate meaningful discussions about sex in real life. Laughter here will be important too: if a participant can later use this crude vocabulary as a comic icebreaker that makes a difficult discussion easier, he or she will have learned something much more useful than, say, the chemical composition of semen.

The humorous driving analogy dispels fear and piety by supplying students with a common vocabulary that brings sex back down to earth and into crude contact. The laughter that accompanies this discovery performs another critical role: it creates community. Each student arrives at the performance with a complex of fears and anxieties that they are certain are theirs alone. The sound of collective laughter tells each participant that in fact their concerns are shared by everyone, which dispels the fear that one is different or alien. Here is a participant commenting on the significance of the collective, communal aspect of laughter:

> *It helped me because before I was really shy about the whole thing. Now that everybody else could laugh about it, I can laugh about it too, and that makes me*

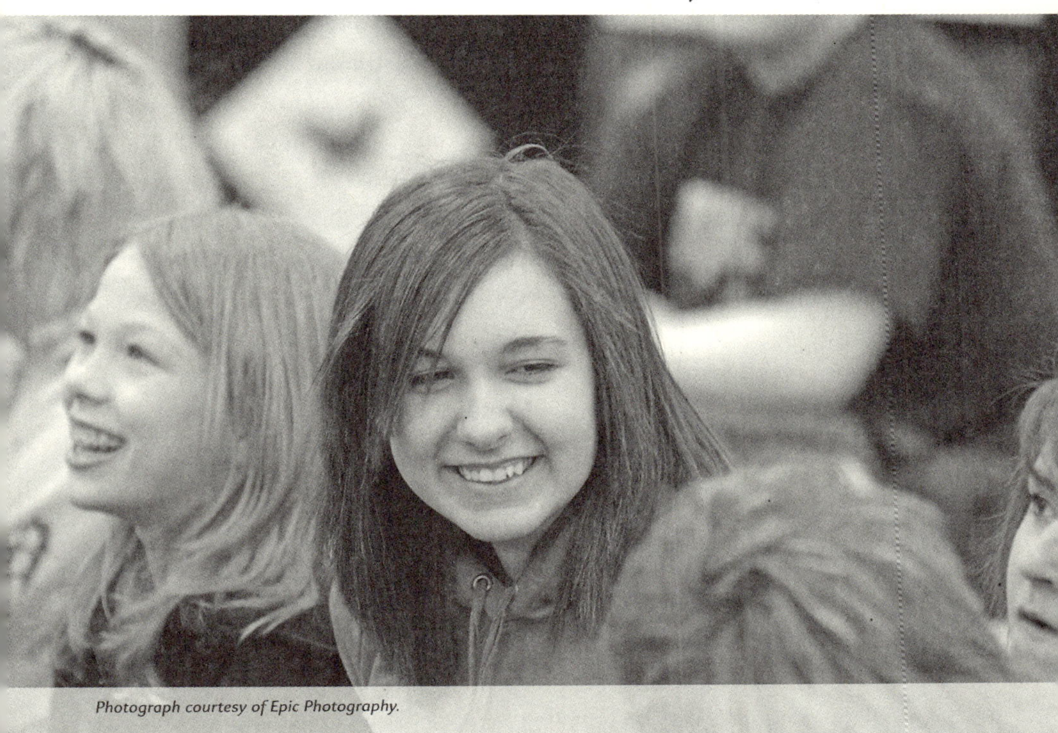
Photograph courtesy of Epic Photography.

feel confident about going into that kind of situation.

—Audience member

The respondent explicitly connects laughter to the confidence (or fearlessness) that Bakhtin claims is the prerequisite for free investigation. His or her claims about everybody else are not only supported by quantitative and qualitative findings, they are immediately and objectively apparent, or rather, audible, to everyone in the room. The sound of laughter permeates the theatre, making the audience keenly aware of their common experience and common problems. This recognition of shared experience allows the play's effect to carry on into the school hallways after the play is over. Laughter constitutes a collective recognition that the fear of being found out as ignorant is shared by everyone. And if so, then there isn't actually any need to fear at all: if everyone is equally ignorant, there is nothing to fear, no need to be shy.

Although I have thus far focused on the fear and piety associated with educational/scientific discourse, a language explicitly parodied in the section of the play that evokes the cheesy film host of sex ed movies sponsored by official culture, *AWTY* also brings the exalted images of popular culture back down to earth and into familiar contact. In Lesson Three, (Chapter 3, page 77) the play deploys the driving metaphor to debunk cultural myths that romanticize and idealize the first time. As their phony names imply, Studley Muffin and Creamy Delight represent a pop culture myth: in reality, no one just instinctively knows how to do it, and that first sexual experiences are very rarely spontaneous and wonderful, and very often fearful, anxious, and hazardous. By lampooning the cultural myth of first sex as wonderful (or even good), the play allows the participants to recognize that they needn't feel anxious about living up to it, because no one ever does.

Similarly, the Clay section toward the end of the play allows students to come into crude contact with popular cultural stereotypes of ideal masculinity and femininity. First, the boys and girls each get to create their ideal fantasy member of the opposite sex, and then each group gets to bring their counterpart's fantasy back down to earth. Both the invitation to fantasize and the subsequent tune-up or realignment generates abundant laughter.[9] Finally, the groups guide their characters through some important crisis moments: meeting, arranging to go on a date, and dealing with a potentially serious sexual conflict. There are no wrong answers. Deliberately bad suggestions, made for the purpose of eliciting laughter, are taken seriously, so that the other group can respond as they would in real life if someone proposed something inappropriate or foolish to them, which, at some point, will almost certainly be the case. If the scene reaches a dead end because of a deliberately dumb suggestion, the characters simply reset, with the help of the audience, until they reach a resolution everyone is happy with. The Clay section exemplifies Bakhtin almost literally, bringing cultural myths down to earth and into "a zone of crude contact where one can finger it familiarly on all sides, turn it upside down, inside out, peer at it from above and below, break open its external shell, look into its centre, doubt it, take it apart, dismember it, lay it bare and expose it, examine it freely and experiment with it" (Bakhtin 1981, 23). The laughter in the Clay section exemplifies an important aspect of the show, as pointed out by performer Ryland Alexander: "The humour comes from the participants themselves and is not entirely written into the play" (Alexander, interview, September 27, 2010).

Rather than being led to the truth by a teacher or authority figure, participants discover laughing matters in serious situations, and the actors take their suggestions and feed them back. The lesson is not dictated, as in conventional classrooms (and indeed conventional theatre) but dialectic, and knowledge is not transmitted—as per commonplace assumptions about what teaching is, still held by many teachers[10]—but constructed by the learners themselves. Alexander describes an example that recurred in many different performances:

> *The amount of times that someone suggested that I put on a condom before my date came over...was staggering. I would then turn the suggestion around on them to let them see the ridiculousness of the situation. I would say something to the effect of okay, so I wake up, have a shower, dry off, put on my socks, put on my condom, put on my underwear, then...etc. Of course I would get a chorus of no from the audience. But until they [see] their suggestions fail, they won't change their views.*

This scenario exemplifies the dialectic of laughter: the performer and the audience experiment with what would happen if we took the knowledge transmitted in a sex ed lesson as sufficient and complete information. After all, the instructions on a condom wrapper (and some sex ed regimes) imply that all we need to do is put on a condom before sexual intercourse. By playfully discovering what happens if we follow the instructions to the letter, the performers and participants discover what happens when knowledge is substituted for learning. Learning is not transmitted (e.g., through the dictum, put on a condom before sex), but constructed through experimentation, laughter, and crude contact.

Discovering laughing matter in sex brings it down to the material plane, dispels the fear around it, and builds the confidence that students need in order to practice safe sexual behaviour (see the health belief model, explained in Chapter 2). The student quoted above makes this connection explicitly clear, "I can laugh about it too, and that makes me feel confident," and this claim is echoed by the quantitative results. After the AWTY Program, students are more confident about talking about sex and asserting sexual boundaries for themselves. One unexpected finding emerging from the study is that while confidence about sexual communication and decision-making skills increased among students who reported being sexually inactive, it decreased among students who reported being active sexually. This doesn't mean that the play erodes the self-confidence of sexually active students; rather, it means that for sexually inactive students, the play demystifies and disarms sex, while sexually active students discover, first, that maybe they aren't doing as well as they thought, and second, since no one else is perfectly confident either as the collective laughter makes evident, it is okay to admit the same about oneself.

Joking about serious topics is often scorned as dumbing it down or willful ignorance, but in fact what Bakhtin calls "coming into crude contact" with the exalted increases self-efficacy precisely by revealing that it is the aura of seriousness, not the topic itself, that makes sex seem so daunting. The play directly represents several of those dreaded situations that some students claim they would rather break up over rather than deal with, such as talking about condoms or sexual boundaries with a partner, and when spectators see, first, that both partners are equally terrified and, second, that even the most awkward conversation is, after all, just an awkward conversation, they realize that talking about sex isn't really such a big deal.

> *I'd probably do what they did in the play and discuss it trying to find a comfort level that is comfortable for both of us. Before I saw the play I'd probably be really uncomfortable talking about that sort of thing but after seeing the play you realize it's not so bad, really.*
>
> *—Audience member*

Comments by participants suggest that laughter does indeed increase confidence and self-efficacy, precisely by making it okay to laugh in the face of these frightening topics. At the same time, the play gives them a useful tool by showing them how to use laughter to defuse a stressful situation.

There is, of course, a type of laughter that is not productive, that which singles out individuals for scorn or mockery, or seeks primarily to disrupt the learning environment. For example, in the vignette I described at the beginning of this chapter, David uses laughter to disrupt a lesson by willfully

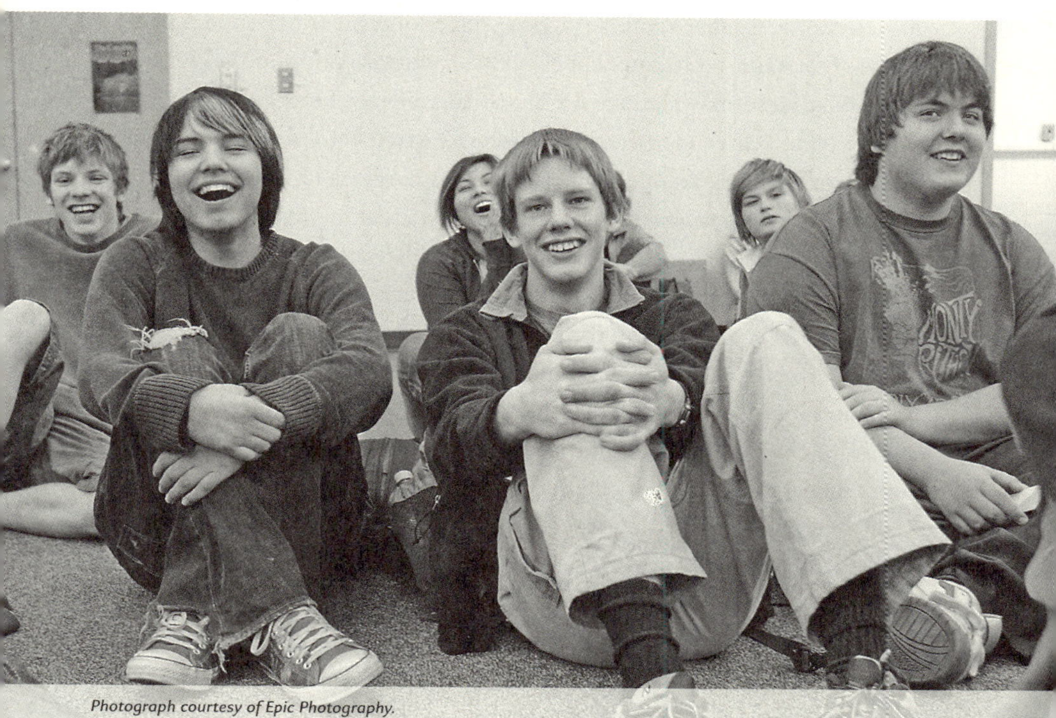
Photograph courtesy of Epic Photography.

misinterpreting the question about who discovered asexual reproduction. However, even this example, seen from Bakhtin's perspective indicates the connection between laughter and learning. First, David's quip reveals, far more efficiently than the teacher's probe, that the students did the assigned reading: their laughter at David's deliberate misinterpretation of "asexual reproduction" proves that they all know its "official" meaning. Second, as is often the case, the students' disruptive laughter reflects their awareness and resentment of the fact that the curriculum has priorities and interests quite different from their own. David has pointed out that what the curriculum expects them to know; "who was the first to..." has more to do with reinforcing the hierarchies that govern the classroom than with scientific learning.[11] The question reveals no knowledge about asexual reproduction; it merely implies that authority and status are based on proximity to knowledge. In other words, it reinforces the hierarchical structure that governs the classroom: the teacher's authority derives from being closer to the source of knowledge. When he attempts to display this authority by humiliating a student, the student shows that real authority derives not from knowing first, but from the ability to put knowledge to productive use. David uses the banal fact of asexual reproduction not to get credit on a test but to expose and resist the dubious legitimacy of classroom hierarchy. His trivial joke thus performs a complex metacognitive lesson (and increases his own social capital in the process). This example shows, first, how even negative laughter constitutes learning and, second, how, in the classroom, it often reflects students' resentment of lessons that serve teachers' interests more than their own.

In AWTY however, the laughter never makes individuals the targets of scorn or mockery. The laughter that prevails during the cheesy film host section, "Puberty and You," for example, acknowledges how sex ed represents adolescent bodies as shamefully undisciplined. As soon as the film host mentions a symptom of puberty, the subjects experience it quite suddenly and to their horror. In the first Clay episode, laughter mocks fantasies produced by popular culture. And while the students could disrupt the play during the participatory sections, they very seldom do.[12] There are several possible reasons for this, but the simplest is that they do not need to; to the extent that disruptive behaviour is an expression of resentment about lessons that don't meet students' needs, this resentment is pre-empted by AWTY because it invites the students to express their needs openly and often. In addition, the performers are not conventional authority figures, nor do they assert conventional authority. Instead, they try to earn trust by taking risks (especially in "Just a Minute," Chapter 3, page 68). In addition, suggestions and participatory comments are directed at the actor/characters, not spectators. Spectators are encouraged to yell suggestions spontaneously and simultaneously, and therefore anonymously.[13] No character or spectator is ever made the target of punitive or judgemental laughter, nor is any participant punished for making a bad or dumb suggestion (although deliberately offensive comments are not tolerated). Performances are generally free of negative laughter, and when the students are confident that no one will be mocked for their ignorance, they participate more, and participation, too, is strongly related to efficacy. Participants have reported that seeing the consequences of their bad suggestions played out in the sandbox mode of the fictional performance is both entertaining and edifying as in Ryland Alexander's example cited above.

Although AWTY possesses a few distinct characteristics not found in most learning environments, its deployment of laughter has broad pedagogical implications: connections between laughter and learning may be productively exploited in any educational setting. It is possible to force students to memorize technical language, names, and dates by impressing upon them the gravity and seriousness of a topic, but if the ultimate goal is to develop self-efficacy, creativity, and critical thinking, students need to make a direct, personal connection with the subject matter in order to recognize it as something familiar rather than exalted. Laughter is also helpful in creating a sense of community and common purpose, and the sense that those present in a classroom, students and teachers alike, are all working together toward a common purpose.

Laughter, in the context of sex education, is as fruitful as it is seemingly unlikely. With apologies to J.K. Rowling, to laugh at that which must not be named (i.e., sex, or the whole thing, as one participant puts it) is not disruptive to learning, it is learning—at least insofar as one hopes that what students will learn about sex is that it is a normal, healthy aspect of their lives that can and should be discussed openly. Laughter signifies that sex has been brought down to earth, where the students can grasp it on their own terms rather than through mystifying medical terminology, the prohibitive (and equally opaque) language of abstinence-based sex education, or the unrealistic, heteronormative, and heavily stereotyped myths consecrated by popular culture. Whereas fear and anxiety create rigid thinking (Break up!), laughter facilitates creative thinking and learning, and builds confidence in self-efficacy. Laughter, in this context, is the sound of students shattering the aura of fear and mystery around sex and coming into crude contact with it, on their own terms. This feeling of control, of being in the driver's seat, as it were, is not only the prerequisite for fearlessness and free investigation, as Bakhtin says; it is also the prerequisite for healthy, positive sexual behaviour.

NOTES

1. Umberto Eco depicts such a debate in his well-known medieval monastic mystery novel, *The Name of the Rose*.

2. Although the technically correct term is sexual health education, I use the term sex ed in this essay to refer generally to the common, though by no means universal, and largely ineffective practices critiqued by our researchers in Chapter 2.

3. There are some gender differences: both boys and girls claim that the play's humour was highly effective in making them feel comfortable and keeping them engaged. However, girls' focus groups often theorized that while the comic content supported their own learning, the boys were drawn into the silliness and took it less seriously. There could be some truth to this or it could simply be indicative of how girls and boys are differently socialized, with girls taking a more normative, suspicious view of humour, at least in regard to its effect on boys. Cultural stereotypes typically propose that females are the more irrational, emotional gender, but the girls' cool-headed observations of their classmates suggest otherwise.

4. If the data are analyzed without the small number of participants (~ 8 per cent) who did not enjoy the humour, positive change (and statistical significance) between pre- and post-treatment increases in every category.

5. One of our researchers observed with some irony that it was almost unfortunate that so few participants disliked the play's humour; their numbers are not large enough to constitute a statistically significant sample.

6. Although, from the perspective of Bloom's taxonomy (1956), humour is valuable because it stimulates the affective domain—we are more likely to retain information and incorporate it into daily praxis when it stimulates us emotionally, not just cognitively. But even this perspective views laughter as something like sugar coating on the bitter pill of information.

7. *Piety* proves a difficult word to define. Many dictionaries refer to it, unhelpfully, as "the act of being pious." But it clearly pertains to reverence and devotion, and thus it connotes an attitude of acceptance rather than questioning.

8. One of the challenges most frequently cited by the actors is authoritarian teachers bent on suppressing laughter and forcing the students to take the play seriously. The actors often must work to pre-empt or neutralize adult surveillance and discipline, and occasionally they encounter a group of students who have had the imperatives of good behaviour so thoroughly impressed upon them that they are reluctant to accept invitations to participate. Most teachers, however, enjoy it as much as the students do, and for those who are familiar with the show, it can represent a welcome break from the usual police work involved in teaching junior high school.

9. In practice, boys can contribute to the fantasy guy and girls can help construct the fantasy girl: the youth are tacitly but subtly encouraged to join whichever group they want.

10. See Ken Bain (2004) whose extensive study of key practices that distinguish the best college teachers shows that excellent college teaching is never based on the model of transmitting information, while mediocre teaching very often is.

11. Of course, privileged status for those who come first is not an anomaly of primary education but rather a ubiquitous cultural prejudice.

12. Or at least, I have heard very few reports to the contrary. The source of disruption most frequently cited by performers is overzealous policing by teachers, not misbehaving by students.

13. The act of uttering a suggestion is quite public, but the students are encouraged to utter their suggestions simultaneously, and the actors are only listening for the suggestions; they make no attempt to identify the individuals whose contributions are chosen. Moreover, many students will inevitably shout out very similar suggestions simultaneously. Therefore, individual participants can shout out contributions with relative anonymity.

11

REZ RIDES

Storytelling Revolution: Reaching Out to Aboriginal Youth

Tracy L. Bear

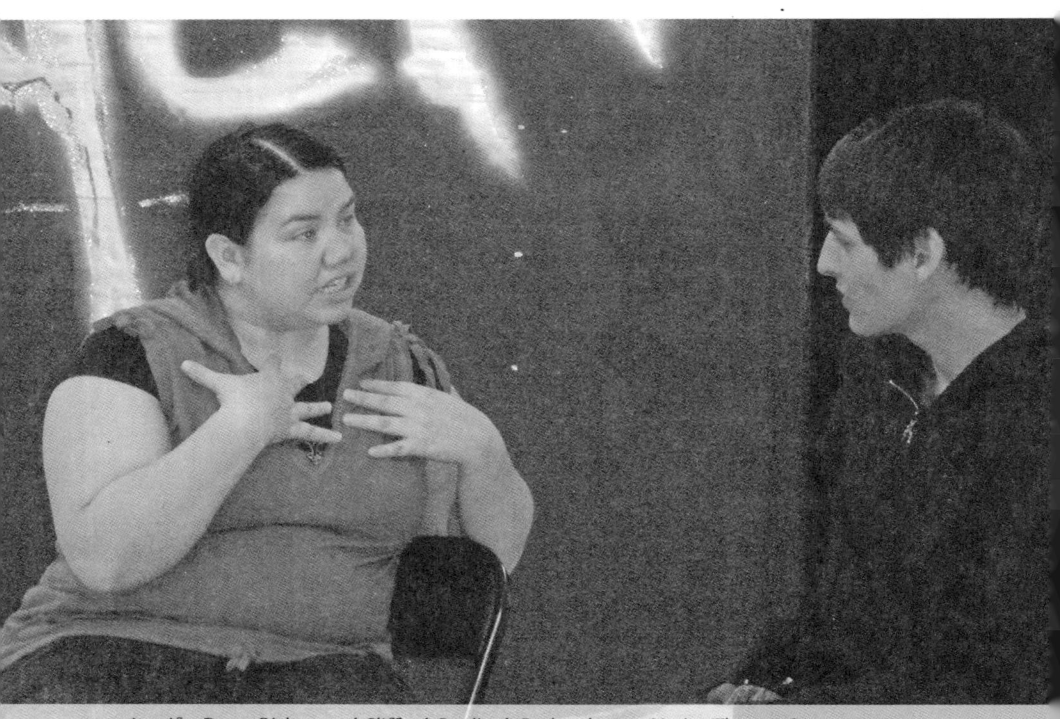

Jennifer Dawn Bishop and Clifford Cardinal, Saskatchewan Native Theatre Company.
Photograph courtesy of Jane Heather.

Tracy L. Bear reflects on quantitative and qualitative research into teen and adult responses to the Aboriginal adaptation of AWTY. She links these findings with theoretical, cultural, and experiential observations and discusses the impacts of culture on reception.

> *From a cultural point of view, I know as an Aboriginal woman growing up that you knew sex was dirty, it was bad, you did not mention it...Seeing kids having the freedom to be able to even just get into a gym and even have a play about sex, I think it's amazing.*
>
> —PARENT OBSERVER

SITTING ON THE HARDWOOD FLOOR of the gymnasium, I glance around at the many young Aboriginal faces. These faces reveal no emotion, these faces are almost hidden and are set deep within their oversized hoodies, many of them are plugged into their music. These grade nines have been informed that they will be watching a play about sex, and, while talking and joking about sex and sexuality is very much a part of everyday conversation with their peers, the simple mention of the word by any authority figure seems to bring about a morose and sullen silence. The music starts to blare and the four young Aboriginal actors (two women and two men) casually but confidently make their way into the throng of teens, chatting and getting a feel for the audience. A mere ten minutes into the ninety-minute play, the hoods slip off and reveal curious smiles. Their body language betrays them as they lean forward to listen intently. Teachers exchange knowing glances, recognizing immediately the telltale signs that their students are completely and utterly engaged. Such is the transformation of every student body that has the opportunity to experience the play *Are We There Yet?*

The appalling rise of HIV/AIDS and STIS within the Aboriginal populations of Canada has triggered a proliferation of sexual health programs and curricula, yet the statistical estimations of this vulnerable population remain bleak (Duran and Walters 2004). Standard or conventional methods of teaching healthy sex and sexuality continue to appear to have little or no effect on the health and safety of Aboriginal youth because barriers that are specific and unique to Aboriginal communities have yet to be fully addressed.

The qualitative and quantitative research analysis of the impact of AWTY and its accompanying health workshop clearly demonstrates this program's effective approach to educating Aboriginal teens and their communities about safe sex and healthy sexuality. The encouraging and powerful evaluation results within the Aboriginal population of Saskatchewan has prompted two investigations: an examination of the distinct issues and barriers that these communities confront when implementing sexual health programs, along with a corollary consideration of the relationship between participatory theatre and the oral traditions of Indigenous storytelling.

Examining the root causes that inhibit the success of sexual health programs in Aboriginal communities requires investigating the intergenerational effects of the historical trauma that continues to impede the progress of teaching and learning of healthy sexuality. Over the past five hundred years, Aboriginal people have endured a significant amount of change and transformation. Of course, civilizations constantly experience shifts and alterations. They grow, adapt, and evolve as circumstances change and situations arise. Language, culture, and societal beliefs are continually influenced by a host of dynamic forces. But not all change is beneficial. Nor does all change equate to progress. The brutal forces of religion, residential schools, and colonialism have been clearly devastating, and, consequently, their undeniable effects resulted in the current crisis in sexual health within Aboriginal communities.[1] Not surprisingly, attitudes of Aboriginal youth and their perceptions of peer norms and self-efficacy reflect how this cultural collision influenced the transmission and circulation of traditional sexual knowledge. Our history influences how we think about our sexual selves and how we convey knowledge about sex and sexuality.

Through stories and storytelling, Indigenous societies transmit essential knowledge critical to survival, and these stories provide a cultural framework for promoting happy, healthy communities. Literature reviews and personal interviews revealed a dearth of effective programs that encourage healthy discussions about sex and sexuality within Aboriginal communities. Aboriginal youth of the ages fourteen to sixteen are targeted with this participatory play and sexuality education workshop. At this age, the youth are first learning to drive, which coincides with increasing sexual awareness and curiosity. It can be argued that youth make life or death choices both behind the wheel of a car and in sexual activities. Employing the metaphor of driving provides an abundance of allegories and traverses the difficult topic of sex, providing a dialectical platform from which to begin to discuss these issues: When do I get to drive? What is driving like? How do I learn about drinking and driving, equipment of different models, and safety rules for the road? While casual observation of audience reaction clearly revealed that teens greatly enjoyed and participated in the play, our qualitative and quantitative data analysis confirmed our supposition that participatory theatre is highly effective in teaching healthy sexuality to teens. Situated within a research project that shows consistently positive quantitative results on the program's impact across three diverse Canadian settings, this chapter principally incorporates 2008 Saskatchewan qualitative data gathered from nine individual interviews and several focus groups. Data from 2007 research in Aboriginal communities revealed significant and interesting trends, which helped focus and guide the interviews with teens and parents for the 2008 research project.

I assert that the simple telling of a story, much like participatory theatre, is the most effective and dynamic method of knowledge transmission. The compelling qualitative and quantitative data demonstrates that this age-old method of learning through stories is still the most effective way to teach. While theatre in education and participatory theatre has gained in popularity as a powerful and innovative mode of knowledge transmission and education in recent decades, I would argue that these concepts of theatre have, in fact, been present for millennia and remain employed within the storytelling traditions of Indigenous peoples. While the custom of storytelling is not restricted to Indigenous peoples, it can be argued that many Indigenous societies value and rely upon oral tradition to a greater extent than Western societies. Unlike many Indigenous societies, which incorporate storytelling and performance to transmit knowledge, Western histories are primarily collected and disseminated through written text. Geraldine Manossa's (2001, 169) article "The Beginning of Cree Performance Culture" examines "the contemporary sociological significance between the viewer, writer and performer. The sharing of cultural knowledge though storytelling is something that occurred prior to contact and perseveres today and continues to shape the realm of Native Performance Culture." Indigenous peoples of North America, such as American Indians, First Nations, Métis, and Inuit, value orality as a means of communicating values and customs and to impart legacies, maternal and paternal lineage, laws, and traditions. Like the turtle depending on the currents of the sea, a prosperous life among Indigenous people hinged upon societies' ability to transmit knowledge from one generation to the next. Leslie Marmon Silko shares this sage advice: "I will tell you something about stories, they aren't just entertainment. Don't be fooled, they are all we have, you see, all we have to fight off illness and death. You don't have anything, if you don't have the stories" (qtd. in Washburn 2006, 115). Since the very first guttural utterances and gestures of our ancient human ancestors, communicating through storytelling has remained not just a cherished and universal practice but an integral element, ensuring survival. An extraordinary example of this intergenerational memory can be found within the Sami reindeer herders in Northern Europe who draw upon traditional stories and ancestral knowledge to identify animal migrations and understand ice and weather patterns (Couzin 2007, 1518).

Much like traditional storytelling, participatory theatre relies on story and personal interaction that includes an honest exchange of ideas and concepts; it is a process that demands genuine human interaction and open communication. Manossa (2001, 78) explains, "Both the listener and the teller are actively involved in the process of storytelling, an exchange occurs... storytelling is a time of sharing." Storytellers gauge the audience's reaction, and like the actors sizing up the mood of the room, storytellers instantly recognize the unspoken language of the body. This highly attuned sensitivity allows the storyteller to instinctively interact with his or audiences. The four Aboriginal actors who conduct themselves as storytellers in the Aboriginal adaptation of AWTY trained and developed extensive experience in audience interaction. The play relies upon the actors' ability to engage the audience and make that crucial connection. Much of the dialogue and forward momentum of the play relies upon this connection between storyteller/actor and the audience; the more engaged the audience becomes, the more powerful the interactions, and our measurements of changes pre- and post-participating in AWTY reinforce the importance of this involvement.

One difference between participatory theatre and storytelling practices is the nature of the reciprocal knowledge exchange and sharing. In participatory theatre, the audience is encouraged to interact overtly and to contribute to the movement of the story. In contrast, when traditional storytellers interact, they are the only ones aware of the dialogue that takes place between themselves and the audience; the conversation is happening, but it is a silent interaction. While the conversation or interaction may outwardly seem one-sided, silent gestures, facial expressions, body movement (or lack of it) defines the way the story unfolds. Like the actors, the storyteller adjusts the pace and timing of the story according to these reactions.

One of the most compelling and powerful examples of listener/teller interactions in the play is the culminating section, referred to as the "Clay" section (Chapter 3, page 88). Thoroughly warmed up and engaged by earlier parts of the performance, teens are divided by gender—females on one side and males on the other. At the start of this sequence, the two female actors preside over the male group while the male actors stand among the female students. The actors explain to their respective groups that they, the audience, are now sculptors and with the integral help of their input, the piece of Clay standing before them will be transformed into the guy or girl of their dreams. The enthusiasm is palpable; eyes flash and wry grins spread throughout the crowd as the girls think about the ultimate man and the boys focus on the perfect woman. The room fills with voices as suggestions hurtle from all sides. From the males' side of the room a voice bellows, "Big boobs!" And from the female side, "Lots of muscles!" Almost no idea goes unheard; evidently, this is not your conventional classroom, nor your conventional play. Ninety per cent of the students, when asked what their impressions were of the play, had a comment on the participatory aspect; this male student (2008 interview) shares his thoughts: "It was pretty cool how, like, you guys talked to the audience and stuff and got them to, like, decide what happened and everything."

The muscle request and breast augmentation are familiar suggestions, so much so that when the actors retreat behind the screen to change into their respective male and female ideals, a fake pair of breasts along with a body suit of phony foam muscles are already included in the costume collection. Once the fantasy Clay has been moulded, the Clay female is sent over to the female students and vice versa for realignments; the students have the opportunity to redesign the Clay into a more familiar model, to be someone they may know. Not surprisingly, each group has much to say, and, once again, students express their opinions and preferences. While two of the actors are carrying out student requests as Clay characters, the other two actors are on the sidelines coaching. These coaches are integral to meeting the audience's need for voice. Literally, these coaches are physically entrenched within the audience itself and are attentively listening to every voice in the audience, verbal and physical. This all-inclusive strategy allows all or most opinions to be represented, and, unlike many conventional classrooms, the quiet voices are given consistent attention and consideration.

Highlighting the Clay sequence in the play reveals significant connections between storytelling and participatory theatre. Much like the line between storyteller and audience, the interface between the students and actors has become blurred. The process becomes an interactive and dialectic journey whose inherent elements are dynamic and fluid. Student feedback through questionnaires and interviews reveal their appreciation for these alternative teaching techniques:

> *Yeah, it's funny. It brings out the funny part and, like, [when] we usually...talk about sex, it's always so serious. In like class, we always have to take notes and all that. We don't actually get out and, like, get involved in it.*
>
> *—Male student*

As this student points out, personal involvement and active participation in their own learning is important to today's students:

> *Think about how much easier it is about confronting this [communicating about condoms with a partner] and thinking better ways to work through things...They can see it in more of a 3D kind of way that you're like...this is ingenious...made me kinda see that the audience was really quite necessary to the whole thing.*
>
> *—Male student*

This student reiterates this sentiment and speaks specifically to his active participation:

> *But a play, it gets you into it, like how we had to basically create the perfect person for ourselves and that sort of stuff. That gets you way deeper into it because you're active then and you're thinking, "Well, how could I make this person someone I would like?"*
>
> *—Male student*

Participatory theatre encourages and allows students the opportunity to contribute to their own learning. The oral culture of storytelling remains the most reliable and trusted technique for learning and is often utilized for sharing an empathetic, communal association with experienced knowledge keepers. Walter Ong (2002, 78–79), in *Orality and Literacy*, speaks to this unification or connection between human minds, invoking Socrates:

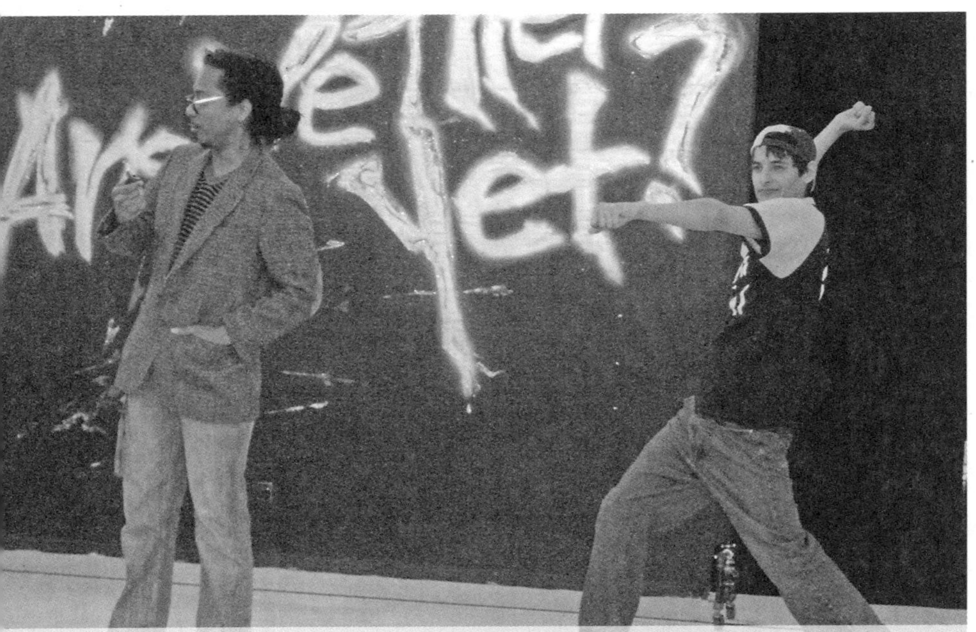

Arron Naytowhow and Clifford Cardinal, Saskatchewan Native Theatre Company.
Photograph courtesy of Jane Heather.

> *Writing, Socrates argues, is inhuman. It attempts to turn living thoughts dwelling in the human mind into mere objects in the physical world. By causing people to rely on what is written rather than what they are able to think, it weakens the power of the mind and of memory. True knowledge can only emerge from a relationship between active human minds.*

The AWTY Program embodies this relationship between active human minds that Ong speaks to; it is the lynch pin to its success. The storytelling model shown in Figure 11.1 demonstrates the intensive groundwork and the complex, rigorous consultative process that happens before any audience interacts with the finished product. While the actors work on the front lines of this knowledge transmission, it is crucial to mention that behind the scenes, the knowledge keepers also include a triadic partnership of the AWTY team at the University of Alberta, community-based Saskatchewan health professionals, and Saskatchewan Native Theatre Company (SNTC), which includes the playwright, artistic director, and the four Aboriginal actors as well as the company's cultural advisors.

Once the Clay people have been revamped (physically and mentally) to both groups' satisfaction, they embark on a new series of events. While students select their Clay characters' names, for the purposes of this chapter, the female is called Charm and the male, Chris. Like directors of a play, the students guide Charm and Chris through a series of life scenarios, beginning with their first encounter. Every aspect of Charm and Chris's relationship is decided upon by the students, from where they meet to their first words to each other. Away from the anxiety and tension of a real-life situation, students are the puppeteers who control and act out scenarios and conversations with a potential partner, helping them through difficult, shy, and sometimes embarrassing moments.

In an attempt to avoid teacher reprimands or authoritative involvement as well as create a safe and fun atmosphere, the actors request that all suggestions must be respectful and appropriate.

Coach A: While they're getting ready we can go over a couple of rules.
Coach B: Number One: Foul. No inappropriate suggestions or comments. You know what they are. (Chapter 3, page 89)

Although they are given these warnings, enthusiastic students have been known to use inappropriate language and/or behaviour, and Coaches use their whistles and call fouls. Fortunately, our audiences are generally self-regulating, as this particular example demonstrates. Saskatoon students had created the two characters and in their first meeting, the male students required that their Clay, Chris, introduce himself to Charm with an offer to "go smoke some weed." While such an inappropriate suggestion would be reprimanded in a conventional classroom, true to the integrity of the play's fundamental participatory philosophies, the actor complied. Chris swaggered up to Charm and in a slow, drawling voice queried, "Hey baby, ya wanna smoke some weed?" Adults need not have worried about the badly chosen suggestion, for the girls' retort was swift and merciless. "Dump his ass!" they yelled. Voices flooded the gym: "Say you're outta here, girl!," "What a loser!," and, "We want a different boy!" Under the play's normal circumstances, Chris and Charm's relationship progresses from this point; they fall in love, discuss condoms, and learn how to communicate about sexual boundaries. This unprecedented turn of events caught everyone off guard, and the talented actors were hard pressed to regain some semblance of order. Eventually, the boys begged for and received a second chance, a do-over. This instance provides a prime example of the power of true participatory theatre and the effectiveness of teaching youth about issues dealing with sex and sexuality. In the drama that unfolded, it was clear that everyone had a voice that had been heard; the actor playing Chris actively listened to the boys' suggestions and carried them through; the actor playing Charm actively listened to the girls' uncompromising answer (which then triggered Charm to shame and humiliate Chris). Finally, confirming their role as active listeners to Charm's (and by proxy the girls') response, the boys requested (and were granted) a second chance.

With apparent ease and effortlessness, the SNTC actors fully engaged with students within a very short amount of time, and while the dynamism of the music, the down-to-earth dialogue and intriguing theme facilitate this connection, we must acknowledge the influence of the powerful cultural tradition of storytelling. A large part of the success of *AWTY* within these Aboriginal communities stems from influential oral storytelling traditions. The prolific utilization of the metaphor stimulates imagination and elucidates concepts that may be difficult to understand or talk about; learning how to drive a car is a safer, more palatable topic than navigating sex and sexuality. This metaphor opens up dialogue, addresses teens' concerns, and gives them space to share their own stories and opinions about sex and sexuality. These participatory theatrical strategies mimic the enduring techniques of Indigenous storytellers. "Storytelling is about sharing the history and knowledge of the land, by recounting how since the beginning of time, we have interacted with it," says Manossa (2001, 178). In "The Artificial Tree," an article based on a five-year exploration, Floyd Favel Starr (1997, 83) defines Native performance culture as the "developing practices of our ancestors." Theatrical traditions are embedded within Indigenous cultures through stories, songs, and dances. Lee Maracle declares that "Anyone who has seen those story dances knows we have a theatrical tradition. Anyone who has watched Basil Johnston perform a story knows that the Ojibway have a theatrical tradition" (qtd. in Manossa 2001, 179). The young Aboriginal actors from SNTC who perform in *AWTY* come from varied backgrounds; some arrive directly from the reserve while others were born and raised in urban centres. Despite their background, SNTC's two programs, Circle of Voices (COV) and the advanced development training of the Ensemble Theatre Arts Program (ETAP), attempt to infuse cultural understanding along with artistic skill development. The actors' initial training in the COV and ETAP programs is the first step of many that prepared them for the *AWTY* production. Kenneth Williams (interview, 2010), the Aboriginal playwright who worked with original playwright Jane Heather on the adaptation, speaks of the journey of these Aboriginal youth into professional and participatory theatre actors: "They had always been led, and now they needed to be the leaders."

For many Indigenous cultures, the significance of storytelling extends far beyond mere entertainment; stories transmit crucial community/family historical knowledge. Qwul'sih'yah'maht (Robina Anne Thomas) speaks to the challenges facing historically marginalized voices in her article "Honouring the Oral Traditions of My Ancestors through Storytelling." Qwul'sih'yah'maht incorporates storytelling as a research methodology and proves the effectiveness of this burgeoning Indigenous epistemology as she utilizes the example of her naming ceremony as the legitimate documentation of reality and history (2005). Historically, criticism leveled by Western historians and archivists comes from the erroneous perception that oral tradition and oral history are mired within the muck of subjectivity and bias, unlike the traditional Western constructs of archival memory, which generate from written evidence and authentic record-keeping. In her book *The Social Life of Stories: Narrative and Knowledge in the Yukon Territory* (1998), Julie Cruikshank addresses the reservations surrounding the validity and consistency of oral history by questioning the reliability of Western European history, invoking Judith Binney's work with Māori oral narratives. Binney asserts that oral history's consistency of factual content outdistances Western European history, which exists only ten to fifteen years before being reinterpreted (Cruikshank 1994, 410). In "Maintaining the Reliability of Aboriginal Oral Records," Shauna McRanor (1997) specifies that Aboriginal voice be included as a legitimate and valid mode of knowledge transmission. Transmitters and keepers of oral history witness ceremonies such as a Tsimshian feast, Haida Gwaii potlatch, or a Qwul'sih'yah'maht's naming ceremony and receive payment for her duties. Such payment demonstrates the weighty responsibility of the witness for her transmission of knowledge as an accurate recording and legitimate documentation of the event. Despite the work of scholars and story keepers from many parts of the world, Qwul'sih'yah'maht continues to struggle against marginalization of her voice. Her resistance to Western ethnocentrism in the academic sphere is symbolic of the fight that oral historians confront. An epistemological paradigm shift is required for Canada to acknowledge and accept Aboriginal oral traditions and knowledge (1997, 76). Evelyn Wareham's article "Our Own Identity, Our Own Taonga, Our Own Self Coming Back: Indigenous Voice in New Zealand Record-Keeping" (2001) also challenges these tactics of silencing and advocates alternative strategies for the inclusion of the Indigenous voice. Unlike any other generation before, we face overwhelming and global influences of the dominant society, which seriously inhibit the retention of our Indigenous culture. This Māori respondent speaks,

> *Many of my children, our mokopuna (grandchildren) don't know their own history, and we don't have easy access to that knowledge because we haven't got kaumatua (elders) left who know it all and can teach us. We are trying very hard to recapture what we have left. It's really important...that information.* (Wareham 2001, 32)

The process of recapturing our stories and harnessing them for teaching opportunities blends well with the consultative process of oral narrative and participatory theatre. The participatory research-based adaptation period gave community members (advisors) a chance to comment on the play, provide advice, and voice concerns. One advisor shared her personal story of sexual assault to the artistic consultation team and relayed how she was able to speak with her community about her traumatic experience. The script changed to incorporate the advisor's story, and while the monologue previously had the character going to a sexual assault clinic, she now went and spoke with her Kohkum (grandmother). The inclusion of a Kohkum in the script has a strong impact on youth, especially when speaking of sexual assault of females by males. Many, if not all, Aboriginal societies highly regard the advice and opinions of Kohkums; co-playwright Kenneth

Williams concurs: "The best way to talk to Aboriginal male youth? Bring in Kohkum" (interview 2010). Further, this inclusion demonstrates the active ongoing process of directly linking the script with its primary audience.

The storytelling model in Figure 11.1 illustrates the dynamic processes of oral narrative traditions and storytelling and the parallel processes of community consultation as this participatory theatre piece developed. It demonstrates the circular movement of oral narrative traditions; the constant contextual reframing and retelling of stories reveal how stories can be used for healing and teaching. The foundational framework of participatory theatre, as practiced in the AWTY adaptation and performances, connects to Aboriginal storytelling traditions; this analogous connection has proven to lead to a remarkably effective method of teaching healthy sex and sexuality to Aboriginal teens.

Neal McLeod (2007, 68) states, "Stories act as the vehicles of cultural transmission by linking one generation to the next and there are many levels to the stories, and many functions to them; they link the past to the present and allow the possibility of cultural transmission, and of coming home in an ideological sense." Stories exist to simultaneously create structure and chaos, they also explain cultural and societal laws and outline invisible borders and unspoken rules. Embedded within stories are complex messages that are part of an interconnected whole. Since one story can have many purposes, the cultural pedagogical approach becomes determined by the audience. For children, some stories operate as urgent warnings or moral lessons, establishing cultural rules and laws. Unforgettable characters such as the evil, cannibalistic beast spirits of Thöxeweya, Windigo, and Quallupilluat haunt my dreams still. Long after the story ends, the blood sucking generations of Thöxeweya's offspring, in the form of the mosquito, continue to remind children of the dangers of staying out after dark. Stories of Quallupilluat speak to Inuit children about the dangers of venturing out alone on the sea ice. Intergenerational family stories also affirm our identities and have the potential to reaffirm and re-establish a sense a belonging to the land, to our ancestors. McLeod asserts that "Our contemporary task is to retrieve tribal narratives and paradigms and to reaffirm our identities in the face of overwhelming pressure of exile and colonialism" (2007, 68). While I agree with McLeod's contention that as Indigenous peoples we have a critical

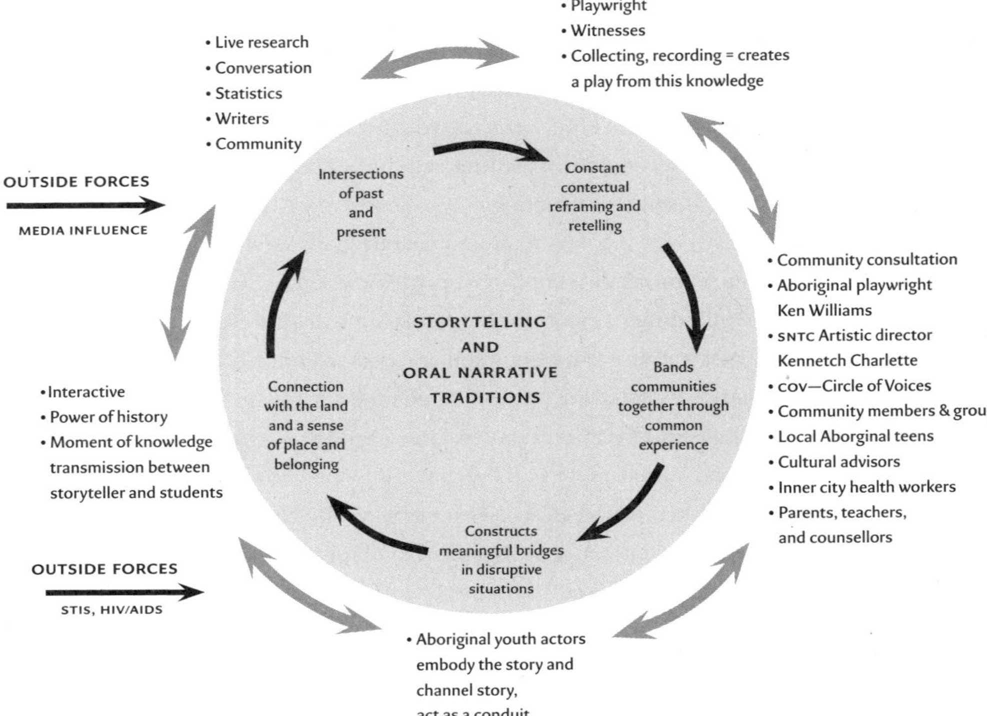

Figure 11.1 Oral Narrative Traditions: A Storytelling Model

responsibility for the retrieval of our stories and tribal narratives, I propose that this retrieval is much better described as a reclamation of our stories.

Seen as the progenitors of the current crisis in Aboriginal sexual health, the assimilationist and colonialist measures of the Canadian government have had tributary trickle down effects in our communities. *Emerging Answers*, a document on teen pregnancy and sexually transmitted diseases, contends that "There are many factors in young people's lives that affect their sexual behaviour; for example, their own sexual drive and desire for intimacy, their families' values, their friends' values and behaviour, their own attitudes and skills, the media, the monitoring of young people by their community, and opportunities for the future in their community emerge for years to come" (Kirby 2007, 7). In keeping with this widely held view, an examination of the historical background of residential schools must be investigated to truly understand the changing attitudes of Aboriginal communities regarding sex and sexuality. Almost exclusively, in a horrendous and appalling respect, Canada's Aboriginal people were forced into a system of legalized subjugation and abuse under the guise of education and civilization. For over a century, until the last residential school, the Gordon Residential School in Saskatchewan, closed in 1996 (Assembly of First Nations 2009), the federal government encouraged the assimilation of the Indian child through legislation and funding. An infamous quote coined during the 1993 Royal Commission on Aboriginal Peoples expresses that residential schools were thought of as internment camps for Indian children (1996). Under threat of arrest and/or imprisonment, parents reluctantly acquiesced to the 1920 legislative demand of compulsory attendance for their children aged seven to fifteen. Several religious orders, including Anglicans, Roman Catholics, Methodists, and Jesuits, dedicated themselves with extraordinary zeal to "killing the Indian in the child."[2] Beginning in the 1980s, accounts from residential school survivors began to infiltrate the mainstream media, illuminating sickening and horrific stories of physical, mental, spiritual, and sexual abuse. On June 11, 2008 Prime Minister Stephen Harper, on behalf of the federal government of Canada, issued an official apology to the former students of the residential school system. He apologized for the removal and isolation of children from a rich and vibrant culture, their families, their language, and their beliefs. Following the public apology within the House of Commons, the Truth and Reconciliation Commission (TRC) was established in July 2009 to create a forum for survivors to tell their stories to begin a stronger and healthier future. The TRC mandate recognizes that "the truth telling and reconciliation process as part of an overall holistic and comprehensive response to the Indian Residential School legacy is a sincere indication and acknowledgement of the injustices and harms experienced by Aboriginal people and the need for continued healing" (2014b). Part of the healing process for many Aboriginal people is the acknowledgement of their experiences, their stories. "The truth of our common experiences will help set our spirits free and pave the way to reconciliation" (2014a); the words of Leslie Marmon Silko echo within this therapeutic storytelling tradition: "they are all we have, you see [stories], all we have to fight off illness and death" (2006, 15). Subsequently, on April 29, 2009, Pope Benedict XVI, expressed sorrow for the abuse suffered by Aboriginal people under the regime of residential schools; the Catholic Church was responsible for administering three-quarters of all residential schools across Canada. Many of the churches responsible for residential schools issued official apologies: the Anglican Church in 1993, the Presbyterian Church in 1994, and United Churches in 1998. It was not until 2009, however, that the Catholic Church, both tardy and tepid, acknowledged responsibility. The Church expressed sorrow, but did not apologize.

While residential schools and church ethos have played an integral role in the perversion of attitudes among Aboriginals toward sex and sexuality, we must also consider the consequences that stem from a succession of colonizers at early contact. Martin Cannon, in "The Regulation of First Nations Sexuality," outlines the array of gender roles and erotic diversity that existed within Indigenous societies at the time of contact with Europeans. Early journals from explorers and missionaries demonstrate a clashing of cultures, especially within the sexual realm, and their claims at this historical conjuncture came from a paternalistic perspective. Cannon (1998, 4) states, "Informed by notions of supremacy, ideologies of racial inferiority and of civilized (hetero) sexual behaviour, the early Europeans saw First Nations (indeed all non-Europeans) as subordinate and underdeveloped entities." The observations and consequent interpretations illustrated in journals and reports spewed forth by British, Spanish, and eventually French colonizers must be understood within the context of their specific sexual culture. In an excellent example involving Cortez, author Vicki Jaimez illustrates how the Spanish commodified and exploited Indigenous sexuality, utilizing native women of Mexico as a means to control the native chiefs (Jaimez in Hayden Taylor 2008, 2). The British also brought with them to the New World inconsistent values of Puritanical virtue and concepts of monogamous marriage/partnerships. These clashing ideologies have directly impacted Aboriginal families' abilities to communicate about sex and continue to reflect today's inhibitions and reticence in discussing sex and sexuality.

The critical need to deliver effective methods of teaching teens about healthy sexuality within urban and rural Aboriginal communities are clearly outlined in the numerous reports and statistics churned out monthly. Articles and texts dating back to the early 1990s call for immediate intervention and action from medical and health organizations and government. One study (Mill et al. 2008a, 2008b) comments that "HIV infection is a serious concern in the Canadian Aboriginal population, particularly among youth; however, there is limited attention to this issue in research literature." The Public Health Agency of Canada reports that Canadian Aboriginal persons are infected at a younger age than non-Aboriginal persons. With an estimated 30 per cent of persons with HIV currently unaware of their status, more information is needed about individuals who are at risk of HIV but have not been tested (2007).

A key strategy in preventing the spread of HIV in Aboriginal communities is the provision of accessible, confidential, and culturally sensitive testing services. In addition, for those who test positive, counselling programs to promote healthy behaviours in the period following infection is recommended. In order to focus prevention activities in the post-infection period, the factors that motivate individuals to have an HIV test and subsequently make decisions about their care and treatment must be investigated. Research is required on issues related to HIV testing in the Canadian population generally (Myers et al. 1999), and the Aboriginal population specifically. Even with these horrific statistics, I contend that another obstacle facing effective sex education is the provincial governments' inability or lack of proactive policies to update woefully inadequate and restrictive grade six to nine health curricula. Both the Saskatchewan and Albertan provincial websites reveal curricula that hasn't been updated for ten years.

Reflecting on best practices calls for an examination of the current sex education milieu. The Saskatchewan curriculum for grades six to nine for health education suggests that HIV/AIDS material be discussed in the following four categories: physical, social, and emotional needs; overcoming stigma; risky behaviours; and present and projected community response to HIV/AIDS (Saskatchewan Education 2009). However, to teach this unit, a school must acquire separate approval from the school division board. It is advised that the local health education liaison committee should be consulted to determine if these potentially controversial topics should be discussed within their communities. Further, the Saskatchewan Education website also states that an elective opting-out policy might be considered for more controversial units (2009). There are two distinct classifications within the curriculum guidelines: those areas that are required and those areas that are optional. Included in the required units for grade nine health curriculum are three topics: dating, chronic illness, and HIV/AIDS education. There are five optional units, but the unit that teaches abstinence, sexuality, transmitted diseases, pregnancy, and contraception has a heavy grey box surrounding the description; this is the only optional unit that must be approved by the school division board before teaching (2009). Ironically, Saskatchewan Education allows their students to learn everything about HIV/AIDS with the exception of how to make healthy decisions to avoid it. Sadly, like Saskatchewan, Alberta Education guidelines for grade nine health education are also more reactive than proactive.

The Canadian province of Alberta, where *AWTY* was first designed, deals with sexuality topics in its health and life skills curriculum. Changes to Alberta's legislation, Bill 44, which was passed in 2009, directly impacted the approach to sex education in schools. The following outcomes for grade nines are available to the general public online through Alberta Learning's website:

> W-9.11 use personal resiliency skills; e.g., seek out appropriate mentor, have a sense of purpose, have clear standards for personal behaviour.
> ***W-9.12 determine safer sex practices; e.g., communicate with partner, maintain abstinence, limit partners, access/use condoms/contraceptives properly.***
> ***W-9.13 identify and describe the responsibilities and resources associated with pregnancy and parenting.***
> ***W-9.14 develop strategies that address factors to prevent or reduce sexual risk; e.g., abstain from drugs and alcohol, date in groups, use assertive behaviour.***

Underneath the outcomes, Alberta Learning relays this message: "Please note that boldfaced and italicized outcomes contain topics related to human sexuality and that parents reserve the right to exempt their children from this instruction" (Alberta Learning 2009, 12). These particular outcomes (and any subject matter that deals with human sexuality) are indeed boldfaced and italicized as a result of Alberta's Bill 44, which gives parents and guardians the option of pulling their children out of class when lessons on sex, religion, or sexual orientation are being taught. A heated seven-hour debate occurred the night previous to the bill's approval, and while people from the gay and lesbian community declare the bill a travesty, Lindsay Blackett, the minister responsible for enacting the bill, states, "People of Alberta are better off for it and we had the courage to actually bring it forward" (qtd. in CBC News 2009).

School boards are legally bound to send parents and guardians a written letter whenever these controversial (but in this author's opinion, essential) topics will be discussed in the classroom. Parents and guardians then have the option of having their child removed from the class. Compounded by the fact that there remains a dearth of effective sexual health education programs that promote healthy communication, talking about boundaries, and the use of condoms to prevent HIV/AIDS, STIS, and unplanned pregnancies, this legislation is bound to have devastating effects on the Aboriginal population. Until recently, with the enactment of Bill 44, Canada's sex education has not been as stifling as most sex education policies in the United States. Many states enforce an abstinence-only curriculum, which has proven futile in eradicating the growing number of teenage pregnancies and STIS (Hubbard, Giese, and Rainey 1998).

The current attitude surrounding sex education in Canada obviously impacts the ability of projects like AWTY to create change. Well-meaning school administrations, teachers, and sexual health co-ordinators fully appreciate the urgency to teach their students about healthy sexuality but are often restricted by policy. The challenges encountered in booking the play and workshop of AWTY in northern Saskatchewan necessitates an exploration into the attitudes toward sex and sexuality within urban and rural Aboriginal populations. The schools that experience the play often request subsequent returns the following year. However, persuading schools that were new to the concept of teaching Aboriginal teens through participatory theatre to bring the play to their community was quite challenging. Often when speaking to the adults responsible for the education of Aboriginal youth, such as parents, communities, school administration, youth counsellors, and teachers, we receive a familiar response; they convey that their students don't respond well to learning venues where there is an expectation to participate. They insist that their kids are too shy or reticent to fully engage with such programs, especially when it pertains to sensitive topics like sex and sexuality. The scene described in the first paragraph of this chapter is not an anomaly; the deep connection of the students with the actors happens every time. By far, these knowledgeable parents and experienced educators are the most habitual and contiguous observers of these youth. Why do they anticipate such reservedness from a group of youth they probably understand better than anyone?

Are We There Yet? challenges preconceived notions about traditional teaching strategies pertaining to sexual health. Misguided perceptions of youth extend to the provincial/territorial governments as well as the federal government. This chapter contends that our Aboriginal (and other) youth are greatly influenced by societal forces that in turn have created a generation of worldly and sexually experienced youth. William Lindsay, an Aboriginal professor at the University of British Columbia, discusses his frustrations with the erroneous moral compass of those who would censure blunt, honest, life-saving information in his article "Gathering Dust Not Saving Lives: The Call for Texts Which Honestly and Straightforwardly Teach Aboriginal Children about HIV/AIDS and Other Important Issues." He states, "Young ones today thus know about sex and some, whether adults want to admit or not, [young ones] participate in it with little regard for the consequences. This is because movies, television programs, music videos, books, and the Internet all present sex as common, acceptable and risk free" (Lindsay 2007, 504). Lindsay's contract work with the provincial government included writing two texts to teach Aboriginal children in the BC school system about HIV/AIDS. While his texts were very well received within academic circles and seen as potentially award-winning, the final texts were rejected on grounds that they were inappropriate (506). Lindsay's discouraging experience offers an excellent illustration of Canadian society unwilling and/or unable to accept our youth's current level of sexual knowledge.

During the community-based development phase of the AWTY project and in individual interviews and focus groups with the play's participants, our research team asked if the play was age-appropriate for grade nines. Unequivocally, youth declared that the play would be beneficial to their younger peers. Although they understood that perhaps these younger students would not grasp the subtler nuances or metaphors within the play, all the students interviewed were in agreement. One student relates:

My brother, he's twelve and he's already curious enough. I'm like sitting in the kitchen and he starts asking mom about birth control and condoms and...his penis and what is it doing?

—Female student

Another student gives this advice:

Well, like [in] this community people get sexually active at quite a young age so it'd better be for, like, grade seven because that's when kids start really getting sexually active...in this town, so it'd be good just to get them, like...because we had a kid in my class who got pregnant in grade eight and she's out now and if she would have had I think more of this stuff, she would have been protected or she wouldn't have had the situation she's in now.

—Female student

Many teachers and parents are not in agreement with the interviewees' sentiment. Lindsay (2007, 505) laments that his inappropriate texts were rejected because "Adult readers did not like my candid descriptions about sexuality, condoms, needles, and the repercussions of HIV/AIDS." There is a large disparity in perceptions among educators, parents, and youth. In their extensive community action research study "Cognitive and Demographic Factors that Predict Self-efficacy to use Condoms in Vulnerable and Marginalized Aboriginal Youth," Shercliffe and co-authors conclude that any intervention program for at risk Aboriginal youth should target younger groups, especially those that have not yet experienced sex (2007, 53). In line with the participatory aspect of AWTY Shercliffe et al. further conclude that "Potentially useful methods to target and increase efficacy when working with Aboriginal groups could include such methods as role playing, and practicing skills" (53). Clearly, delivering truly successful programs and effective educational material for teaching youth about sex and sexuality must not only consider the input from a diverse base of knowledge and experience, but these knowledge transmitters must also possess the courage to be candidly honest in direct and accurate terms. To continue to do otherwise ensures serious and devastating consequences.

Aboriginal peoples' historical legacy with government and church results in a continued blanket of silence and shame that inhibits the transmission of healthy sexual knowledge. Students repeatedly demonstrate that they have extensive knowledge about how the use of condoms prevents pregnancy, STIS, and HIV/AIDS, but research and recent statistics reveal they aren't using them in real-world situations. Several studies reveal familiar explanations, and youth utilize the same justifications repeatedly as to why they don't use condoms; they report a loss of sensation, the embarrassment and silliness of condoms, condoms aren't readily available, condoms are too expensive, and, finally, they aren't able to communicate to their partner their wishes to use condoms. According to Brian Joseph Gilley (2006, 559) in his article, "'Snag Bags': Adapting Condoms to Community Values in Native American Communities," "Indigenous people have the lowest documented condom use rates." Gilley worked with two large HIV/AIDS awareness organizations in the western United States that distributed condoms in concentrated areas of Aboriginal people, places such as powwows, round dances, ceremonies, and other social occasions. The term *snagging* refers to Aboriginal or Native American youth who meet in these arenas and involve themselves sexually with one another on a non-committal and short-term basis. Trysts such as these obviously reflect a high risk for unplanned pregnancies, STIS, and HIV/AIDS, and are targeted by prevention programs. However, these HIV/AIDS field workers found that their booth at these cultural events was conspicuously avoided and any attempts at handing out condoms were met with great resistance (562–63). Gilley surmises that the cultural values within contemporary Native communities inhibits public displays or discussions about sexuality. He quotes an HIV counsellor: "The young people are more receptive to accepting condoms, but not in front of the elders. Adults, especially if they were raised by dominant Christian society, they don't discuss sex, they don't discuss condoms. It is a topic that is never brought up" (563). A workable and simple solution came about when the workers started putting condoms, lubricant, and STI and HIV/AIDS literature in a plain brown paper bag. These became known as "snag bags," and this story illuminates two important points: first, there is very much a cultural stigma attached to discussing or even acknowledging sex in a public arena; second, by considering the historical significance and cultural frameworks and by thinking outside the box, sex education programmers were able to find a simple solution to a previously perplexing problem.

The silence, shame, and stigma attached to discussing AIDS/HIV, STIS, unplanned pregnancies, and FASD (fetal alcohol spectrum disorder) prohibits open dialogue; people in small communities are suffering in silence with diagnoses of HIV/AIDS. They refuse to tap into valuable resources, including medication and mental health support, due to the stigma surrounding this devastating disease. Urban centres are also plagued with untreated cases; Saskatchewan Northern Inter-Tribal Health Association's communicable disease control nurse speaks to this population who suffers in silence.

Sometimes it's very difficult to convince people in positions of leadership or authority that the rates of STIS in their communities are real issues. Health educator Wendy McPhail commented,

> *We recently found out that in Saskatoon they had five deaths in six months all related to undiagnosed HIV. All those deaths were Aboriginal, they weren't even diagnosed... they had no opportunity to receive medication to extend their lives. They were somebody's children, living on the street, living who knows where...that to me is absolutely atrocious, how is this happening? (interview, 2007)*

Familiar with homophobic attitudes on and off reserve, playwright Kenneth Williams reveals, "Guys are sleeping and breeding as much as they can with anyone they can to prove they weren't gay" (interview, 2010). Aboriginal families are not alone; this cloud of shame and silence often surrounds both Aboriginal and non-Aboriginal communities and families alike when discussing sex and sexuality.

What are the factors contributing to this silence? Gilley's "Snag Bags" article outlines stigma attached to sex: "School administrators feared upsetting parents and the community with programs that dealt with sexuality and STDS in candid ways, while community members who felt strongly about pushing safe sex agendas were seen as being divisive" (563). Shame has traditionally been utilized as a way of managing community and cultural behaviour. This shame must be taken into account when creating and implementing sexual education and prevention programs. AWTY incorporates community meetings to challenge this vacuum of dialogue and discussion within the community. Snippets of the play are performed for the community prior to the play being delivered within the classrooms, and often this approach alleviates many concerns expressed by community members. Despite the proliferation of silences, AWTY generates much discussion and dialogue about the issues and challenges within the community with regards to sexual health and brings to the forefront an issue foolishly avoided by provincial curriculum.

In conclusion, and perhaps best stated by Suzanne Fournier and Ernie Crey (2006, 144),

> *Aboriginal children, regarded as the very future of their societies, were considered integral members of the family who learned by listening, watching and carrying out tasks suited to their age, sex and social standing. The economic and social survival of Indigenous societies depended on the transmission of a vast amount of spiritual and practical knowledge from elders to the young, through an exclusively oral tradition.*

Despite the many challenges of social and political barriers to teaching healthy sexuality to our Aboriginal youth, Are We There Yet?, an innovative and distinct program, has proven to be a significant and powerful influence on Aboriginal youth and their communities. The use of participatory theatre revolutionizes storytelling and transforms the way we convey knowledge. We share stories for countless reasons; they consist of cultural knowledge and tribal narratives that link the past with the present and the future. Indigenous communities use oral narratives to reaffirm identities, convey cultural rules and laws, and strengthen our sense of belonging to the land and our ancestors. Quite literally, our lives depend upon the stories we are told. Yet, in today's dangerous realm of sex and sexuality, we stumble with our words when we speak to our children. Kenneth Williams recalls an elder's reaction after seeing the play for the first time: "The power of the play was evident, an elder spoke up and said, 'We need this in our community, not just our children...some adults need this'" (interview, 2010). Through the play AWTY many have witnessed or participated in honest and candid dialogue about healthy sex and sexuality. Our children are benefitting from this revolution in storytelling. With the rising incidences of HIV/AIDS, STIS, and unplanned pregnancies in Aboriginal communities we must (re)embrace storytelling as a valuable weapon to teach our children about healthy sex and sexuality and lift up this heavy blanket of shame and silence.

NOTES

1. "Current crisis" refers to the alarming rise of HIV/AIDS and STIs in Aboriginal communities. These statistics are outlined later in the chapter.
2. This phrase is commonly attributed to Duncan Campbell Scott. Although there is debate about the origin of the quotation, Scott and the sentiment are rightly viewed as central to the brutal Indian residential schools in Canada.

12

MODIFIED RIDE

Experiments and Explorations in Adaptation

CONTENTS

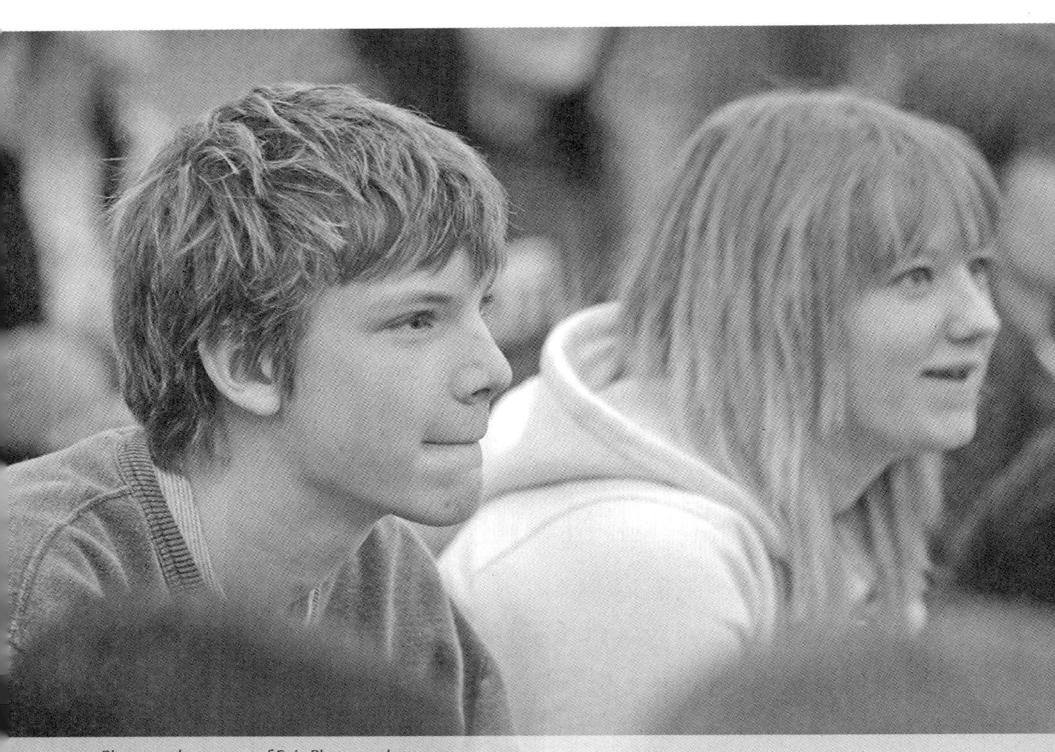

Photograph courtesy of Epic Photography.

The playwright reflects on opportunities and dilemmas that arose as the play was adapted with various artists and for various communities.

> *The strength of the performance...is that gradually the audience comes to embrace and have ownership over the performance and the production. Likewise in rehearsal, if you can encourage the actors to own the material and own their process so that they're comfortable doing things, then you're way ahead of the game. Everyone's different, but ownership, ownership of the process and of the program itself is key to the success of the play.*
>
> —JARED MATSUNAGA-TURNBULL,
> *AWTY* ACTOR AND DIRECTOR,
> CONCRETE THEATRE

DURING THE INITIAL WRITING OF THE SCRIPT and over the years that *Are We There Yet?* has been produced, many parts of the script have changed. The original producing company, Concrete Theatre, and I had the unusual luxury of testing material over several years and with many teens. The song that included all the slang names I could think of for body parts and sexual intercourse was cut in the first week of the first script workshop. In one case, the introductory participation was changed, tested, and proved to be more effective than the original choice. A larger change was the addition of a longer and more detailed participation for the Mac character (Chapter 3, page 81) and the scene leading up to this participation was substantially rewritten. In the early productions, several different issues were considered and tried for the final part of Clay ("Step Five: Dealing with a Relationship Crisis," Chapter 3, page 92). In each case, we were looking for answers to these questions: What kinds of scenes lead to the deepest and most expansive participations? And given that there are many kinds of teens in the audience and we want to be as inclusive as possible, is the balance correct between different kinds of teens: male/female, sexually active/not sexually active, LGBTQ/heterosexual, etcetera?

Some actors returned to perform the show over many years and, in conjunction with experienced directors and stage managers, had very articulate and detailed advice about what was working or not working in the play. Their commitment to the topic, the participation, and the audience were invaluable to me and created a deeply collaborative team approach to clarifying, rewriting, and adding material to make the play as clear and impactful as possible. Actors in this kind of show aren't just the conduit for a playwright or a director's vision; they are often profoundly invested in the content, the form, and the intention. A school tour is arduous. Shows start at 9:00 a.m. or earlier and getting in a cold van at 7:30 to set up in a cavernous, chilly gym and prepare to pour on the energy required to engage grumpy fourteen-year-olds is no picnic. One actor said he got himself going by telling himself every morning, "I could make a difference in a kid's life today."

If an invested actor, with a lot of shows under his or her belt, told me a scene or a participation wasn't working or something was missing, I would absolutely trust his or her knowledge and understanding. They know this audience and they work on the front line.

The research and adaptation project that we embarked on in 2005 brought many other invested adults (artists, teachers, parents, health educators, theatre administrators, grad students, and family studies and sexuality academics) into the mix. We have actively and avidly sought and listened to responses from all, about the play and the program. Many thoughtful and thorough comments have been made in response to what is in the play, but often comments focus upon what is not in the play. It's been exhilarating and often challenging to respond to the myriad of absences that have been identified. In most cases, the absence of a particular character or situation was a choice (usually a difficult one), and not an oversight, but the funded and long-term research project attached to this program, in addition to creating opportunities to adapt to varying cultural situations, allowed each choice to be revisited and rethought.

All aspects of the various adaptations to the play, the health partnership, and the nature of community involvement offered opportunities to go back to the reasoning behind script and production choices and test their current validity. What a gift! In this chapter, I discuss some of the gaps in the play, how we tried to address them in the past, what we tried in different communities, and what might be possible in the future adaptations. It's teens and sex, it's controversial, and content is and always will be a conundrum.

The Content Conundrum

There are a number of content and a few form issues that have and continue to be problematic. Adults identify these content issues as:

- Lack of enough LGBTQ content
- Lack of child sexual abuse content
- The boys all want it, the girls all don't (lack of sexually aggressive girl character)
- Lack of asexual teen or teen committed to complete abstinence
- Lack of mentally or physically disabled character

Some of these content issues have been a conundrum since the play was first conceived, some have been identified by many adults, some by only one or two.

The LGBTQ Issue

The lack of significant LGBTQ (lesbian, gay, bisexual, trans*, queer/questioning) content in *AWTY* has been an ongoing issue for theatre artists and health educators. The most obvious place to include a LGBT or Q character is in the monologue sequence (Chapter 3, page 83). The intention of that section is to tell survivor stories in order to acknowledge some of the sexual things that can go wrong for young people and model how some can move beyond these incidences. Each character is looking back at an experience they had when they were younger and describes, in first person, direct to audience, what happened to them, the consequences of a sexual experience they had, and what helped them to address the event. In keeping with the car metaphor, this is the crash portion of the play. As we knew that some audience members have already had a crash experience, it was important to name some, state that people can recover from crashes and encourage, through character, getting help.

In the initial research and writing, a number of crash possibilities emerged. I wrote six different monologues, including one from a young lesbian, a teen who faced an unintended pregnancy, an older woman with a very checkered sexual past including STIs, promiscuity, and the sex trade. The three that Concrete Theatre and I ultimately chose to use in the play were an attempt to represent as many kinds of youth as possible and the most common kinds of sexual crashes they might experience. Given that the play could only accommodate (we thought) three scenarios, these were difficult choices.

Serendipitously, the first pilot of the play in 1998 was rehearsed at the Gay and Lesbian Drop-In Centre in Edmonton and staff (and other LGBTQ adults) were invited to an early, test presentation. Anxious about the lack of LGBTQ material in the play, I asked these audience members to comment. Five things emerged from that conversation:

1. Everything in the play's teaching points applies equally to homosexual and heterosexual relationships, e.g., establishing and communicating

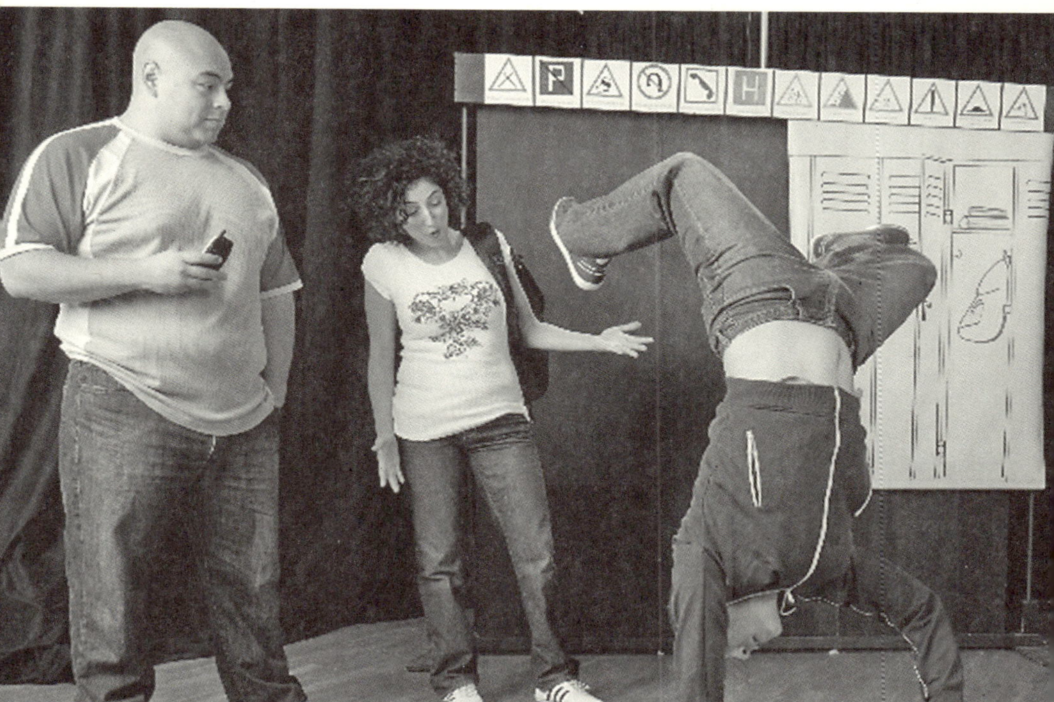

When is the right time to talk about condoms?
Pedro Chamale, Azin Sadr, and Raes Calvert, Neworld Theatre. Photograph courtesy of Tim Matheson.

sexual boundaries, negotiating condom use, establishing a relationship, and negotiating a crisis in a relationship.

2. Metaphor, humour, tone, and non-participatory scenes work for teens of all sexual orientations.
3. Overt homosexuality in the play might prevent it from being performed in the schools.
4. The short appearance of a gay character in the "How do I raise condom use with my partner?" section was enough code for the LGBTQ teens in the audience. As one person said, "The straights won't get it and the gay kids will, we certainly all got it."
5. Mentioning at the beginning of Clay that the focus will be on a girl–guy relationship but that it could also apply to a homosexual relationship

would also signal to the queer kids without asking them to out themselves or giving a reason for schools and parents to block the program.

> *I think something about* Are We There Yet? *that I really connected with was that it had a queer component, that this show was talking about sexual boundaries and, negotiating that, and wasn't afraid to include all different types of sexuality. That it wasn't just focused on the heterosexual kids in the class. The queer youth in the class could connect to the stories, and connect to the energy in what was being presented in that room. I would say that some of my most connected experiences with the show were with queer youth, and kids that would be brave enough to vocalize what they thought.*
>
> —*Nathan Cuckow,* AWTY *actor,*
> *Concrete Theatre*

Our collective fears about the power of angry parents and nervous schools were not imaginary. In the mid-1980s, Edmonton's Catalyst Theatre's production of *Feeling Yes, Feeling No* (a play about sexual abuse prevention for kindergarten to grade six students) had provoked a spate of outraged letters from parents in the newspaper, and although the play was not cancelled, it reminded schools that to book the show was risky. This tension and balance between getting to the audience with real stories and characters' dilemmas about sex, and keeping the most conservative parents (and teachers) off our backs, was a factor in the decisions we made about content. Around the LGBTQ issue, we created codes that allowed us to slip under the wire. We could not code all the content, however. In the early years of producing the play in Edmonton, individual principals in Catholic schools slid the show into their schools. However, the content came to the attention of Catholic School Board administration and the obvious endorsement of condom use could not be disguised. A few years into running the program, AWTY was no longer welcome at Catholic schools.

The decision not to include the lesbian monologue or the unplanned pregnancy or the thirty-year-old with the checkered past or the HIV-positive character was our attempt to calculate our risk, make sure (as much as possible) that we could get to the audience, and cover as much territory as we could, knowing we were leaving some audience members out. Other factors also influenced our choices. The unplanned pregnancy would lead to a debate about abortion, too big for the current play; the HIV character had few places to go in terms of story, either they were worried and had not been tested or they were positive and...became a cautionary tale about safer sex? Perhaps that item was sufficiently covered in other parts of the play. We wondered, could the HIV character be gay? But decided this was too stereotypical about both gay men and people with HIV, particularly if this was the only gay character in the play.

Another factor was, and continues to be, time. The play requires a full ninety minutes to be performed, and any additional material would require something else to be cut. It was difficult to figure out what could be taken out to make room for other material.

Artistic director Marcus Youssef of Neworld Theatre and sexual health educator Kenji Maeda were keen to address this lack in the Vancouver adaptation. They felt that in 2009 the time was right to include more LGBTQ content and that the community, adults, and teens, was ready as well. The research project associated with this play was once again allowing us to explore, expand, and improve the project. I offered five possible spots where rewrites or additions could be made.

1. Non-participatory sections: For example, "Studley Muffin and Creamy Delight" (Chapter 3, page 77) could be same-sex; "Puberty and You" (page 71) could have three actors so when the instructor says, "and they begin to notice each other," actors can look at the same and opposite sexes; Ben and Fern in the stand-up bed could be same-sex (page 79).
2. Participatory sections, "Just a Minute" (Chapter 3, page 68): one of the actors could tell a same-sex story in this early participation; Delphi and Marcel (page 72) could be same-sex, Carol Ann and Mac (page 79) could be same-sex, Clay characters (page 88) could be same-sex.
3. The Clay section: keep the couple girl/guy but when one does not want to have sex again they confess to their team that they are gay/lesbian or questioning. In that case, the participation would become focused on how to come out, not how to renegotiate a sexual boundary, but it could work.
4. Add a monologue.
5. Make Annabel or Josie (monologue characters, Chapter 3, page 83) a male.

Youssef and Maeda decided a new monologue would be best. I offered several possible topics, including gay bashing and bullying, sexual assault, online exploitation, and coming out. They chose a male coming out story as the topic of the monologue. I think the most significant question in the process of these decisions was, "What is the most important thing that LGBTQ teens in the audience need to hear in this play?" The answer was: "They don't need to hear anything different from what other teens hear, they need to be acknowledged."

As the characters in the monologues are young adults telling a story from younger years, I conducted community research with several twenty-ish gay men of my acquaintance. I asked them to think back to grade nine. It was a great pleasure to talk to these confident, grown-up men and ask them what it was like and what they would have liked to have heard when they were fourteen. "If you could go back now what would you say to your younger self?" Not surprisingly, much of what they had to say is very similar to the messages of the "It Gets Better" campaign.[1] Research participants were very enthusiastic about getting a chance to talk to young men through this monologue.

Youssef and Maeda worked through several drafts with me until we were satisfied and ready to test it. The monologue was performed in the Vancouver adaptation and has been incorporated into the Edmonton production as well. The inclusion of this new character and story addresses (to some extent) a long-term problem in the play. Both Concrete Theatre and Neworld Theatre were very pleased and excited to try the monologue and reach out to students who had formerly been underrepresented. The positive effects of inclusion and identification are documented in the research. The more that youth identify with and empathize with the characters on stage, the more they are impacted by play and its intentions.

Each company discovered, however, some of the difficulties the monologue presents. First, it can give permission for audience members to shout out homophobic remarks, which can make it emotionally rough for the actor, and could revictimize LGBTQ audience members. The companies needed to be prepared for this and developed strategies to communicate the stance of the production and company on these responses and ways to continue to encourage participation while simultaneously enforcing the no put-downs rule of participation. In some cases, acting companies have made a call during particular performances about whether to do the Mateo monologue or not. This decision has been made based on how vicious and vocal the homophobic remarks have been before the show and during the participations leading up to the monologues.

Second, the monologue impacts the audience, but it also impacts the actor. It requires a male actor (gay, straight, or other) to inhabit a character that is often seen by audiences as the actor telling their own, true story. This audience perception can be awkward for the actor and unearth unexpected reactions within themselves. There are two factors at work here: returning to junior high school and playing the audience catapults an actor back into their own adolescent experience at school with all the attendant anxieties about popularity and pecking order. If the actor feels the cool kids think they are telling their own personal story about coming out and are turning against them, it can make the actor distance himself from the material as part of a survival at school strategy. Additionally, participation depends upon audiences' empathy with and recognition of characters, and actors are keen to ensure audiences are on their side. If the character is being targeted by homophobic bullying, actors/characters have to find ways to stand up for themselves and, by proxy, for the silent LGBTQ teens in the audience. This can alienate other sections of the audience.

Third, in smaller urban, rural, and even some large urban schools, a homophobic culture and lack of LGBTQ services for youth may mean that encouraging LGBTQ teens to be themselves and come out is dangerous advice. The actor playing Mateo in one of the Edmonton productions remarked that, in some cases, it might be best to tell youth to stay in the closet until they can get to a bigger city.

Fourth, as the Vancouver production operates in a school structure that only allows eighty minutes for the play, the company performs only two of the four possible monologues in each performance. This is not a problem per se, but a creative solution to time constraints and the desire to include the Mateo monologue as often as possible. All producing companies and health partners (current and future) live with the fact that the experiences and issues of some teens will not be represented in AWTY.

The addition of a gay character to the play has been satisfying to theatre artists and companies, health partners, and other adults. We are confident it is also helpful and satisfying to LGBTQ teens in our audience but we can't know because we can't ask. Because we cannot ask teens in schools to self-identify as LGBTQ (except in the anonymously provided demographic information in the questionnaire), we cannot research many aspects of the response of this particular group. We know, however, that in addition to the vocalized homophobia, teens also approach the actor playing this character after the show. Often they want to know if the monologue is true; they seem to want to know if the actor is gay. Actors can only respond by saying they don't answer personal questions. The teen and the actor speak through the character, referral to the health partner, and the information about agencies mentioned in the play and on the help card. We believe that the experience of seeing an Aboriginal actor in the play, described by Sheldon Elter, is what is happening for LGBTQ teens when they see and hear Mateo.

> *Immediately after shows I'd get Aboriginal kids coming up. Sometimes it would be simple, they just want to say hi. They'd have trouble looking me in the eye, they're extremely shy. But they get to come up and be brave for just a moment. Basically I think they're saying, "I identify with you." Then it becomes human. Suddenly it becomes accessible for them. It allows them to feel, "I feel the same as you; if you're in these situations I can identify with you." It changes the way they viewed the show. You could see that suddenly it's like, "oh cool, there's a guy who's possibly related to me," or "that's the same race as me who is in this show."*
>
> —*Sheldon Elter,* AWTY *actor,*
> *Concrete Theatre*

Progress is being made (if agonizingly slowly), and we are moving to a more open and equal environment for LGBTQ people but we aren't completely there yet. The Mateo monologue is an important addition to AWTY and it is hoped that it helps LGBTQ youth to feel included and acknowledged in what is often a lonely, confusing, dangerous, and painful time in their lives. For some, Mateo, though fictional, may be the first live, gay, adult they have ever seen or heard speak overtly about his sexuality. The character signals that there is support and help available, in the room when the show is performed, if not (or not yet) in their community.

Child Sexual Abuse

The desire to include this issue in the play was expressed most urgently in Saskatchewan during the adaptation for Aboriginal communities. This was not the first time I had encountered this content conundrum. While working with youth in a small isolated northern Aboriginal community some years ago, the issue also emerged. Sex is a taboo subject in many Aboriginal communities and certainly in the community I was working in. The groups I worked with could talk about alcohol abuse, dating and love, suicide, school, and the terrible choices that they made to leave family and tradition to get a white education, racism in school and the media, and family violence, but sex? No. Two group members did come to me privately to say the word abuse in my ear. After some probing and some listening, it became clear they were talking about child sexual abuse that each of them had suffered and that a family member was the perpetrator. They wanted to do a scene about it, they could barely speak. My response to them was based upon my experience doing *Feeling Yes, Feeling No* (a sexual abuse prevention program for K–6). Because I had acted in that show, I knew what to say when someone disclosed: "I believe you. It's not your fault. I'm glad you told me. I'm sorry this happened to you." But the last one stuck in my throat, "and I'm going to get you some help." The two group members and I knew there would be no help for them if they disclosed in this community. There would only be grief. "This is important," I said, "this is huge, this is happening, but we can't do a scene about it." Not yet.

Sexual abuse of children is a destroyer, and every day we stay silent another child is broken, another adult inflicts a wound that also wounds him. What blocked this suggestion for me is the consequences of exposing child sexual abuse. Who will pick up the pieces? Who will look after the victims? Who will take charge of the disruption and the change? Who has the courage and the resources to deal with the fallout? Who in the community? A group of teens or a theatre company does not have the skills or the capacity to deal with child sexual abuse. The need to deal with this issue or even talk about this issue in Aboriginal communities is extreme, as it is in many communities here and around the globe.

I resisted pressure to include a scene or monologue about child sexual abuse during the community research part of the Aboriginal adaptation of AWTY for quite some time. Some members of the community youth and adults pressed very hard for the inclusion of this issue. In each case, it seemed to me, the drive to have their own experience and pain acknowledged was undeniable. My fears were not a good enough reason to keep saying no. It began to seem that colonial paternalism was fuelling my reluctance, and that my commitment to community engagement and ownership was false. I wrote three monologues and sent them to my co-writer, Kenneth T. Williams. His response was swift and blunt. I had written monologues about victims and perps. All three pieces involved victims disclosing and getting help and support from family, community, and elders to move toward healing. Ken said to me:

> *We can't, it isn't true. We would like, in the Aboriginal community, to have family and elders that are ready to take this on but in too many places we don't, not yet. Particularly in the rural areas, the people and the systems are not in place to deal with the flood of current and past victims. Victims of priests and residential school, yes, but victims of family members, no. It's not on, we can't name this, and we can't lie and say kids will get help.*

So, for this show, and the work I did with Aboriginal youth twenty-five years ago, child sexual abuse within communities remains a secret that everybody knows.

The key point is not that child sexual abuse should never be raised in a possible future adaptation of this play. If significant community support systems were in place, the play (or a version of it) that contained a character that had been a victim of child sexual abuse could be an important part of helping victims and preventing future abuse. Any community might identify this, or some other issue that is not addressed in the play, as crucial. A good deal of careful thought and planning to ensure youth audiences get the assistance they need would be required. Then material would need to be tested. Planning, strategizing, and organizing is a crucial step but testing with audiences and other community members would be equally important. Theatre is visceral and potent and you don't really know what you have on your hands until an audience is present.

The process of developing the material and community supports to confront the issue of child abuse would be long and would require resources to do it well. But it could be done and would be a remarkable project, with potential to have impact locally, nationally, and internationally.

The ethics and politics of what research is taken up or buried in a play created from community research are complex and wrenching. The decision to not include a scene or monologue about child sexual abuse haunts me. Maybe we should have included something even if we had reservations. Maybe that is part of theatre's job, maybe you have to have the courage to break it open and run, to begin the process. Maybe some kids disclose because of a play and get ignored or vilified, maybe that's the price you pay. Maybe somebody gets help who has been silent and in pain. It is my hope that an Aboriginal playwright, together with appropriate community health partners to provide the necessary follow through and support work, takes this on and makes it move.

The Sexually Aggressive Girl

This issue has come up occasionally over the years but we were able to begin to examine it during the participatory research period with Saskatchewan Native Theatre Company (SNTC). We spent four weeks over a period of four months investigating what the AWTY Program should become in this setting. Of all the adaptation processes, it was here we had the most extended contact with artists and community. Perhaps because of the luxurious amount of time, the conversation about what else could/should be included in the play was most extensive. When the topic arose, a new participatory scene was written to look at the issue of aggressive girls. This theme was identified by the artistic director at SNTC and a community health worker as an issue for young men. In the scene, a young man (Tyrone) is hotly pursued by a young woman (Inez) but he is not at ease with how quickly she wants to move into a sexual relationship. He goes to the audience. The participation was intended to elicit advice from the audience about how he could gracefully handle this situation without humiliating the girl or himself. The scene was framed in such a way that the hot pursuit of Tyrone was public (at a dance) and observed by peers. The second part of the participation was to be about peer pressure.

The company had a chance to work on the scene while waiting for another event to take place. When the actor got to the point of needing advice from the audience, the director wondered aloud if the character was gay. He made this remark not as an audience member but as a dramaturge, as a discovery: Ah! *this* is what the scene is really about. This was an interesting turn of events. I had developed notes for this participation, clearly stating that this was bound to be a response from the audience and that the actor would need to deflect this solution if the participation was to really dig into the issue of aggressive girls. However, in the hurry of the moment, the artistic director focused on getting the scene up and so the LGBTQ content surfaced. Community members and health educators in Saskatchewan had never mentioned the lack of LGBTQ material in the play, although an actor had. Now, by accident or design, the issue emerged. In discovering the subtext of the character, the issue they had wanted to address disappeared and the "I am gay or questioning" issue took over.

Even this small test drive raised many questions. Is "aggressive girls" a real issue? Should the scene instead be a way to raise homosexuality? Did the community not raise the lack of LGBTQ material during the adaptation process because it is not an issue in this Aboriginal community or because it is deeply buried, much more deeply than child sexual abuse?

Later, the two playwrights discussed what had happened with this first and quite casual look at a draft scene. If we continued to develop this scene, would we want to change the issue to *how can I come out*? Is that the most significant issue for the community, even if they didn't mention it? If we went that way with the scene, would we signal that the only reason a boy might decline a sexual advance is because he is gay? If we wanted to keep this scene as participation about aggressive girls, how can the actor deflect the suggestion that he is gay in order to focus the audience? What can an actor playing a straight character say except, "I'm not"? Doth he protest too much? What is the centre of the issue? Whose issue is it? How significant an issue is it? What about the girl character? Is there participation for her? Why does she not get the signals from this guy? What's her deal? Was she sexually abused as a child? Is this self-destructive behaviour at fourteen? Or is she exercising her right to her sexual power? What research do we need to do to find out? Is this the right scene for either topic? What is the sexual health, healthy decision-making direction for this scene?

Although we never got back to this scene, the initial steps we took and the questions that were generated helped us reflect upon a model for creating and testing new material.

The Asexual and/or Totally Abstinent Teen

This teen exists and is making a healthy sexual choice. The two adults who felt and expressed the need for an abstinent character to be represented appeared to do so for the same reason adults feel a LGBTQ needs to be represented—so that these teens are acknowledged. However, these groups also have quite different things to deal with. A LGBTQ teen is not making a choice about their sexual orientation, and they need to be acknowledged because their identity issues are often painful, whether public or private. The issues abstinent teens face only become issues if they want or are being pressured to change their sexual boundaries. If that happens before marriage, there is a great deal in the play about these issues.

If research showed that an important issue or character was present in the community but missing from the play, the process outlined above when developing the aggressive girl scene or the new gay character and monologue could be employed. I was invited to meet and work on an adaptation of *AWTY* with a theatre company in Maryland a few years ago. In this community, the abstinent teen was very important for some of the adults who were considering supporting the project. They wanted this role model on stage. I was only able to do a bit of research, but one of the issues a youth identified was a process of taking a vow of abstinence, publically, in a ceremony with her dad and a few years later starting to have sex. She felt enormous guilt and alienation from her family because she had let them down and broken her vow. She also felt unable to get or ask her partner for condoms or other ways to protect herself because she was not supposed to be having sex. Being damned and going to hell was also part of the package. I can see an interesting and worthwhile scene about a teen like this in a community with abstinence-only sexuality education in schools.

A Character with Mental or Physical Disabilities

These teens are a particularly vulnerable and underserved group. In the past, when thinking about representation and acknowledgement, only two possible solutions seemed to present themselves: cast an actor with a disability or have an able bodied actor play a character with a disability. Neither of these is a particularly satisfactory solution. An actor in a wheelchair might address some acknowledgement issues but would require a number of questions to be answered, such as which sexuality issues are the same as for other teens and which are different? Is an able bodied actor in a wheelchair sufficiently inclusive or just tokenism? An actor with a disability could certainly be cast in the play but what of the current scenes would need to be adapted and what new scenes would need to be added to address specific circumstances in an honest and thorough way? This research project has allowed us to keep asking, what needs to be adapted here, for this community? We have seen several different health educator/theatre company partnerships, each developed to suit a particular community, their geography, health systems, and needs. Theatre companies and artists have developed new material and cast actors that would resonate most deeply with the teens in their community. The variety of adjustments and adaptations for specific communities opens up some enticing possibilities for considering how to address the needs of this particular community. In a way, the research has bumped the needle and puts it in another groove. The adaptation that might work best to address the issues of teens with disabilities may be to the theatre company. There are a growing number of disability arts companies in Europe and North America and it would be thrilling if any were interested in adapting and producing AWTY.

As we know from the adaptations that we have undertaken so far, casting the play in such a way that the actors and the audience share cultures and/or ethnicity has huge impact on the participations, and on identification and impact. Could disability arts theatre artists and companies perform this play with teens in their community? The play does require highly skilled and trained actors, but such actors are now emerging in other abled companies. To address the specific issues of teens with impairments would require new material. The same participatory community research process could be employed to determine what key issues are missing from the play for this group and what could be retained as applicable to that community. Some of my previous research with this community indicates that the issue of sexual abuse by caregivers might be very important, as well as the general misconception that teens with impairments are asexual or inappropriately sexual.

Who Else Is Missing?

There are many other groups of teens that are not represented in the play, and their issues around sexuality and relationships are not explored. These groups include immigrant and new Canadian teens, homeless teens, addicted teens, teens with mental health issues, teens in state care, and teens in the sex trade. These teens are in our schools and in our audiences and their lives and issues are not directly explored, but they could be.

Form and Structure

In addition to content issues, the form of the play has also raised questions and prompted experiments and explorations. Theatre artists, other adults, and in some cases members of the youth audiences, quite often raise three form or structural questions:

1. Why does it need to be live? What about a DVD?
2. Can't students perform this? Why does it need to be done by trained adult actors?
3. Why split the genders for Clay? This is awkward for the LGBTQ teens and reinforces a false gender binary.

The DVD

Elsewhere in this book we have made the argument for live theatre. The main arguments for a DVD are that theatre is expensive and time-consuming, it cannot reach all the teens that need a program like this, and even if a DVD cannot replace live theatre and participation, it is better than nothing. These are legitimate arguments for a DVD version of the play. The strongest argument for a live participatory theatre event comes from the audience. Their relationship with the actors is visceral and immediate.

Because, I mean, teenagers do act like that and they can relate to the people on stage, and the people, like the actors at the play, I think they knew what we felt and stuff and they could...like, they knew our feelings about it so it was easier to really relate and understand what they were saying about sex.

—Audience member

Coming to their school to talk to them signals seriousness and care. The audience loves the actors and it is reciprocated.

If you're very very old, like teacher old, it's kind of hard to relate to them. Cuz you think it was a long time ago, like a different environment for them, perhaps. So it's better with the play and the actors.

—Audience member

The audience sees people who are intimate and sexual together: Delphi and Marcel actually kiss, in front of them, right there in their gym; Mac and Carol Ann are about to have sex (albeit under a blanket); and Ben and Fern have had sex. The current generation is screen saturated and savvy; their whole world is shaped by how they take in information and interact with screens. But they know the difference between live theatre and cameras.

When the couples were making out, I wouldn't really think they would do that but they did and they were honest. Like, they thought we were mature enough to see that.

—Audience member

There is not currently a screen technology that can reproduce the kind of in-the-moment deep participation upon which this play rests. Factors such as identification with the characters and recognition of the situations impact the degree of participation, which in turn impacts the change and learning that the teens experience. As the technology grows and changes and we get closer and closer to the holodeck, virtual participation may be able to capture more of the "humans in the room" quality that is such an important element of the success of the play.

Students Perform for Students

From time to time, there are requests to get the script for students to perform the play for other students. Often this request comes from high school teachers with senior drama students who are looking for socially relevant and useful theatre. In most cases, schools and teachers are involved in a variety of peer educator programs and philosophies. These circumstances might be very conducive to producing the play, but there are a few caveats. The play is part of a program that includes a sexual health educator, sexuality training for actors, and some familiarity with participation or participation training. It would, of course, be quite possible to produce the play or parts of the play without these things in place. This book includes the text of the play, in addition to other information about all aspects of the program and the research, but it is up to individual readers to use the book as they see fit. The well-being of the youth in the audience and the youth on stage will perhaps be the main consideration in how the information here is used and disseminated.

Splitting Genders for the Clay Section of the Play

Occasionally, in performance, a teen audience member is not sure where to go when the actors split the audience into gender groups. Gender is not a binary; it is a spectrum, but this part of the play is shaped by a binary. Actors in the Concrete Theatre production have had some experience with this issue and handled it by being alert to the possibility, watching for a student who was reluctant to go with the girls or the boys and quietly inviting them to join the group of their choice. In Vancouver, when Neworld Theatre was preparing their second production, this issue came up again. I asked Adrienne Wong, who directed the show, to talk about what happened and what they did.

> **Jane Heather**: *What prompted the decision to try creating teams not based on gender?*
> **Adrienne Wong**: *As we were heading into the final stages of rehearsal for Neworld's 2010 fall production of* Are We There Yet?, *some interesting conversations started to surface about how gender and sexuality plays out in the show for* LGTBQ *youth. During one of our runs with an invited (adult) audience, we began dividing the audience for the Clay participation with girls on one side and guys on the other. One guest raised his hand and said, "What about me, where do I go?" This question prompted a conversa-*

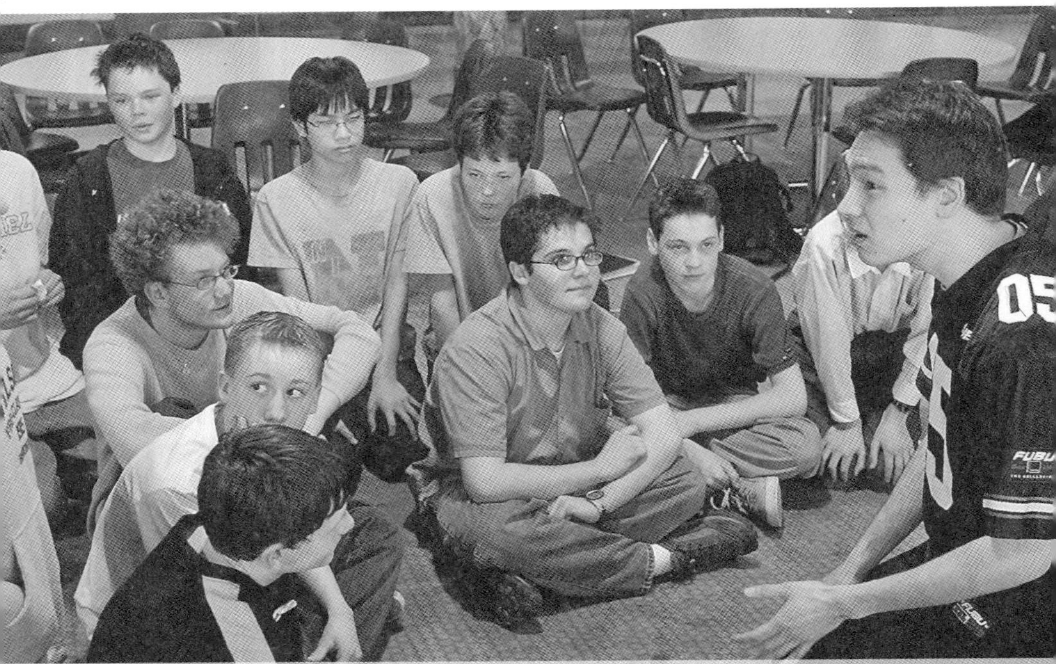

What should I say to her?
Jared Matsunaga-Turnbull, Concrete Theatre. Photograph courtesy of Epic Photography.

tion about how we can help LGTBQ *youth to navigate the Clay section. We don't expect youth to be as confident and outspoken as our adult audience member, and at the same time we don't want to inadvertently out anyone.*

One of the key reasons to have test audiences is to surface issues that may come up before the show is performed in the schools. All the possible things that might come up can never be covered in rehearsal. When issues arise, the opportunity to test a solution with an audience is ideal.

Adrienne: *Knowing that we had a preview audience of high school youth the next day, we developed a plan to change the way the audience was divided. We sought a means to divide the audience in a way that allows the participants to choose where they want to go rather than having a division imposed on them based on sex. So the coaches* *would say something like, "Over here we're going to create a fantasy guy. Who wants to help me create a fantasy guy? Come over here!" And the same with the girl. Youth would then have the freedom to choose where they wanted to go based on their desire to create a fantasy girl or guy. We tried it out at a school the next day. Initially, as the performers were dividing the group, the teachers approached Kenji, the sexual health facilitator touring with the show, and me. Both teachers had seen the show before and expressed their approval for this new way of making the groups that wasn't based on sex. "I hope there's students from both sexes in both groups," said one teacher.*

A sensitive, observant teacher can be a very useful and important resource for the theatre company. They often know their students very well and are alert to how they might respond. Visiting the same schools more than once can build an informed and supportive network for the theatre company, another boon for the program.

Jane: *What happened?*

Adrienne: *As the scene played on, it became very clear that what we were gaining by creating space for LGTBQ youth meant losing some of the qualities that drive the scenes forward. Some observations:*

1. *While the groups were mixed gender, they were very different in size, with ten students creating the fantasy girl and twenty-five students creating fantasy guy. Social cliques tended to stay together, and it appeared as if all the cool kids were in the big group and the less confident students were in the smaller group.*
2. *There were a lot of differing opinions and perspectives about the qualities of the fantasy characters. Female Clay was both a bad ass (a guy's suggestion) and benevolent (a girl's suggestion). She had a v-shaped waist (guy's suggestion) and liked to wear pants more than skirts (girl's suggestion). The actors observed that it was difficult to include all the voices: "If we listened to the girls, we shut the boys up, if we listened to the boys, we shut the girls up." When the fantasy female entered, Evelyn and Azin (performers) both expressed they felt they had to either disregard or blow out of proportion the girls' suggestions to play the stereotype.*
3. *Having both sexes giving suggestions in the same group may have caused some students to self-censor. The teachers also noticed that the students were less vocal and engaged with their characters than they had been in our previous visit last season. As a result it was very hard to move the scene forward. Over the course of*

the relationship negotiation for the realistic Clay characters, the students eventually ran out of suggestions for male Clay. One guy said outright, "we don't have any more advice for you."

4. *We lost the excitement of building a fantasy.*

Adrienne: *When we returned to the studio, we had a long discussion about how the Clay worked, the importance of the fantasy Clay section, what purpose it serves, both within the rhythm of the show and in the ideas we are asking the students to engage with. We discarded our notion of finding other means of splitting the group into two smaller groups. Some options (counting off students 1-2-1-2) would break up cliques, but were time-consuming. A fast solution like splitting the room in half would maintain the social dynamics of groups who choose to sit next to each other. And neither of these methods would address the reality we had encountered: that the students seem freer expressing themselves in a group of just girls or just guys. We decided it was important and useful for each group to feel like they identified with their Clay character, male or female, and that this sense of identification was more about self than it was about sexual orientation or desire.*

Jane: *Do you have other thoughts about how to split the audience for the Clay section?*

Adrienne: *Changing the structure was like herding cats; by taking care of one cat, six more darted off behind us! But we still wanted to make a change to at least acknowledge what could be a difficult moment in the show for* LGTBQ *youth. Our conversation zeroed in on how we talk about with the fantasy Clay. Referring to fantasy Clay as "an ideal, fantasy girl or guy" implies, for us, a desired partner, girlfriend, boyfriend. Could we, we wondered, still bring in questions about gender stereotyping without linking it to desire?*

Would this provide enough space for queer or questioning youth to not feel excluded from an assumption of desire? It's this personalized desire that we felt was part of creating the presumption that girls like guys and guys like girls. What if, instead of focusing on your fantasy X, we asked students to focus on the perfect X? Would we get the same generalizations and stereotypes that make fantasy Clay so fun to play if we worked outside of a framework based on sexual attraction?

We tried out this new solution the following day with our second preview audience. The scene played out with the fun and playfulness we expected. The change in wording was subtle, and maybe only registered by the company working on the show. It's hard to say how much the change impacted the students' experience. The solution is imperfect, though. To address one problem would mean changing the architecture of a scene that works so well as it is.

The real impact of our investigation was on the heightened sensitivity the performers felt toward the issues and anxieties of queer and questioning youth. The discussion also helped the performers to develop strategies and language they could use if something came up. It helped them to feel like they had the tools to engage with the uncertainty of audience participation on tour.

I like how they separated the boys from the girls because if we would have been all combined it would have been harder for like, us to say what we wanted to.

—Audience member

THERE ARE MANY OTHER QUESTIONS AND COMMENTS that the play has provoked. These include:

1. Can the interracial dating in the play be addressed? The cast is often diverse and the two couples in the play are almost always of different races.
2. Is the Josie character/monologue too stereotypical? This thirteen-year-old character is promiscuous, and has anonymous, unprotected sex at parties while drinking. Does she (or another character) need room to reclaim or own her promiscuity?
3. Does there need to be more in the play about anal sex?

These questions demonstrate the range of opinion about the play and the experience of adapting, and adjusting the play for community circumstances may demonstrate ways to address these concerns. The play is very adaptation-friendly. Any number of scenes or monologues could be cut in order to add things that are not currently in the play but urgent for a particular community. Community research would be required to find out what the issue is for teens and the stories around that issue that are significant for the audience. A script workshop, similar to any new play workshop, would also be required, but the dramaturgical questions would include many that a conventional workshop might not (such as the questions above). Research with teens, critical and analytical thinking about intention, careful choices about what can be cut from the play in order to make room for a new scene, capacity to support teens once an issue is raised, among others, would all be part of the adaptation or creating new material process. The health education partner would be consulted about the issue and the key teaching points. Teens would need to be involved throughout the process and invited to be a test audience, ideally, several times before material was incorporated.

Adaptation could be a solution to incorporate many of the kinds of teens and issues that are not currently in the play, but, in some cases, the solution is probably another play or many other plays. The best possible outcome of this project would be that the things we discovered could be used by others to create additional inventive, creative, inclusive plays and programs to help the teens and communities they care about.

> *Like when I have a problem or whatever now I'm not scared anymore to say something that I'm thinking or be like, "Oh god, I don't think I should tell him that."... Like, the person you're in a relationship with has a right to know what you're thinking because they're probably thinking the same thing.*
>
> *—Audience member*

NOTE

1. The "It Gets Better Canada" campaign is readily available on YouTube.

13

IT'S THE WHEEL THING

What Can Theatre Do? And How Do We Know?

CONTENTS

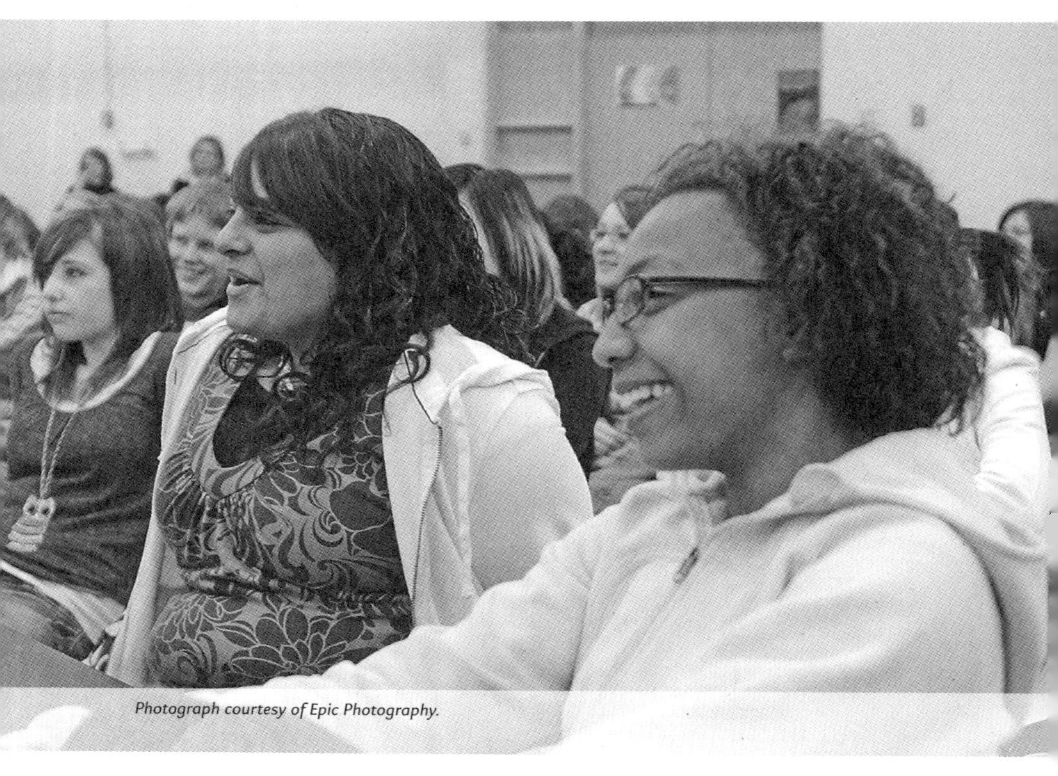

Photograph courtesy of Epic Photography.

This project gave us the opportunity to test long-held theories of why and how theatre connects with audience members. Theatre artists and social scientists collaborated to develop ways to measure the theatre experience objectively.

> *The situations were actually real and the characters that they made weren't actually fake. I don't know—I could just relate to it.*
>
> —AUDIENCE MEMBER

THEATRE ARTISTS COMMITTED TO USING THEATRE for social transformation work largely on faith. We believe in what our eyes, ears, and emotions tell us—that audiences come away from theatre that is relevant not only moved but also willing to look at the world differently, willing to act differently. We hold on to anecdotes of impact, we sense a change in people who interact with our work, we believe we make a difference. In recent decades, theatre researchers most commonly considered theatre's impact via lenses and concepts provided by cultural and performance studies, while research based in the social sciences, both qualitative and quantitative, was applied primarily to theatre for education projects, often in response to funders' needs for proof of efficacy.[1]

But can we combine the insights of humanities, fine arts, and social science research methods to learn something further about how theatre works and what theatre can do? The alliance of researchers and community partners created by the Are We There Yet? research program aimed to discover new knowledge about theatre's impact and sought to determine ways to understand and assess theatre both thoroughly and usefully. Because of this research context (a six-year, well-funded alliance that includes theatre and social science researchers, theatre artists, and sexual health experts), we sought to dig deeper than a single program assessment can. These conditions created the opportunity to investigate not only the efficacy and impact of the project itself but indeed the ways that theatre can be understood.

We started with a very successful play. *AWTY* was produced nine times from 1998 to 2005. From 2006 to 2013, the play was mounted thirteen times by four different Canadian theatre companies.

We (the theatre artists) asked social science researchers to create ways to measure the impact of this play. They did so, using theories about how people learn and mature, and how to define and measure people's capacity for supporting safe and respectful sexual relationships. (See Chapter 9 for a description of the methodologies, theories, and findings of research into the relative impact of the play as a tool for sexuality education.) But the social scientists also asked: Why do we think theatre is a good way to reach teens on this subject? What theory supports the use of theatre? What theories are the bases of theatre? Of this kind of theatre? In answering these questions, we offered for reconsideration our basic truths about how drama and theatre work. We started here:

> *[When participating in a theatre event], audience members recognize the character(s) and their dilemmas and identify with the people portrayed. And because they can watch rather than live the experience, they also objectify the problems, and in so doing begin to be able to think critically about possible solutions or alternate actions. The combining of empathetic involvement with the opportunity to observe, analyse and form opinions regarding characters' actions creates a condition where audience members want to think; they have the opportunity to problem solve in a safe but vital environment. (Prentki and Selman 2000, 8)*

So, with our social science partners, we created a set of questions for our audiences that we hoped would interrogate these ideas as well as provide insight into the particular play and production. These questions could be grouped into some basic concepts about how theatre works and about how audiences and theatre interact, through pleasure, identification, and distancing. While perhaps not all aspects of each of these concepts are measurable, we thought it was important to invite our audiences to reflect on the quality of their experience. The social scientists approached this challenge from a mixed methods design, which allowed for qualitative responses (interviews, focus groups, and structured observations) to complement quantitative findings (a questionnaire using numerical scales). In the first year of conducting quantitative and qualitative evaluation of audience response, our research partners told us that "these theatre questions really hang together." This sounded exciting, but what did it mean? The theatre questions "loaded together on the same construct." We theatre types were none the wiser; this interdisciplinary project spends a lot of time translating for one another. In lay terms, this means that the theatre questions met the following criteria: they were valid; they were testing what we wanted to be testing. For example, three different questions that assess audience's sense of pleasure were answered consistently. Further, they were reliable or, in other words, repeatable; audience members gave consistent answers to quite different questions that were meant to measure the same thing.

So, we had a good set of questions in that they were valid (tested what we hoped to be testing) and we had a good delivery system in that they were reliable (individual audience members responded consistently to related questions). We had to know more. Were these questions proving to be important tests of our basic theories about theatre? What follows is a discussion of core theories regarding how theatre works, intercut with what has been revealed to date when social science tests these theories with specific audiences. While we recognize response to a theatre experience is largely holistic, we separated components of this experience for the purpose of this study and experimented with varying forms of analysis. We think that there is value beyond assessment of a single project; with these sets of questions we are finding some ways to interrogate our field's truths about live theatre.

Pleasure

Pleasure is an undertheorized and undervalued aspect of theatre's power.[2] Of course, there are many levels of pleasure, and we start here with the kind derived from entertainment. However, when considering pleasure, we need to think about it in the plural—the pleasures of humour, arousal of emotions, empathy, or a moment's reflection, of recognition, insight, of being transported to a new or strange place, of being endowed with intelligence, of taking power. All these and more are parts of this phenomena.[3] Pleasure leads to openness, creativity, receptiveness. When these conditions are in place, people want to engage with the performance, the play and its ideas, as well as with other members of the audience. Brecht (1964, 180) notes that "the theatre's broadest function is to give pleasure. It is the noblest function that we have found for theatre."

Some of the elements in AWTY that are crucial to spectators' pleasure are its metaphor, humour, the variety and energy provided by its wide ranging and quick changing styles, and its direct contact with its audience. The central metaphor, comparing learning about sex with learning to drive, has the teen audience (and adults who see the play) laughing hard. Audiences enjoy the metaphor, and especially catching on to the metaphor. This aha moment can give them pleasure, a sense of complicity; they like being in on the joke along with the actors. They enjoy the respect that is offered, finding pleasure in being presumed to be intelligent and capable. The capacity for theatre to offer the audience a chance to make connections and apply them is a feature that contributes to audiences' sense of empowerment. Traditionally, theatre has used dramatic irony to endow audiences with wisdom; they enjoy knowing something that a character doesn't. In this play, audiences are offered this metaphor to enjoy, to extend, and to endow with meaning. From this point in the play onwards, audience and actors use a common shorthand—the driving metaphor—to reference stages of gaining knowledge about safer sex. The metaphor is fun, can be used in many ways, and engages the audiences; it is one of the elements most often cited as particularly enjoyable in audience interviews and focus groups.

> *Yeah, it makes it more comfortable for students rather than just saying this is the parts of the body just pointing out, it's like they made it funny. Like the glove compartment and the gear shift, headlights (laughter) and, like, how they put it... it was...like, comfortable...they made a comparison with driving. We're comfortable with talking about driving—so they made it comfortable to talk with before they even started talking about it.*
>
> *—Audience member*

This play has a number of challenges to overcome if it is to give its audience pleasure. The play is presented in schools and is about sex. Audiences arrive quite sure that it will be boring, or at best good for them. They also presume it will be careful. The topic is touchy or embarrassing. Talking about sex is. The metaphor, the play's use of direct address, and the overt and accepting participation the play employs soon dispel their fears—laughs of surprise as well as humour soon take over the school gym. Picture students sprawled across the floor. Picture them minutes later laughing, leaning forward, engaged. That's pleasure.

This "attainment of a humorous attitude" (Critchley 2002, 41) has been considered central to making meaning and to development and expression of imagination. Philosopher and art theorist Susanne Langer (1953) finds humour to be one of theatre's "most useful and natural elements" (346), stating that "the feeling of comedy...[is] a feeling of heightened vitality,

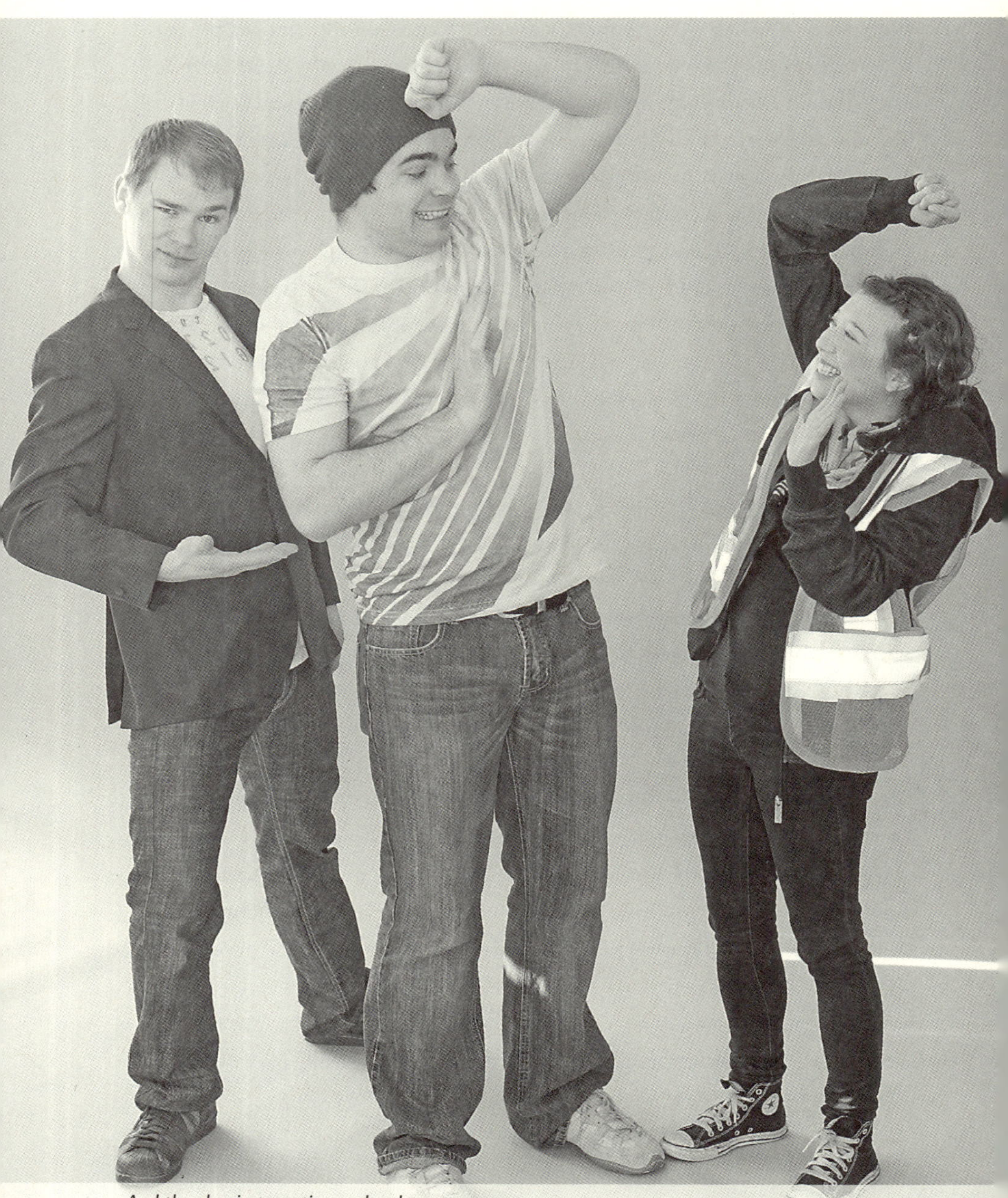

And they begin to notice each other
Cole Humeny, Garett Spelliscy, and Ming Hudson, Concrete Theatre. *Photograph courtesy of Epic Photography.*

challenged wit and will" (348–49). Bakhtin (1984, 23) in particular captures the importance of laughter to the artists who strive to create an outstanding experience with this play:

> *Laughter has the remarkable power of making an object come up close, of drawing it into a zone of crude contact where one can finger it familiarly on all sides, turn it upside down, inside out, peer at it from above and below, break open its external shell, look into its centre, doubt it, take it apart, dismember it, lay it bare and expose it, examine it freely and experiment with it.*

Pleasure was measured through three items on our questionnaire. We started simply; teens were asked to indicate how much they agreed or disagreed with the statements: "I enjoyed the play," and "I liked the humour in the play." The answers to these two items have a high internal consistency and reliability, meaning that these two items measure the same general construct (pleasure). A large percentage of students indicated they enjoyed the play (92 per cent), and enjoyed the humour in the play (93 per cent).

Qualitative research yielded similar results. There was unanimous agreement among those interviewed that the play's format was an effective and fun way to learn about sex. When asked to think about the play and state the first thing that came to mind, students most frequently responded that the play was funny, fun, and humorous, or, in other words, pleasureful. Further, the humorous and pleasurable atmosphere was reported by the audience to increase their level of attention during the play. Various comments were made about the power of the play and its ability to keep their interest as well as make an impression: "It was funny and you remember things that are funny better than just general information" (Audience member).

They also spoke about the impact of the humour. Some expressed that the production's open and humorous style helped them to feel more confident and comfortable about the topic. They felt more able to discuss things openly when they hadn't before:

It helped me because like before I was like really shy about the whole thing. Now that everybody else could laugh about it, I can laugh about it too, and...kind of... made me feel confident about going into that kind of situation.

—Audience member

Bahktin would agree with this teenager: "Laughter demolishes fear and piety before an object, before a world, making of it an object of familiar contact and thus clearing the ground for an absolutely free investigation of it. Laughter is a vital factor in laying down that prerequisite for fearlessness without which it would be impossible to approach the world realistically" (1984, 23).

Responses demonstrate that audiences, in this case teens, remember information and engage with ideas when they are presented in a manner that evokes a pleasurable response. One respondent stated, "Guys don't typically take things very seriously in grade nine." The researcher followed up, "But do you think they took the play seriously?" The respondent replied, "They took the information in. [The actors] just made it more fun." Another student stated, "We had fun, [laughter]—but we still learned at the same time." "Sex I guess...it was pretty funny. It's good acting yeah when they let the audience get into it a lot" (Audience member).

A finding that is most important to the theatre artists is that those who found the play pleasurable also increased communication skills around this sensitive topic. As outlined in Chapter 9, the quantitative survey included theatre questions plus a variety of question groups that measured impact of the play's themes on audience members, themes such as self-efficacy and capacity to name and communicate boundaries. Audience members who found the play pleasurable also significantly increased in their sexual decision-making skills. For the group who experienced pleasure when watching the play, sexual communication changed significantly from before (pre) to after experiencing the program (post). These audience members felt that they were more able to communicate about sexual issues. Those who were less pleased with the play-going experience showed no significant change, and the only significant change for the control group (a similar age group who did not participate in AWTY) was a decrease of perceived ability to communicate about boundaries.

This finding (the more pleasure, the more impact on certain outcomes) is a pattern that continues through the measurements of the impact of other theatre concepts (identification and participation). It suggests to theatre artists that the better the theatre, the greater the real impact of a theme or project's intent.[4] It suggests to theatre creators with social agendas the importance of balancing pleasure, identification, and opportunity for reflection and analysis. The challenge is to create the best mix of these experiences.

Later in our multi-year study we added to the ways the quantitative data was analyzed, employing causal modelling to further understand the links between the makeup of our audiences,[5] the theories of theatre we were using, and the measures of impact. This kind of analysis is used to test theories of what will create change and to predict impact. A lot of factors can affect the degree of change someone undergoes as a result of an experience, including gender, race, age, learning styles, family situation, among others. Causal modelling allowed us to find out what the key influencers were. For example, using this approach, we asked: Is pleasure a significant intervening variable? Or, in other words, does it actually matter to the project's impact whether our audiences experience pleasure? This analysis showed pleasure to be the most important variable in our audience members' changes in perceived capacity for communication about sexuality and perceived sexual decision making.

In observing the audiences for this play, a couple of complications to the concept of the value of pleasure arise. We have observed the danger of too much pleasure. For example, when actors and audiences got on a roll in the interactive sequences, enjoying too much fun silliness, the more serious intentions of a section have been lost to hilarity; these choices are performers' judgement calls in the participatory sequences. Rehearsals and debriefs must seek to define the best balance of fun and the more serious payoffs that emerge from the pleasure of identification and emotional engagement. One day an actor had the audience rolling in the aisles with a joke about squirrel stomping. Unfortunately, the scene's central struggle how to communicate about renegotiating sexual boundaries never quite got the attention it needed. While participants in interviews and focus groups volunteer their enjoyment of the humour, and while humour energizes and builds comfort and openness, it is the contrast and balance with more serious situations and dilemmas that create a deep pleasure. Audience members are delighted, open to the experience, and then respond to more complex aspects of life. We noted, for example, that after the humour, audience members often highlight the play's serious monologues, which involve direct address and stories of recovering from difficult sexual experiences. The pleasure of empathy and recognition play a role here, a topic we will return to.

> *Ummm, the one where they kind of did the monologue, like the support group almost. And you just had to talk about things like I think if something like that did happen to someone, it's better to express it and know what you've done wrong and know what happened to you so other people can help you, instead of just bottling it up inside. Right. Cuz it just makes it worse.*
>
> *—Audience member*

> *No, my friends and I did talk a lot about the, like, the way that the guys said, I didn't realize that I was sexually assaulting her because he was just pushing it. We talked about [how] that happens a lot but you don't realize how serious it is, you just kinda think, oh yeah, I just pushed it a little bit, but you don't realize that it's actual sexual assault.*
>
> *—Audience member*

Identification: Recognition to Engagement

As we know, much of theatre's power is tied to levels of identification. Artists aim to engage their audience intellectually and emotionally, and one of the most powerful ways to do this is to focus their attention on a character, build empathetic involvement with the character(s), then put them at risk. Audiences care what happens and this builds emotional engagement. The higher the stakes, the more the engagement. Theatre theory helps us to understand the steps to building this quality. Make a character worthy of our concern, we care more. Make a character attractive, we engage. Add a foible, they are human, so more like us. Put them at risk, we care what happens.

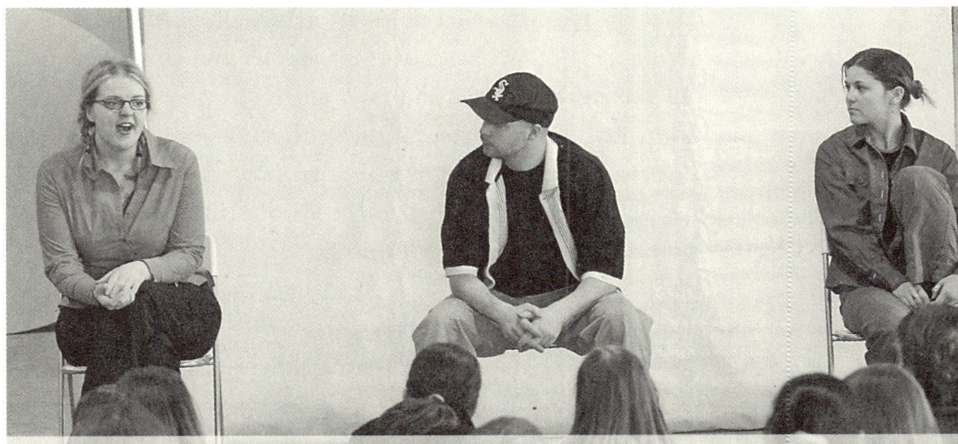

Sometimes I see eyes that say, "It happened to me too"
Jana O'Connor, Bob Rasko, and Shannon Larson, Concrete Theatre. Photograph courtesy of Epic Photography.

Since Aristotle, identification with the characters on stage has been understood as a key quality of theatre and central to enjoyment and emotional impact on audiences. Despite attacks on this concept, empathetic involvement with characters and their fates is understood as integral to the theatrical experience (Langer 1953, Carlson 1993). Jonathan Levy (2005) proposes that emotion is the essential and possibly the only positive thing that theatre provides. David Krasner (2006) suggests that theatre audiences empathize through identification, compassion, sympathy, and understanding (258) and goes on to argue that audiences "think, feel, reason, and empathize simultaneously" (263). An argument for a local, culturally specific (and live) theatre that tells stories that are directly meaningful in specific and local situations is a familiar one in many parts of this globalized world. Indigenous and relevant art, born out of local perceptions, is seen by many to matter. In Canada, we see this insight expressed in our arts policies (with substantial funding linked to production of Canadian work) and more specifically in the calls for adequate representation of our culturally diverse set of voices. Taking this argument for identification further, we join the worldwide network of popular theatre and community-based practitioners and theorists and argue that, for greatest impact, we must create characters who are like the audience ("they could be me") and put them in situations "that could happen to people I know." Based in these notions, AWTY was adapted for each cultural setting in which it was produced—rural, Aboriginal, and urban—and is updated and made specific each year it is played.

It is of interest to note that even Aristotle, currently out of favour with those concerned with bringing greater democracy to our stages, looked for, as Angela Curran (2001, 169) offers, "a kind of affinity between the audience and the characters who act and suffer." However, Aristotle worked in a context that he understood to have a homogenous audience, one of common perceptions. While, as Curran suggests, Aristotle's theories required that he have an "idealized spectator" in mind, this notion can be transposed to support current conceptions of theatre artist/activists who create theatre for and with particularized audiences.[6] AWTY sets out to reach a specific age group, and some of the evaluation research investigates its audiences' responses not only as one aggregate group but also from specific segments of that audience.[7]

Providing characters that are recognizable to a specific audience leads to a new depth of engagement. Identification is higher and empathetic involvement is possibly greater. The stakes are intensely familiar; characters that are like me are at risk, in situations I identify with and care about. Jeanne Klein (2005) argues that there is "a causal sequence whereby observers first determine social realism by whether a character portrayal appears socially normative (like most people I know)," then judge "how similar a character's identifiable traits are in relation to personal experiences." She proposes that "if characters survive this perceived similarity test, the viewers may identify with attractive characters and want to be like these ideals." She goes on to claim that "if they feel highly capable of assuming the character's identity...or performing the same activities and they expect to achieve the same rewarded consequences as the character, then they may likely adopt the character's prosocial and/or antisocial behaviours in similar situations." She further suggestions that "empathy (i.e., sharing the same thoughts and emotions)...generates subsequent altruistic behaviours" (49–50).

Are We There Yet? takes a related but inverted tack, inviting audiences to shift characters' opinions and actions through direct intervention. The production employs a variety of theatrical techniques to grab the attention of its audience, enticing them to delight in the novelty of its humour, interaction, and bold improvisational spirit, all of which ready them to invest and engage in the more true-to-life elements of the play. Teens reported being able relate to the characters and situations. They believed that the scenarios represented issues that they may face (or have already faced).

> *It opened a window to show me what was actually out there in the world and what can happen to me and what I should be prepared for if I should want to do stuff like that.*
>
> —*Audience member*

This authentic fiction makes it easy to apply the information to their own lives and see the potential for using the information in future relationships/situations. For example, one audience member connected it to her relationship at the time and realized that she was not in a good situation:

> *I saw the play and then I saw a couple of things he did to me in the play and that was pretty much what ended the relationship, I couldn't stay in it after that, all my friends in grade nine saw the play and so they were pushing me to break up with him after that, but before I saw it, I think I knew what was going on. I just didn't want to admit it and it was a little bit hard to ignore after I saw the play.*
>
> —*Audience member*

Another realized she hadn't dealt with some issues surrounding sexual abuse and went to a counsellor after seeing the play:

> *I...learned a lot, like, I found it really neat that I learned about [indecipherable] approaching someone about, like talking to them about that. Um...the...whole issue with, like, sorta, like, the girl that got raped, it...I didn't relate...I got molested and I...kind of...it's [indecipherable] and I had to go talk to the counsellor after that because there was some stuff I had never dealt with and hadn't told anybody and so that was...it was feeling in that way, I thought, I dealt with, that was...yeah.*
>
> —*Audience member*

On our second try at finding ways to measure audience members' emotional engagement, we used two constructs (groups of related questions) to investigate Identification and Empathetic Involvement. The former covers the extent to which individuals recognized and believed the realness of the characters and their dilemmas. Items include: "I believe that teens find themselves in situations like the ones that were shown in the play," and "the characters in the play seemed real to me." The Empathetic Involvement scale focuses on audience members' feelings for the characters and what they are going through; because of the interactive nature of the play, we asked about their sense of stakes and audience impact. Items include: "I felt the characters needed our advice"; "I hoped the characters would solve their problems"; and "one or more of the characters learned something because of the audience's advice."

Again, we see that the greater the identification and empathetic involvement, the greater the impact the piece had on its audiences in terms of the play's goals. Sexual communication and sexual decision making changed significantly from before to after the play for the group who identified with the play. Youth felt that they were more able to communicate about sexual issues and thought they were better able to make decisions about sexuality. Audience members who empathized with characters in the play felt more able to communicate about sexual issues and about their boundaries. In contrast, the control group, those who did not participate in AWTY experienced next to no change during this period, except in communicating boundaries, which significantly decreased, and there was a little but not statistically significant change for participants who reported less empathy for characters; this insight encourages the artists to consider the range and diversity of characters and the nuances of characterizations they portray in this multi-character piece.

When the social science team further assessed this theory,[8] we found that identification with the play's characters and situations emerged as being more important than a myriad of other factors (including learning style, gender, etc.). Audience members who identified the most showed the greatest change in perceived decision-making skills.

When participants were asked in interviews and focus groups why they wanted to give the characters advice, a few recurrent themes emerged. The majority gave advice because they felt that either the character needed it or that they wanted to help the relationship and/or character. Linking back to the "pleasure factor," respondents also indicated that giving advice made the play entertaining and fun, that they had advice to give and wanted to guide the characters to make better decisions. As with the metaphor's impact, we detect audience pleasure in the acknowledgement of their expertise and insights:

> *Because I wanted to help them out with advice they didn't know, so they could sort out their problems without breaking up.*
>
> —*Audience member*

Participants also reported that being able to relate to the situations that the characters were going through and identify with them contributed to their decision to give advice:

> *Because I felt a part of the issue. Kids my age were going through the same thing and I would like to learn more.*
>
> —*Audience member*

> *Because I've been through the same stuff and it didn't go well.*
>
> —*Audience member*

> *I felt bad for them, I wanted to help because I felt like that could be me.*
>
> —*Audience member*

We argue that if the audience does not see themselves on stage in some capacity, whether it is in the characters or in the situations depicted, the show will remain presentational and removed from their real lives. Just another sex ed lesson. Similarly, we argue that locally created theatre that represents lives and concerns of that culture will have a special level of impact. Theatre is a live and ideally, a local art. It is through identification with the people and events on stage that the audience members can see how they fit in the picture, and this engaged recognition can then extend into an exploration of their own lives. This powerful medium becomes theirs.[9] As Mary Spratt and Benji Leung (2000, 223) highlighted in their reflection not on theatre but on peer education, "familiarity and relevance of subject matter allow students to bring their own life experience and knowledge to bear." Jill Dolan (2001) also proposes that theatre becomes a site for social transformation when it engages with participants on a specific and local level. Here, the power of the theatre lies less in the universal and rests on the audience members' ability to form momentary communities. The youth arrive distracted, wary, goofy. They are invited to laugh, together and with the actors. They are invited to participate with actors. They are invited to engage with characters and situations they recognize. The community of audience members is involved, together, looking for active strategies for their real lives, and all the while, they are meaningfully involved precisely because of their pleasure in engaging with the material. In AWTY performances, communities are built through a range of experience: common pleasures (common humour, common vernacular), silences of shared empathy for characters who are in trouble, as well as through invested, collaborative problem solving.

Distancing

However, Brecht (1964a, 190) and others challenge theatre artists to make more of the theatre than providing a good night out.

> *We need a type of theatre which not only releases the feelings, insights and impulses possible within the particular historical field of human relations in which the action takes place, but employs and encourages those thoughts and feelings which help transform the field itself.*

Brecht (1964b, 71) famously argued,

> *The theatre-goer in conventional dramatic theatre says: Yes, I've felt that way, too. That's the way I am. That's life. That's the way it will always be. The suffering of this or that person grips me because there is no escape for him. That's great art—Everything is self-evident. I am made to cry with those who cry, and laugh with those who laugh. But the theatre-goer in the epic theatre says: I would never have thought that. You can't*

do that. That's very strange, practically unbelievable. That has to stop. The suffering of this or that person grips me because there is an escape for him. That's great art—nothing is self-evident. I am made to laugh about those who cry, and cry about those who laugh.

In the play, distancing is accomplished through a variety of theatrical devices, including the juxtaposition of theatrical styles and points of view, the use of multiple characters and actor/character transformations, actors' informal interaction with the audience as themselves before and after the show, and direct audience address. While the audiences' identification and empathetic engagement is sought by the artists, so too is a "critical social reflection leading to social change that Brecht sees as central to theatre" (Curran 2001, 171). In our view, the forms that AWTY employs build engagement, as well as break it.

I think it definitely delivered that message but I think they took it one step further. I think it showed kids how to be real and how to be yourself. Through taking their advice, through the participatory aspect of the play, taking their advice and showing it to them, and I was seeing themselves outside of themselves.

—*Teacher*

Fiction

Some community and popular theatre sets out to represent individuals' own stories. We think that this method misses a powerful opportunity, the power of fiction. Shauna Butterwick and Jan Selman (2003, 56) highlight the importance of this element:

There is a power that is possible in experiencing theatre and drama because of the use of fiction. Observers (and participants) can recognize and identify with characters and events, yet at the same time objectify them. With this identification comes a sense of relevance, engagement and urgency, while the objectification offers an opportunity to analyse, strategize and test alternatives.

Using fiction, when paired with certain staging devices such as direct address and audience participation, links the audience members with the dramatized stories. This creates a state that enables both engagement and a capacity for critical assessment: "The language of theatre can produce a quality of double-seeing that permits the state Augusto Boal calls metaxis: the stage of belonging completely and simultaneously to two different, autonomous worlds: the image of reality and the reality of the image" (Salverson 1996, 187). *AWTY*, although working from a script that is fictional, employs the experiences and, later, the expertise of the audience as it deals directly with issues relevant and immediately pertaining to the audiences' lives. Maxine Greene (1995, 4) writes about the importance of encounters with the arts and how they offer new possibilities for understanding: "the extent to which we grasp another's world depends on our existing ability to make poetic use of our imagination."

The fact that these stories are not the actual stories of the youth creates a safe space within which the participants can try out ideas and make suggestions. These are stories to use rather than real life. Here authenticity becomes vital. If an audience member does not see the characters and situations as authentic, identification is impossible. However, if there is no distance between the audience and the stories, which fictionality provides, identification steps into the real, which in turn, moves the audience away from critical and active engagement with ideas. So, while participatory theatre presents and elicits people's stories and anchors discussions in lived experience, it also creates a distancing that is part of the process of building deep and uninhibited identification.

There is complication here: two-thirds of the way through this ever-changing, overtly theatrical play, the actors perform three monologues from characters who have each moved through a sexual crisis and on to greater health or insight. The monologues are about things that can go wrong, and about seeking help and moving on; characters (and actors) are more revealed. In the midst of fun, lively theatre, with much laughter and verbal participation, we can suddenly hear a pin drop. The entire tone and nature of audience engagement changes. Despite all the signs and signifiers that remind audiences that these are actors with multiple roles, change up of styles, freeze action, and more, invariably audience members ask: Were these people real?

Is that really your story? They ask it during the performance, after the show, and much later in interviews and focus groups. Many are not really sure. Arguably, audience members are experiencing an ambiguous, liminal state that the theatre offers, full of potential. In this moment, many in our audiences shift their level of empathy, identification, attention, and commitment. They open themselves to these characters' experiences, and to the dilemmas and complications of the rest of the play.

As we have seen, AWTY delights the audience members, then switches gears and involves them empathetically with characters and their dilemmas; characters then break that reality by turning to the audience. The juxtaposition activates the audience, allowing them to think critically about what they are seeing reflected. This criticality not only engages the audience members as active participants in the show but also works to spark their imaginations and "stimulate creativity of thought by encouraging more flexible thinking" (Chapman and Foot 1976, xxviii). Perhaps this quality of involvement, born out of combinations of entertainment and pleasure, identification, and distancing devices, is better termed heightened engagement. AWTY carefully avoids, and indeed attacks in various ways, separation of audience from the actions on stage and from the actors; it skews and interrupts these presentational models, making immediate the relationship between actor and audience in a way not imagined by Aristotle or even Brecht.

Participation

While the play utilizes a variety of distancing devices, interrupting the emotional identification and providing conditions for critical analysis, the social science-based evaluation focused on assessing the impact of one of these: the play's use of direct participation.

Recognition and engagement (*This is relevant and I care*) combined with the opportunity to observe and assess, plus the opportunity to apply this within the play's participatory form, leads to active problem solving for someone like me. We suggest that participation and the freedom born of fiction combine to address Brecht's primary quibble with the use of empathy in the theatre; as Curran (2001, 174) suggests, his primary concern was "by identifying with the protagonist and sharing his feelings, the viewer is locked into the perspective of the character" and barred from "the 'freedom to consider' everything relevant to understanding the character's situation." Participation, when handled with depth and critical consciousness by actor and playwright, does indeed encourage spectators to reflect critically and provides another step toward a process of change. In addition to pleasure, involvement, and critical distance, a play such as this one creates opportunity, within the theatrical event, for praxis, for an opportunity for audiences to recognize and exercise agency.

Dramaturgically, this play puts characters in complicated situations that drive to a moment of crisis. In this moment of intense dilemma, a character turns to the audience for help. The stakes are high; the dilemmas are real. A teenage girl doesn't know how to bring up condoms with her boyfriend so runs away:

> *Now I don't know what to do. I'm meeting Mac in a few minutes at the mall. What should I tell him?* [the Audience advises Carol Ann and she tries to do what they suggest] *(Chapter 3, page 81)*

A teenage male tries to duck wearing a condom:

> *Everybody knows it's just not as good for the guy. Like it reduces the sensation, that's what my brother says. And we don't have diseases so maybe we don't need them...*[The Audience and Mac explore this; Mac throws up a lot of blocks, then eventually comes to the nub of his issue]...*What if she sees you and you aren't...what she expected? What if everything just...fades away? What if she laughs? I don't know. I don't think I can do it.* [They advise Mac] *(Chapter 3, page 81)*

Audiences can assess options, try strategies out, see them actively tested. They see results immediately, revise, and try other options. They also hear others' ideas, and consider how these relate to their lives.

Praxis, as promoted by educational theorist Paulo Freire (1983), can be defined as the marriage of action and reflection. Specific to theatre, praxis requires audiences to engage (care), reflect (distance, assess options) and select (advise). AWTY builds this space; spectators move from a climate of

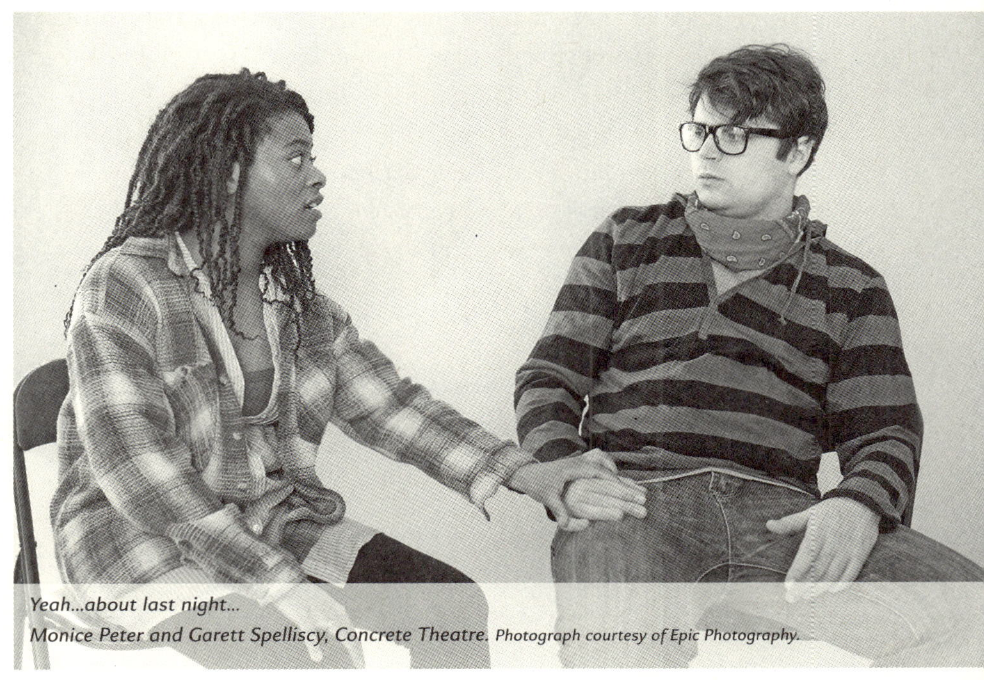

Yeah...about last night...
Monice Peter and Garett Spelliscy, Concrete Theatre. Photograph courtesy of Epic Photography.

simply watching to one of playing. They are implicated in the action and meaning making. By identifying, they can metaphorically place themselves in the action, but through participation, they can move from the idea of real life to the actual exploration of it. The space created by the actors is one that fosters openness, freedom of thought, and active engagement. The audience members feel as though they are implicated in the action and in the themes and storylines that are played out in front of them.

Participation was measured by three items, including: "I participated in the play by providing advice or ideas to a character"; "I felt comfortable about participating in the play in the latter part of the performance"; and "I participated in the play by listening." Naturally, more audience members reported participating in the play by listening (88 per cent) than by providing advice or ideas to a character (64 per cent). A majority felt more comfortable participating in the play in the latter part (69 per cent). Those who participated in the play were most likely to enjoy the play (pleasure), feel empathetic involvement with the characters, and identify with the characters and

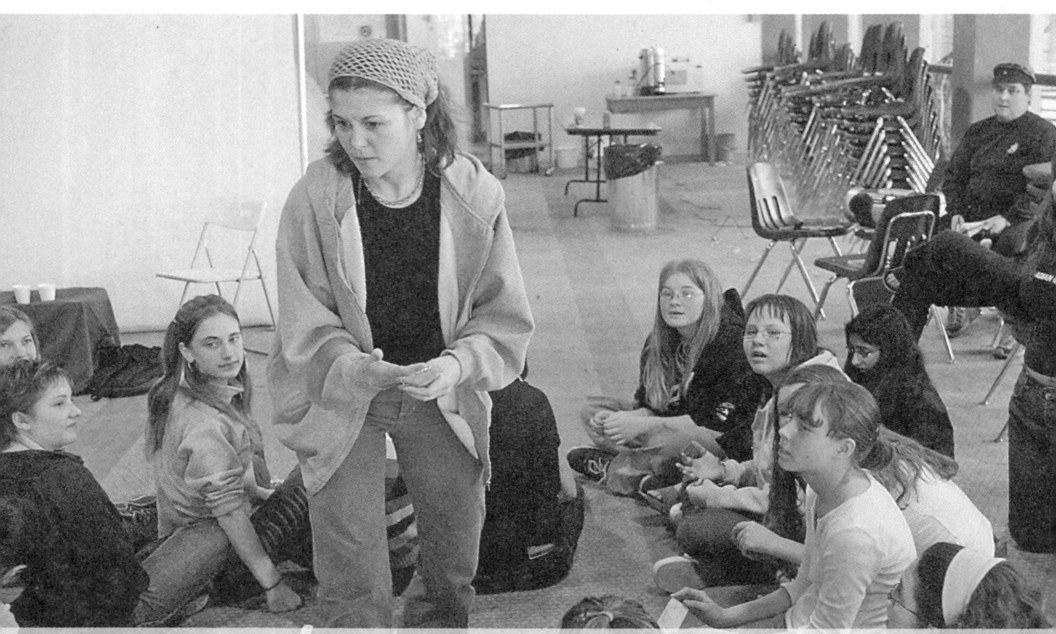

What can I say to him?
Shannon Larson, Concrete Theatre. Photograph courtesy of Epic Photography.

situations in the play. Their participation took the form of active listening through to giving direct advice to the characters.

More to the point, the audience members who reported participating in the play also demonstrated greater increases in their capacity to make use of the safer sex strategies proposed by audience members as well as by the script and characters in the play. Audience members felt that they were more able to communicate about sexual issues, make sexual decisions and communicate about their boundaries, and they increased in self-efficacy in the area of sexuality after experiencing the program. Data analysis demonstrates that level of participation (as compared with other variables) was the most important predictor of change in perceived ability to communicate boundaries and change in sexual risk-taking behaviour.[10] One-on-one interviews and focus groups revealed that teens felt the participation to be an important and fun component of the play, allowing for their own voices to be heard and their opinions incorporated into the scenes.

You can put the play and you could kind of...plug it into your real life, basically. You could take the situations and have them help you.

—Audience member

[I was] able to participate, not just sit there passively while the teacher tells you stuff. *—Audience member*

Participants were asked if they think they got more out of it by participating than if they did not:

Yeah, I do. I really do because you got to interact and it's more interesting when... cuz people can relate to it and it's so much easier to take things in and to use it in real life when you see something relatable...

—Audience member

All audience members who were interviewed responded positively to the interactive aspect of the play. They felt that it allowed them to interact and feel more comfortable overall, and they liked that they could hear what others were thinking. They stated that the participation gave them a chance to voice their opinions, express themselves, and try things out. They liked the idea of testing things and that they could see what happened without having to live through real-life consequences.

I think it helped me, like, think, thought-wise I think it gave me more ways to approach different situations and for how I'd feel, I think it helped me feel more like opinionated, like more stronger with my opinion that I could hold it and I think it would help me be able to say no easier.

—Audience member

So, our social science colleagues can demonstrate that each of three concepts central to theories of theatre, its reception, and impact-pleasure, empathic involvement, and distancing had a significant and powerful affect on its audience. These findings suggest there is value in giving close consideration to the mix of these qualities in plays and productions, and challenge those of us who may be inclined to downplay one element or the other in our theatre work. Further, these cross-disciplinary studies also show that audience members who had higher response scores on the total theatre scale exhibited significant change in all but one component of the outcomes that were measured.[11] Audiences felt better able to communicate about sexuality and boundaries, more able to say no, and that they would be more in control of sexual situations after seeing the play. This was in contrast to the youth in the control group, who, over a similar period of time, did not change significantly, or in the case of one important area, capacity to communicate boundaries, felt they decreased in ability.

Of course, there are some limitations to this study. We cannot leap from these findings to implications for all theatre and all theatre makers. *AWTY*, the case study, focuses on youth and the sexually charged experiences and relationships that they encounter and care about. While the audience is far from homogenous, these conditions enabled a focused study of a fairly goal-oriented theatre piece, an approach that may not be possible with many theatrical events.[12] However, when examining what can theatre do, the combination of the analysis of outcomes beside the investigation of audiences' experience of what theatre artists, philosophers, and theorists argue are central to theatre's power (pleasure, engagement, and distance) appears to provide some answers. While new answers and questions emerge, I hope that this work contributes to a pressing need to argue for theatre's concrete contributions to society, as well as to discussions of theatre quality and capacity.

We are living in a time of great questioning of theatre. Artists restlessly search for essential theatre, theatre that compels and has impact. We search for a theatre that satisfies our understandings of the postmodern, multivalued, globalized, mediatized, and digitized conditions in which we live and work and create. We want to make challenging, riveting theatre, and theatre that audiences want. And we debate what, if any, kind of theatre can do that. Kurt Lancaster (1997, 76), referencing critics from Aristotle to Turner and Brecht to Bennett, proposes that at this juncture, people seek a theatre that rediscovers, in today's terms, "participatory communal relationships between spectator and performer." This play, and the measurements that capture some understandings of impact as it relates to pleasure, identification, and participation, seem to suggest one route. The audience starts cool and protected; an hour later, they are huddled in a theatrical frame that elicits urgent, impassioned debate with one another and with the theatrical event. Perhaps, then, there is a theatre that will re-take the central and socially transformative role we imagine.

NOTES

1. For a useful discussion of approaches to measuring impact of applied and/or theatre in education, see Lynn Dalrymple (2006) and Michael Etherton and Tim Prentki (2006).
2. While many reference Horace's *Ars Poetica*, a richer look at the levels of pleasure within the experience of theatre (and their impact) is needed, particularly in this rather depoliticized post-dramatic theatrical age. See one example in Chapter 10.
3. For a useful discussion of the role and range of kinds of pleasure experienced in the theatre, see Ubersfeld's, "The Pleasure of the Spectator" (1982).
4. Of course, there are attendant dangers to this claim, such as the risk of defining "better" as pleasing to everyone.
5. See more about causal modelling as a powerful approach to analyzing data in Chapter 9.
6. See, for example, Ross Kidd's "Popular Theatre, Conscientization, and Popular Organization" (1985) and Tim Prentki's "Introduction to Poetics of Representation," in *The Applied Theatre Reader*, edited by Tim Prentki and Sheila Preston (New York: Routledge, 2009), 19–21.
7. For more detail, see Chapter 9.
8. This analysis used a causal modelling approach.
9. These beliefs led to decisions to adapt and assess the play and program in three other cultural communities; see Chapter 7 for a discussion of adaptations.
10. Causal modelling was used to explore the most dominant influences on audiences and to control for other factors that may influence this analysis.
11. The total theatre scale is an amalgam of the responses to all the theatre questions on the quantitative survey. Youth who had higher scores on the total theatre scale exhibited significant change in all areas but sexual decision making.
12. See other publications from the AWTY CURA research program, which examine diversity within the audience and discuss variations in response depending upon factors including learning styles (e.g., Munro et al. 2007; Munro et al. 2009).

14

WHERE ARE WE NOW? ARE WE THERE YET?

CONTENTS

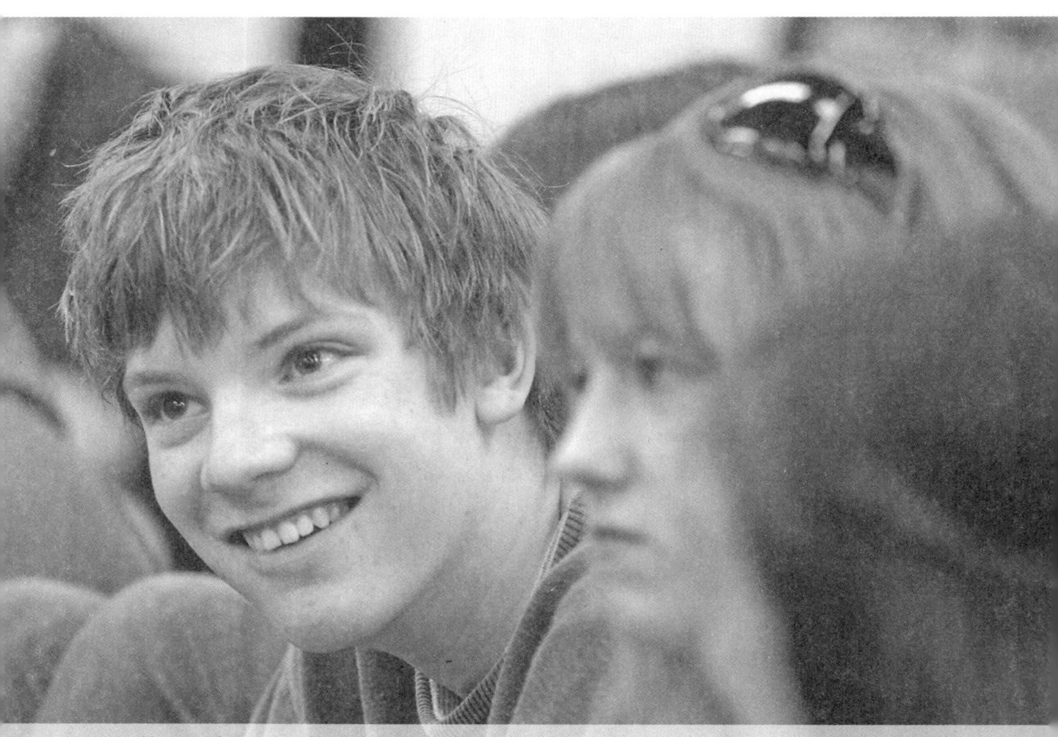

Photograph courtesy of Epic Photography

Principles and findings extracted from this interdisciplinary research program about ways to make theatre vital, relevant, and part of real change are collected here and (re)considered in light of a radically different context.

THE ARE WE THERE YET? PROGRAM IS UNIQUE in two ways: first, in its longevity; and second, as it is the subject of an extensive, interdisciplinary examination and evaluation. The former allowed the development of profound expertise; the latter enabled a rigorous process that proves the program works. With this book we endeavour to put all the pieces together in one place: the expertise, the proof, and the tools. The book is intended for use by others who see a need to find ways to use theatre for change.

This research project allowed us to take a long, thoughtful look at a complex artistic, social, and educational intervention. Our basic questions about theatre, participation, community and strategic partnerships, and adaptation of interventionist art for varying contexts have, through this project, been explored, sharpened, and largely answered. Does this theatre and workshop program make change? Yes. Qualifiers and caveats abound, but we think we have been able to extract some principles that should be applied to other topics and other contexts. We believe, and have largely shown, that when these principles are applied fully through processes of participatory engagement, a project has impact and will contribute to meaningful change for people.

Five Key Principles, Five Key Questions

1. Discover Community Context (Research and Adaptation)
2. Build Partnerships
3. Evolve Theatre Forms from Context
4. Invest in Training
5. Aim for Sustainability

With these principles in mind, five questions are essential to explore, rather than presume.

1. Who is the audience?
2. Who are the community partners?

3. Who are the theatre artists/performers?
4. Who trains the actors and community partners?
5. Who supports the program?

By way of concluding this discussion, we re-open these questions and test the principles by applying them, albeit theoretically for the time being, to a new situation. Principal investigator of this research program and co-writer Jan Selman was living and working in Kenya through the final stages of writing this book, and as a result of her contacts and conversations with artists and activists there, a thread of an idea emerged. We sought to apply long-held principles and some new insights about adaptation, partnership, and the value of participatory theatre interventions to another, extremely different context. Could they hold up when applied in vastly differing circumstances? We hope the following brief investigation might serve to pull together, test, and extend some of the insights gained through the AWTY CURA processes.

We start from an assumption that were we to develop the project in this very different context, we may find that radical adaptation is required, or that we need to start completely afresh. While starting with this understanding, we lay out a set of questions below, questions that taken cumulatively ask:

Could AWTY be successfully adapted in Kenya?

This speculation and question catalyzes a flood of others, some of which follow.

Is this a crazy and/or stupid idea?

The only answer to this question, initially, is *maybe*. A *maybe* might become a *no* or a *yes* at any point in an adaptation and partnership building process. However, once we considered the first question and acknowledged the second, we let others flow. Each question implies a number of others. Although they appear here in a linear manner, each question branches and connects to another or another set of questions. Some questions that appear late in the following list might need to be addressed very early. The list is not a blueprint or a formula but an attempt to think widely and openly, to imagine a future project in another context.

We place ourselves in a specific but, for us, largely unfamiliar location, time, and situation to explore these questions. We imagine that in future we might build a useful project in Kenya. We wonder if some emerging relationships and insights may be the starting place for a serious exploration of whether or how an adaptation of this project may have a role to play here. There are many questions to answer.

1. Discover Community Context (Research and Adaptation)

Who has issued the invitation to explore this possibility? Who are the first people or organizations that need to be involved?

An invitation to begin a conversation is crucial. It must be genuine and requires a personal face-to-face relationship of trust between an AWTY team member and a Kenyan who is grounded in his or her communities. Jan made such a connection with a young and remarkable activist, Raphael Omondi, and she explored the possibility of an invitation to begin a conversation. Everything about such a process is delicate but not impossible. Historical and contemporary contexts impact every aspect of the relationship and the possible conversations.

A long and filthy history of colonization, imposed solutions, and exploitation of the Global South by the Global North is part of the context for any imagined partnership. Colonial era atrocities are common in former colonies but the current situation in Kenya is particularly raw. Snapshot: In April 2011, four Kenyans, three men and one woman aged in their seventies and eighties, launched a human rights claim against the British government. Almost half a century after their country gained independence from Britain, these people have claimed they were tortured and sexually assaulted in British-run detention camps during the 1950s Mau Mau uprising (Cobain and Walker 2011). The Kenya Human Rights Commission has said ninety thousand Kenyans were executed, tortured, or maimed during the crackdown and 160,000 were detained in appalling conditions.

In addition to the colonial history and the recent court cases (there are others), the topic is also delicate: teens and sex. When we consider all the daunting differences in culture, race, age, gender, and more between the two

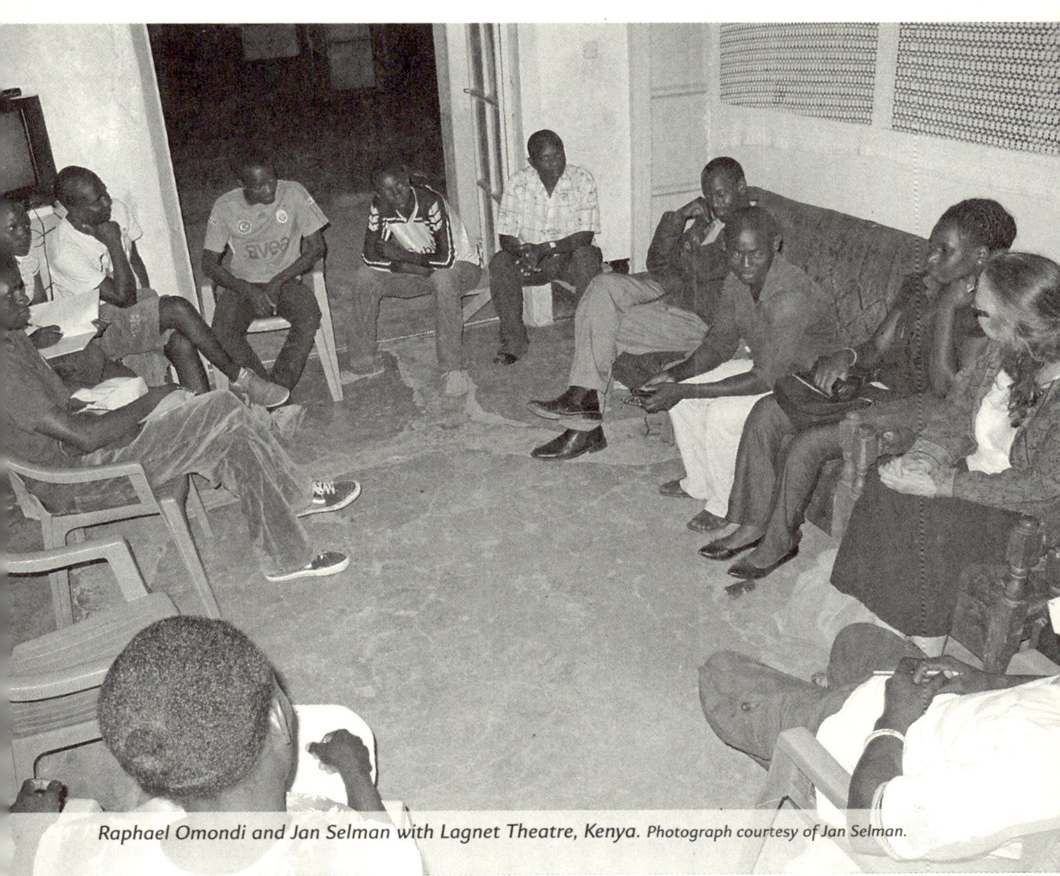

Raphael Omondi and Jan Selman with Lagnet Theatre, Kenya. Photograph courtesy of Jan Selman.

people who might explore this idea, all the unknown and perhaps unknowable Kenyan and Canadian attitudes, customs, issues, and cultural rules about teens and sex, and all the suddenly preposterous things (such as the title of the play and the driving metaphor) that need to be explained before an invitation could be offered, we are tempted to give up. Given all the possible pitfalls, the answer to, "Is this a crazy/stupid idea?" is obviously "Yes!" However, time, human connection, and a growing sense of common intention keep the possibility alive. Perhaps we can look to Gramsci (1994, 299) for encouragement, who enjoined us to live without illusions yet not become disillusioned.

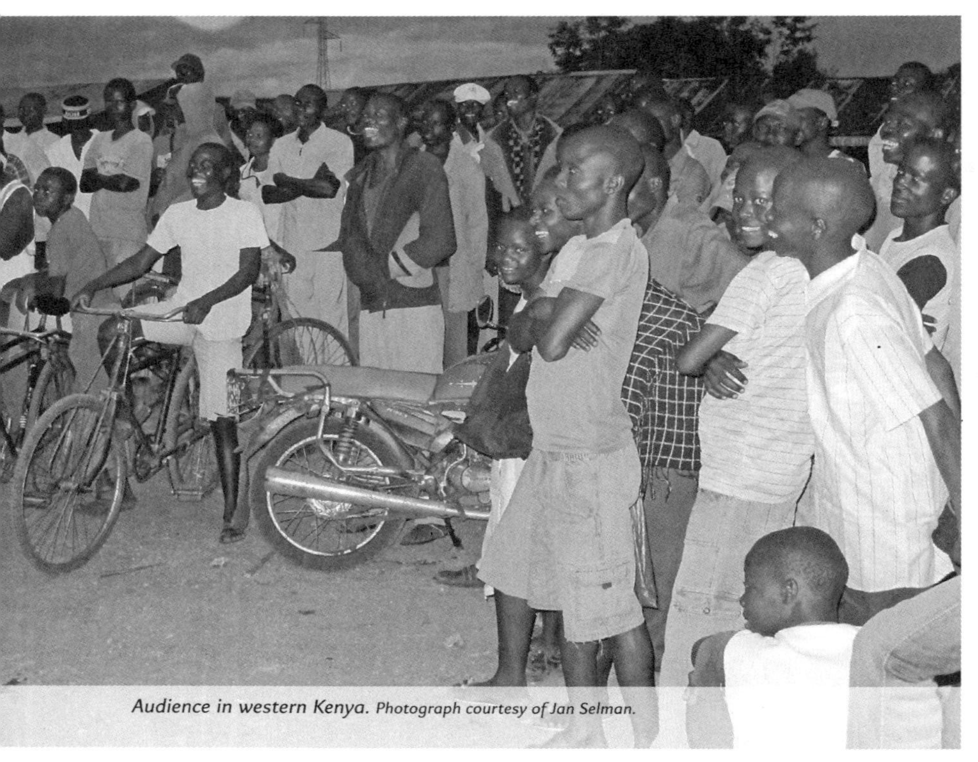

Audience in western Kenya. *Photograph courtesy of Jan Selman.*

Beginning the Conversation

Raphael Omondi's organization, Pamoja Youth Foundation, worked with a consortium of NGOs and others on a remarkable project on sexual safety, including rape prevention. So, asking about the foundation's work put one aspect of our topic on the table. The campaign's name is Sita Kimya, loosely translated as We Will Not Be Silent. The initiative relates to Pamoja's platform, an organization that is run by, for, and with youth. As the organization's website explains, "[It] works to better the life chances and quality of living by improving their talents. In doing so, Pamoja Youth Foundation aims to help in the transformation of youths from lives of crime and drug abuse to self-reliance and into people who promote peace and justice in the globalized world" (2013).

Another important moment of connection to the topic of sex education arose as Jan and Raphael, over the course of several conversations, talked about Pamoja Youth Foundation. This time, current affairs played a role in opening the subject:

> *Raphael told me that recent research had revealed that circumcised men are less likely to contract HIV/AIDS than those who are not circumcised. He said that this highly promoted finding is leading some men to believe that if they are circumcised they can have unprotected sex! We shared our dismay.*
>
> —*Jan Selman, June 9, 2011*

If the first crucial step was taken and an invitation to discuss this project was offered, many other questions immediately tumble out. Jan and Raphael eventually decided to meet to discuss the AWTY project in the context of thinking about this book.

> *A driver who I know and trust drove me to Kibera, Nairobi's famous slum, famous for its size and its issues. We drive down the hill, past the field where evangelists hold meetings and temporary markets set up, and into the one and only road that takes us into this huge community. From afar one can see a chaos of roofs, which cover a wide hillside stretching down to the river. I remember a painting of kids by the river, shanty buildings behind. But here, in the middle, the road is jammed with people, buses, taxis, trucks. Stalls stretch along the roadside, at first apparently makeshift, selling second-hand everything, others fruit and vegetables. It is noisy. Crowded. A bus with a huge open side window, blaring music, clogs the road. It is promoting an upcoming football game. More stalls, giving way to more permanent looking grill windowed stores. We park and Peter Kariuki, the much-trusted driver, walks me down wet earthen tracks between, to my eye, a chaos of small floorless homes, to a gate, a cement walkway, a door. Raphael is across the way, charging his computer. Two padlocks later, we settle around his desk, watch a snippet of AWTY on his computer, Carol Ann's monologue and part of her interaction with the Edmonton teen audience.*
>
> —*Jan Selman, June 9, 2011*

Raphael responds to the piece:

> *It's a kind of...what I call street education, what sometimes I refer to as street university, the reason being, like, you are getting the information to both the educated and illiterate people. They are participating and feeling they are part and parcel of what is happening...A lot is coming from the audiences, they are the ones giving the options, "Why don't you try this, why don't you do this?" And the character is actually putting their advice into action and seeing whether it is working out or not, and is coming back to the self same person and saying, "Hey, what should I do?" So in one way the character is not working with a fixed mind. She has a lot of options to explore and for that I think this is perfect...Kids are the best teachers...here you can be working with open-minded people.*
>
> —*Raphael Omondi, director, Pamoja Youth Foundation, Nairobi, Kenya, March 5, 2011*

Sex Education

Where/how do teens learn about sex? Radio? tv? Peers? Parents? Websites? Is there sex ed in schools?
Understanding the current delivery system is necessary to have a deep understanding of how an alternate delivery system might augment or disrupt the status quo. We believe and can show that the AWTY Program can make change in Canadian contexts, but in this new context, we need to ask, change from what?

What sex ed is currently delivered to youth in schools? Youth not in schools? Is there a consistent message and consistent program? How is it delivered?
These questions dig deeper into the current content and form of sex education.

What is urgent? Can we assume: HIV, gender violence, including coercive sex and other abuse? Early intercourse and/or pregnancy? Support for unwed mothers? Parenting by youth?

Creation or adaptation of a project would be impossible without a clear understanding of the crucial issues identified by all the stakeholders in the community, but most particularly by teens. Partnership with a youth foundation, run by youth and for youth, makes some sense, and would be a departure from the school-centred original *AWTY*.

What do teens say about sex and sex ed? What does the culture say?
Significant participatory community-based research would be required to find out what youth know, where the knowledge gaps are, what they want to know, and how and with whom they want to learn it. Our research tells us participatory theatre, performed by young actors that reflect the audience, is an excellent vehicle for sexuality education. A new context would require new research to test those findings. The community of youth is the co-researcher in this process. We wonder too whether a process of development such as in the *AWTY* adaptation with Saskatchewan Native Theatre Company may be a useful model. It involved a team of Aboriginal youth artists as well as the director and writers in meetings and workshops with younger teens as the project was made specific to their communities.

What is taboo?
Sexuality education with teens raises hot button issues, but within that there are some buttons that are inflamed (such as homosexuality and abortion). Are there subjects that are so forbidden that to raise them would risk censure or expulsion? We know that until recently homosexuality was illegal in Kenya. Where the Canadian adaptations responded to the increasing acceptability of this topic in the schools, could a Kenyan project?

What roles do religion(s) play in shaping this project?

Who is in the audience? What age group is the primary audience?

> *What is happening is we are talking about the kids. Some of the kids are teenagers. Some of the kids are parents, sixteen years, fathers, mothers, yeah. So the target is from about fifteen to twenty-five years old. The reason being that they [kids] are never com-*

fortable to ask questions of their parents. So if you are providing something like this it will be able to build the kids' self-esteem...because if a kid will be able to get the courage to ask a certain question...if they ask and you're telling them "that's a stupid question." [If you don't reach the parents and the kids]...it's like having a football team and you concentrate so much on the players you forget about the coach.

—*Raphael Omondi, July 23, 2011*

What are the popular culture, traditional culture, urban culture, and rural cultural messages about sex? Advertising, Internet, film, tv, comics? What/who are youth watching and listening to?

How does gender impact culture and audience make-up? What about language, religion, ethnicity?

How homogeneous is this audience? Will they have common experiences?

Should we consider creating and performing separate shows for each gender?

Where is the audience? Is this a Kibera project? If a project is a good idea, where should the project be situated? Why?

National Statistics about HIV infection each year they are getting at least 15 per cent infected with the virus. So living in a world of HIV and AIDS, what shall we do? Make sure the new generation that is coming will reduce the prevalence. So what is needed to be done is the sexual education. And we cannot say that now we have done enough sexual education. If you ask me and I work in the civil society, where there is a lot of sexual education is in town. Go to rural. You were there. Did you see even a single NGO signboard? There was nothing, and compared to here, it is everywhere. Go to the rural. They will tell you here in town there is 99 per cent sexual education. It's not even 99, because Nairobi's not Kenya, town is not Kenya.

—*Raphael Omondi, July 23, 2011*

In schools? In the village square?

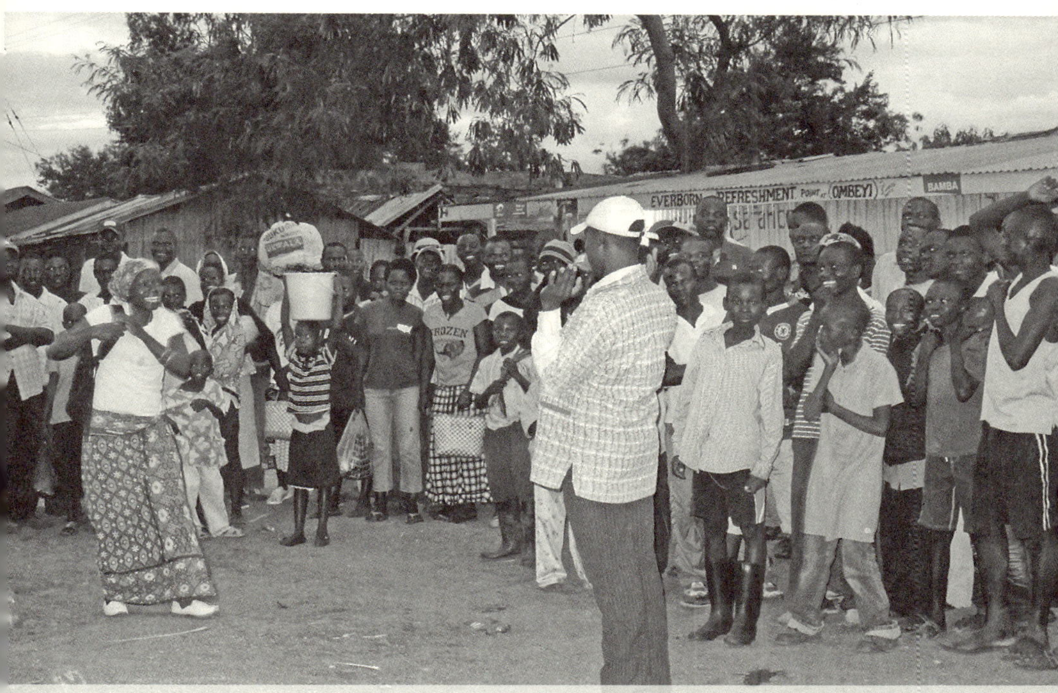

Lagnet Theatre performs at a Village Market, Kenya. Photograph courtesy of Jan Selman.

A project like this should be the first project to start breaking the barriers between the parents and the kids, between the religious leaders and the congregation and I think if this was implemented in Africa, not in town, in town there has been a lot of NGO *funding a lot of sex education projects, but if you go to rural areas you don't have anything happening there. And I think that this kind of project would be perfect in the rural...in schools it will work perfect. Take the same project to churches in the community will work. I believe it will.*

—*Raphael Omondi, July 23, 2011*

Sex education is happening in the schools in Siaya,[1] *it is but it is "you should not do sex." But what they are forgetting is what happens when students move out of the school. Out of the church. They are meeting their sexual partners...so whether you are telling them it is bad or not, so the pastor may say "it is bad" and they are saying, "hey, let me test what is bad and see whether it is bad or good." So whether they like it or not, it is something that is happening. The level of sexual education is too minimal. And what about the brothers and sisters that have never had the opportunity to be in a class, what happens to them?...And in the subject social science that is talking about sex, it is not even a topic, it is a sub, sub, topic.*

—Raphael Omondi, July 23, 2011

What other sex ed (usually HIV) theatre projects have there been? In Kenya? Elsewhere?

The best-known and longest running project is Theatre for Life in Johannesburg, which has been in operation since 1987 (AREPP 2010). What can be learned from their experience, research, and evaluation? And is that relevant to the Kenyan context?

2. *Build Partnerships*

Who decides about the content and delivery of sex ed for teens? Individual teachers? Are there local, regional, or national curricular guidelines? Do parents make these decisions? Religious figures?

Education always has an agenda. School and state agendas may be in conflict with parental or religious agendas. The politics of sexuality and sexuality education must be uncovered in order to know where the power resides and how that might impact a program. This set of questions would help establish who has a stake in maintaining the status quo and who might need to be convinced of the value of a program such as AWTY.

I learned (from a wonderfully committed young woman who is making a difference in one school on this issue) that in many schools girls must stay home each month during their menstrual period. They cannot afford and do not have pads. Often their mothers miss work for the same reason. So every month they miss school, or work, sit in the dark at home in the corner, I am told. This is a feminist issue, a social inclusion issue, an equity issue. The government plans to support supplying all girls in school with these, but time drags by with no action.

—Jan Selman, June 6, 2011

This conversation added to the process of uncovering potential partners, and who may initiate an action, and even who may actually make some meaningful change.

If there is dissatisfaction about current sex ed in schools, where is dissatisfaction coming from? Teens? Schools? Health providers? Teachers? Parents? Government? NGOs?

Si Kahn (1970), noted civil rights, labour, and community organizer, advised community organizers to meet with community trouble makers as a first step toward creating community alliances. Seeking out and working with those who feel a different approach to sex education should be considered would be a very valuable way to gain insight into how people perceive the issues and possible problems around the current situation. It could be that every stakeholder is perfectly satisfied with the current approach to sex ed for teens. Or it could be that many feel abstinence only, ABC ("Abstinence, Be faithful, and Condoms as a last resort") are the best messages for youth in Kenya. We cannot assume there is dissatisfaction, but if there is, we would want to know as much as we could about it.

Many believe more strategies are needed to respond to HIV/AIDS and other sex-related issues. One recent response to community conditions was Sita Kimya. This sexual violence awareness and prevention program was a very large initiative in East Africa, with many strands and many players. While press reports suggest that in Kenya it focused on men's role in sexual violence,[2] the project was more widely based. Pamoja Youth Foundation, for example, focused on a festival in Kibera that raised awareness and mobilized participants but also promoted a range of public communications and, significantly, took direct action around ensuring those who reported sexual assault were supported throughout their interactions with hospitals and police (Raphael Omondi, March 5, 2011).

What are the cultural and political factors, local, national, and international? For example, will organizations support comprehensive sexual education? How has US funding policy shifted from the abstinence-only Bush era? Where is the US Agency for International Development on this issue now?

This is a lifelong and ongoing investigation but every piece of information would be valuable and would shape the project.

What organizations are already involved in sex ed? Youth organizations? Women's organizations? Health organizations? NGOs? Community development organizations? Artists? Are there popular singers who sing about safer sex? Theatre organizations?

> *While in Kenya, I have been quite inundated with commentary on problems of opportunistic art programs and opportunistic NGO activity. Concerns from artists and activists include: one issue work, thin art, one shot activities, final reports that claim great improvements followed by grant applications that decry the conditions on the same issue. The urban arts community is very suspicious of and largely rejects the theatre for development approach; a new label and differing processes are required. There is a lot of activity which uses arts in education and community initiatives. I am told there is some great work as well as work with little meaning or impact. There are a lot of committed people and there is a lot of cynicism.*
>
> *—Jan Selman, July 30, 2011*

What groups might provide leadership for a project in this context? Is there an appropriate link to make with a group that is already doing participatory work?

Youth, women, health and community organizations, and activists may already be working in the area of comprehensive sexuality education for youth. Artists, particularly musicians, are significant cultural forces in many communities and an alliance with artists who promote or support comprehensive sexuality education would expand the range of the project.

> *I am struck with the energy and commitments and insights of youth activists here.*
>
> *—Jan Selman, May 25, 2011*

We also must remember how our project, during our adaptation processes, clarified the pressing need to invest in building comfort and self-knowledge around this sensitive topic, for all those engaged—actors and other artists, health educators, and certainly arts administrators. A commitment to workshops in naming and clarifying attitudes to sex and sex-positive work must certainly apply as we reconsider the nature of the project leadership in this new context.

3. Evolve Theatre Forms from Context

All of these questions about the play and the participation would be examined through participatory community-based research.

Who are the theatre artists/performers?

In Canada, each adaptation kept the original model's engagement of young adult, trained actors who as much as possible reflected the culture and social experiences of their audiences. Would this choice be appropriate here, or will performers be needed who are even more closely allied to each community?

> *I recently met with three community-based theatre companies in rural western Kenya. Each was quite different, each met with me and talked shop (theatre making, goals, and relationships with their communities and survival). Each performed something, two in their work areas and one in a village market...There are some remarkable talents, with outstanding work in large characterizations that were expressive, humorous and loving of each portrayal...The groups are embedded in their home communities and the groups have members who are community educators, specialists in various themes (women's organizing, youth development, social analysis) as well as actors, dancers, musicians. Some of great talent.*
>
> —*Jan Selman, June 1, 2012*

With the many ethnic and language groups in Kenya, does the cast need to change for each region? Will the play be in Swahili, English, or each home language? Are the answers to these questions the same in the city and rural areas? Should the play be multilingual?

What are the metaphors of coming of age that might replace the car and driving metaphor?

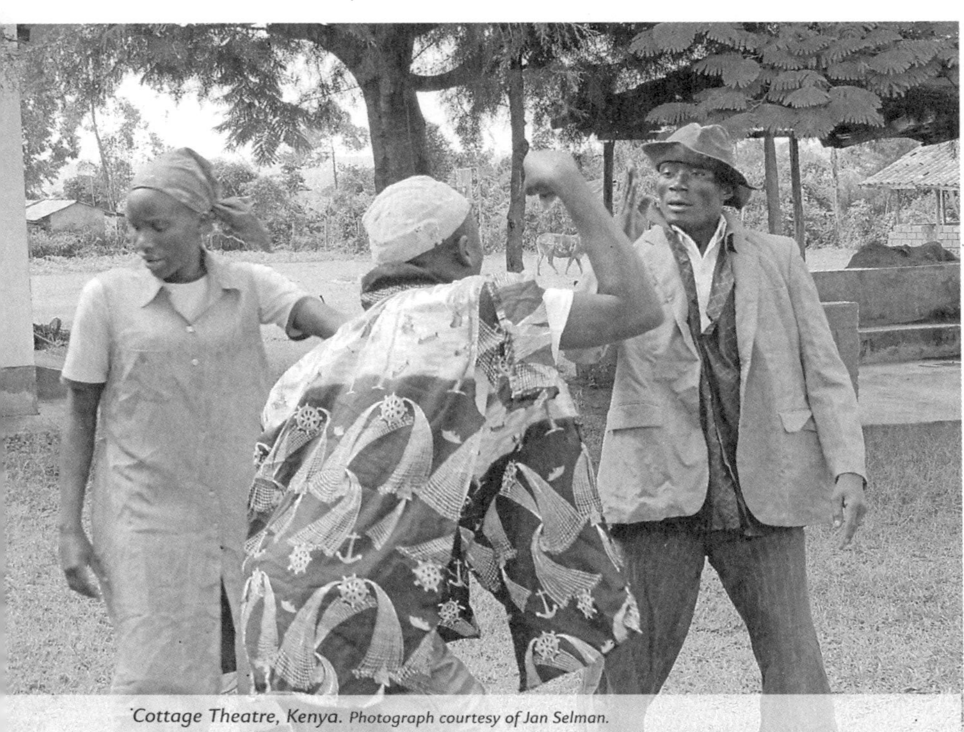

Cottage Theatre, Kenya. Photograph courtesy of Jan Selman.

> *While car ownership is growing, most of the people we would be trying to reach have no car, nor is there one in the family. It is not the metaphor for coming of age that it is in North America. When I first ever mentioned this project to Raphael I started there: the play is called* Are We There Yet? *I suddenly thought: I have to explain this title, the metaphor. This was not the place to start.*
>
> —*Jan Selman, August 8, 2011*

In the original, there are three key teaching points: establishing and communicating personal boundaries, negotiating condom use with a partner, negotiating a change in personal boundary. **Are these the correct points? What other ones might be important?**

Humour is key, so what's funny?
This is only discovered by being in the midst of the future audience for some time.

What performance style is required to catch Kenyan youth in the beginning of the twenty-first century? Is this the same or different from region to region, community to community? Should we rethink and revise, for this context, the dramaturgical principle of character-based participation, where characters who are like the audience are put into crises and dilemmas? Should we imagine and create scenes with multiple characters that interact with and ask advice of blended audiences? What do we gain and lose? Who gains voice and agency and who may not?

4. Invest in Training

Based in the work to date, we believe that getting ready to create a new version will likely require at least a one-month to six-week workshop with young actors and others, as well as with youth and other representatives of a project's future audiences, to answer some of these questions and develop material. Will the project need to provide basic actor training as well as participatory theatre and sex ed training?

Who should provide that training?

Is the theatre company also the health partner? Is the health partner also the theatre company?

5. Aim for Sustainability

How can the project be built with sustainability in mind?
If we were able to answer this long list of initial questions and still felt the answer to, "Is this a crazy and/or stupid idea?" was, "no," we may want to look around for a prestigious public person who would support and lend their weight to the project. This question might come up much earlier in the project:

Who supports the program? Who needs to be on board to make a pilot happen? Who will help? Who is likely to block? Where is the power? For example, if Desmond Tutu supports the program, would that help? Who is Desmond in Kenya? Is it a woman? What about Ngugi wa Thiongo? Could we get him on board? Should we?

Who else could help? Who are the visual artists, performers, musicians, or others who should be involved in some way?

The following question would also come up early and often during the process, perhaps very early:

Where is the money? Bill Gates? Warren Buffet? Bono? The Aga Khan Development Network? Common Ground? Universities? Government? ngos? Grassroots International, Unity Theatre Trust? C.A.R.E? Swedish International Development Agency (SIDA)?

How can the impact be measured and what approach should be taken to assessment?

Constant Questions and Iterative Processes

The following questions would also be very important and would need to be asked and answered regularly, as the answers would change or refine over time.

What are the goals and intentions?

Do we have any role in this? Is our role to offer this book and walk away?

Is this the right topic? Are there other topics or issues that are more urgent in this context?
Jan asked Raphael this question. Without hesitation, without a breath, he responded: “corruption.”

People don't know their rights, they don't have information. So government officers are giving the bursaries to their family members. It is the way of life. So people need the information, so the people can start demanding for their rights. So you can go to that office and ask for your rights. So you say you dropped out of school because you don't have the money. You can know you can go to that person and know that that is your money. That person will give you money...if you don't know your rights then you don't know you can deny things a person is doing. But if you know your rights you know you have a freedom of movement, you know you are not supposed to be somewhere because you are a Luo or Kikuyu, then you can know, "this is my constitutional right." Freedom of expression to ask people, "What are you doing with our money? We elected you to do this or this and you are not."

The other issue that people should talk about is corruption. We have a lot of money but there is nothing happening. Where is our money? Immediately people start asking these kinds of questions I think the whole development will change.

...You should not fear. These offices are to serve you. People can learn how to ask so people will assist...This is democracy. Making a decision is part of the democratic process. You have that power to ask questions...It is my right to ask questions.

—Raphael Omondi, July 23, 2011

As this project comes to a close we ask ourselves, do the principles we articulated and tested in Canadian settings hold beyond here, in new circumstances? Exploring this from the middle, as we step into a new context, we think that there is a priority principle. Those wanting to engage and make a difference through art and partnering for change need to walk these questions, not merely ask them. We must invest in relationships and listen as well as ask, in action. The listening includes deep curiosity. The walking includes a search for points of common intention. It includes taking time, letting time help build relationships. Just as participatory theatre is most meaningful when performers and playwrights are open, curious, and committed to hearing silent and spoken perspectives from all, so too, is project development. The capacity to listen flexibly, to hear and change because of how the answers emerge is paramount.

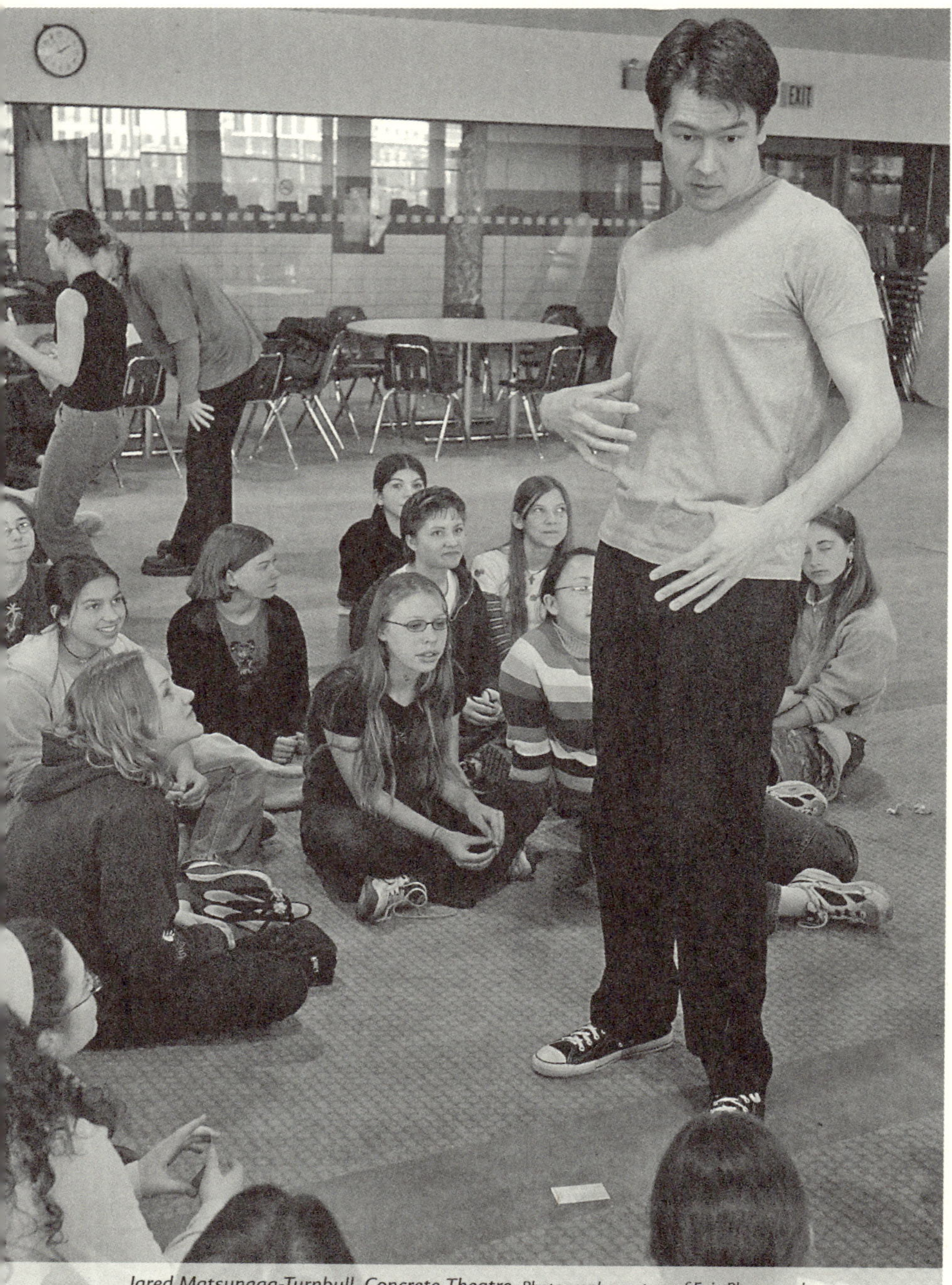

Jared Matsunaga-Turnbull, Concrete Theatre. *Photograph courtesy of Epic Photography.*

NOTES

1. Siaya is a district in Nyanza, a province in western Kenya. It is mainly rural and people mainly live on subsistence farming.
2. See, for example, a comparative report called *Chewy Chunks* (2011) on two projects, Sita Kimya and a second called Mrembo. (http://chewychunks.wordpress.com/2011/07/25/comparing-two-rape-prevention-programs/). Both programs were considered successful, though very different; both used storytelling for research and action.

APPENDICES

1 *Theatre*

1. Script Adaptation: The Hal Monologue, Aboriginal Example
2. Rehearsing the Play: A Template Schedule
3. The Goals of the Play
4. Animating Audiences: A Cheat Sheet of Techniques for Rehearsal
5. When Audiences Suggest "Compromise" to Marcel and Delphi

2 *Sexual Health*

1. Resources: The AWTY Workshop Manual and DVD
2. The Teen Workshop
3. Teens' Anonymous Questions

3 *Community Meeting*

1. The AWTY Community Meeting: Sample Outline
2. Sample Participatory Scene for Adults

4 *Promoting the Are We There Yet? Program*

1. Copy for Promoting the AWTY Program
2. Adapting Promotional Materials

5 *The Are We There Yet? Community-University Research Alliance Partners*

APPENDIX 1

Theatre

1. Script Adaptation: The Hal Monologue, Aboriginal Example

Hal: I'm Hal, nineteen. First off I'm not a pervert or anything. I'm not some big rapist or stalker okay? I'm just a normal guy. Well, you just do what everybody does. In grade seven all the guys snap the girl's bras. You stand around outside the school and yell stuff at them as they walk by: "Whoa baby look at the size of those...,you've got the biggest...back pack I ever saw on a girl." You get the picture. It was like a competition, who could get a good one off, make everybody laugh. I knew it didn't make the girls feel very good, most of them, well I guess all of them but...they never said. In high school all the guys ever talked about was scoring. Scoring, scoring, nailing her tonight. Man if those guys scored as much as they said they did...I knew they were lying but I didn't know how much. I was sixteen, still a virgin, and really horny all the time. So I started seeing this girl that everybody said was easy. She wasn't but I tried everything, bought her stuff, told her I loved her, told her I was going to die if I didn't get laid. And one night we did it. I forced her. I didn't like, use violence or threats, I just pressured her until she gave up. She didn't want to, but she didn't want to break up either. So I won. But it didn't feel like I won, and we broke up anyway.

One day, they have this workshop at school about sexual assault. They made all of us go. I didn't want to. I never assaulted anyone, why did I have to go? And then I see my Kohkum and I wonder what she's doing here. Well, she gets up in front of everyone and she starts telling a story about something that happened to her when she was in school. About a boy she liked...and about what happened when he wanted to and she didn't. And how it had changed her. Man, I hated that guy. I wanted to kill him for doing that to my Kohkum.

Then it hit me. I was no different than that guy. I sexually assaulted my girlfriend in grade eleven. I wish I hadn't. I wish I could go back and tell her. I'd tell her that I'm sorry. I hope she'd forgive me but I don't know if she would. This last winter I helped coach the wrestling team at my old school. And I tell the guys: "Think about how you'd like to be treated and treat girls like that. Why not try to find a way to behave around them so they feel good about themselves and their bodies, instead of like it's open season and any jerk can make a comment about them or hit on them any time?" And you know what? I think they're getting it.

2. Rehearsing the Play: A Template Schedule

Lengths of the rehearsal period will change in varying settings and should be driven to some degree by two questions:

- How much training in participation will the company require? (Or has anyone done this play or another that uses animating in role before?)
- How many workshops and test audiences will you be able to arrange (for participation practice)?

Here is a template provided by Concrete Theatre, who have produced the play many times.

Rehearsal Template (Three weeks/eighteen days)

Are We There Yet? by Jane Heather. Template prepared by Concrete Theatre.

Week One: The Project and the Script

Day One:

- Meet and greet
- Contract and other administrative business
- Discussion of the project: partners, background, history, participatory theatre, philosophy and goals of the project
- First read through
- Viewing and discussion of archival video (to introduce what the show does with an audience, provides intro to participatory theatre)
- Reflections on when and how we first learned about sex, related issues and sharing
- Discussion coming out of first day

Day Two:

- Reading/viewing current teen sexuality resources
- Discussion and brainstorming list of teen resources, culture: pop culture, music, movies, TV, expressions, fashion, games, websites, etc.; list is ongoing
- Table work-through of script
- First session with sexual health educators on sexuality information

Day Three:

- Brainstorm list of fears, concerns, hopes, and dreams about doing the show; list is ongoing
- Start blocking non-participatory sections

Day Four:

- Continue blocking
- Practice basic facilitation skills in context, e.g., gathers for just a minute, traits for Clay
- Costume inventory/measurements
- Brainstorm list of sex language, sex terms, and slang; list is ongoing
- Teen research/character observation at a mall, etc.

Day Five:

- First facilitation training workshop: introduction to participation and hands-on introduction to basic participatory skills gathering
- Start work-through of play, including beginning work on participations
- Develop outlines for "Just a Minute" stories
- Character hot seats to flesh out character back stories

Day Six:

- Continue work-through
- Stumble through working/talking roughly through participations as well
- Debrief the week

Week Two: Participations

Day Seven:

- Off-book day
- Work monologues: Hot seat monologue characters
- Run (review)
- Participations: Delphi and Marcel

Day Eight:

- Continue work on monologues
- Participations: Mac and Carol Ann
- Shopping for costumes as needed, more teen observation

Day Nine:

- Participations: Living Clay
- Full run with participations

Day Ten:

- Participations
- Second facilitation/participation workshop: Work-through of questions, problem areas in participations, working on skills to deepen

Day Eleven:

- Work sections as needed

- Run participation sections
- Shopping as needed: Costume and props for Living Clay

Day Twelve:

- Run throughs with debriefs of participation
- Work sections as needed
- Debrief the week

Week Three: Test Audiences

Day Thirteen:

- Italian run
- Invited run for health educators, chance to work them in
- Second session with health educators, to cover disclosure training, practice, and role-play for disclosures
- Debrief day, notes from run

Day Fourteen:

- Work notes from previous run
- Full run with notes
- Discussion of tour protocol, roles, and responsibilities of actors and stage manager on the road, etiquette in schools, safety issues, plan for set up, and strike
- Preparation for test audience number one
- Pack up and load van

Day Fifteen:

- Test audience number one. Audience should be a known easy audience, not too large. A university class is a very good audience; they can be asked to respond to the show as grade nines
- Debrief and notes from run

Day Sixteen:

- Work notes and all participations
- Preparation for test audience number two

Day Seventeen:

- Test audience number two. Audience should be a little tougher, larger, teens
- Debrief and notes

Day Eighteen:

- Friends and family invited dress
- Revisit fears, concerns, hopes, and dreams list
- Discussion of process for debriefing shows on tour to continue strengthening the show, review roles and responsibilities
- Rehearsal of pack of van
- Pack up and load the van

3. The Goals of the Play

As the research program started, the playwright prepared these goals upon the request of the social science-based evaluators.

The immediate, short-term goal of this project is to create a safe, loving, respectful, fun place for youth and adults to discuss sex together. The play's initial task is to carve out such a space in the cacophony of voices where a kid can listen, speak, and be heard. This is the groundwork necessary to achieve the medium term goals, which are:

- To provide information about sexuality, sexual health, and sexual decision making
- To provide information about the agencies and organizations that provide services to adolescents and to encourage them to use these services
- To identify, practice, and develop the communication skills necessary for the healthy sexual choices. These include:
  –Naming and negotiating personal boundaries with a partner
  –Naming and negotiating condom use with a partner
  –Negotiating a change in personal boundaries

- To encourage youth to reflect upon the consequences of uninformed, poor decisions related to sexuality and sexual choice
- To encourage youth to analyze:
  –The negative impact of sexism on sexual attitudes and choices
  –The media's impact on sexual attitudes and choices
  –The inadequate sex education in school on sexual attitudes and choices
  –Their peers' influence on sexual attitudes and choices

The long-term goals are behaviour change, delayed onset of intercourse, reduction in STDs, STIs, and unplanned, unwanted pregnancies.

4. Animating Audiences: A Cheat Sheet of Techniques for Rehearsal

Developed by Jan Selman

Preparation

- Agenda clarification: What is each interaction supposed to accomplish?
- Building the scene to set up the participation hot moments, first questions/statements to the audience
- Character development
- Know your audience: What kind of people/kind of interactions will they respond to/respect?
- Greeting the audience to build rapport, to learn about them, to make contact

Participation Techniques

Successful, honest audience animation is rooted in curiosity and character need.

1. *Gather = Brainstorm via "Yes And" (and Sometimes "Yes But")*

- For lots of ideas
- For inclusion

- For atmosphere
- To build comfort with participation
- It is non-critical, non-judgemental

Methods:

- Ways to say "Yes And":
  –Anything else?
  –Do you agree?
  –What a neat idea!
  –I never thought of that!
- Repeat or paraphrase
- Summarize, then: "Anything missing?" or "Does that cover it?"
- Translate into character's language and emotion:
  e.g., "Do you agree?" = "Really?" = "You're kidding!"
- Set up with a closed (yes/no) question then broaden with an open question (Why? Why not? What other choices are there? etc.)
  e.g., "Oh, should I try it?" (Answer yes/no). Then, "Why do you think so?"
- Physicalize—energize across the space
- To widen a gather:
  –Who agrees/disagrees?
  –What about the boys/girls, section back there, etc.?
  –Any other ideas?

2. *Deepen = Extend Ideas via "Yes But," "Why?" and Block*

Used to probe, deepen the thinking, acknowledge differing points of view, acknowledge and elicit emotion, circumstances, etc. (to get beyond "the right answer").

Explore:

- Consequences (Yes but...)
- Costs (social, emotional...)
- Circumstances (complications)
- How to do it *really* (go beyond the easy, learned answer; e.g., they say, "Communicate," you say, "What should I say?" or "How?" or "I want to but he won't listen.")

- Deal with a character/person's reality (no "magic")
- Move beyond "magic" fixes

Methods:

- Translating into character's language and emotion. For example:
  –Yes But = agree, then have a second thought, such as
  –"Yeah that sounds great...but how could I make her do that?"
  –"Wow! What a great idea...but she'll dump me when she finds out, won't she?"

(Note: complete playing the "Yes" before moving to the "But.")

  –Why = "I don't understand," "Why should I," "You've got to be kidding."
  –Block = "No, I couldn't ever," "S/he's too..."
  –Stories: based in character backstory, used for "Yes And," "Yes But," and "Blocking," and even for "Why"?
- Great ways to block, which deepen, are theatrical, can suit a specific character:
  –Character chooses the wrong answer (so the audience corrects and explains)
  –Play out/try a suggestion, it fails, ask audience why or give up (so they egg you on or explain what went wrong) now what? (NB: both actors need to create this; you don't need to make it easy to succeed.)
  –Alternative: when the suggestion fails, character blames the audience, "Gee thanks a lot!" They'll say you did it wrong...etc. "They" are the "Expert!"

3. *Acknowledge Audience*

To build rapport and future openness to participation:

- Thank them, with a word, gesture, or expression
- Summarize
- I would but I can't/don't dare
- Make a decision to try...
- Use their exact words or directions
- Succeed, using their advice
- Keep a connecting thread with them throughout
- A glance as you leave

4. *Focus Audience on the Task*

- As you start a participation: What is the audience's task?
- Restate the question or problem
- Play the character objective ("I need to know what to say to him.")
- Clarify the stakes or urgency ("I need to tell him something or else...")
- Summarize: then say, "anything else?"
- As you move from participation to trying the suggestions, help them watch/care:
  –So they root for you (involvement/empathy): What would be a success?
  –"It will be hard but..."
  –"I'll see if..."

5. *Play Out Suggestions to Test Them, Theatricalize*

- Start to go and play the suggestion, but stop yourself: "But what if..."
- Improvise a bad idea
- Improvise a good idea
- Actually start to use advice but then give up: "It's too hard," "I'm too scared," "It wasn't what I expected."
- Work together (with your scene partner) to:
  –Make it hard, face obstacles
  –Make it easy, succeed
- While playing a scene, check-ins with audience via looks or comments ("Is this what you meant?," "Shall I really do it?," "It worked!," "Gulp.")
- To deepen: Try something, it fails, ask audience why/give up so they egg you on or explain what went wrong, now what?

6. *Classic Problems to Grapple with, Practice ahead of Time in Rehearsal*

- No one will talk, silence
  –Enjoy it
  –Confidence comes from having the second question prepared
  –Have a fall back (e.g., "Okay, I'll try..." Give the wrong answer.)
- They talk very quietly
- An answer is very long
- Everyone talks at once

- Same few dominate, so widen the conversation
  –"Do you agree?"
  –"What about you?"
  –"I need to hear from the guys"
- Lose energy between participation and scenes
  –Leave on a peak
  –Use a summary to get you into the scene, use summary to build anticipation
  –Blend the two styles (check back in scenes, try stuff out on the spot during participations, theatricalize the discussions)
- The right answer is given early in a participation
  –Add a complication: "Yes but..." "Do I have to?," "But what if..." etc.

5. When Audiences Suggest "Compromise" to Marcel and Delphi

(Chapter 3, page 76)
Although this sequence is participatory and therefore improvised, in rehearsal the actor playing Instructor Two finds it useful to follow this outline. Audiences often suggest "compromise" or the equivalent, such as "she's got to move her line." The actor playing Instructor Two needs to help the audience work through the consequences of compromise without dismissing the idea. A visual representation of "compromise" helps audiences "see" and process the suggestion. In the rare case when compromise is not suggested, the actor still needs to work through this option.

Instructor Two: Okay, compromise. What does compromise mean? (AUDIENCES *may or may not come up with a definition, e.g., "meet in the middle." If an audience gives a definition use it, if not use this one.*) Find a middle place? Meet in the middle? Is that what you mean? (AUDIENCE *agrees.*) Let's take a look at this. Marcel's personal boundary is here. (*Place your hand level, about one foot above your head.*) So Marcel is comfortable with all the things they might do together up to here (*While saying this line, move your hand from below your waist up to the level you established as* MARCEL'S *personal boundary.*) and Delphi's is here (*Place your hand level with your* *waist.*). She's comfortable with everything up to here. (*Again, start your gesture about mid-thigh and, as you speak the line, bring your hand up to the position you have established as* DELPHI'S *personal boundary.*) If they find a middle place, meet in the middle, compromise, (*Choose two of these, including "compromise."*) they both move their personal boundaries (*Demonstrate by moving top hand and bottom hand to the same level, at about chest height.*) to here, is that what you mean?

Check with audience that they are following. You can also demonstrate the hand move again as you, and the audience, think about what this means. The actor can wait at this point to see if audience responds; if they do not, they need another clarification, such as:

Instructor Two: How do you feel about that? (Or:) Is that going to work? (*Hand demonstration again. If the* AUDIENCE *says "no," follow with an open question.*) Why not? (*If they say "yes," follow up with a specific question:*) For both of them? How might Marcel feel about that? (*Move hand to demonstrate.*) What about Delphi? What's happening for her? (*Move hand to demonstrate.*) How is he going to feel? How is she going to feel? (AUDIENCES *will usually name that both of them will be unhappy or uncomfortable with this solution.*) So Delphi will be uncomfortable (*Use* AUDIENCE'S *exact words.*) and Marcel will not be very happy (*Use* AUDIENCE'S *exact words.*) either. What else can they do? (*The* AUDIENCE *offers suggestions. Common solutions include:* MARCEL *will have to wait,* MARCEL *will have to come to her level, maybe over time when they know each other better they can move up together.*)

Deflecting the "break up" suggestion

Sometimes audiences will say, "He needs to find a girlfriend who will be more at his level." Actors can remind the audience that the characters said they want to stay together and can check with the Marcel and Delphi characters that this is so. In that case, the suggestion to find a new girlfriend will be redirected to "making this work, being patient, waiting," etc. Some audiences will identify the pitfalls of compromise much earlier in the participation. Some need a few more "hand demonstrations" and more probing about the consequences for both characters. Once these issues are resolved Instructor Two wraps up with Marcel and Delphi:

Instructor Two: So you two heard all that? Seems like you're going to have to talk about this. And Marcel? You're going to have to respect Delphi's boundary. Are you ready to try that?

APPENDIX 2

Sexual Health

1. Resources

As part of the Community-University Research Alliance activities, Options Sexual Health and particularly Brian Parker worked with several groups as they prepared to participate in the Are We There Yet? Program—the play and workshop. Out of these experiences, a manual and accompanying DVD was prepared, both highly recommended for health partners.

The Manual

A Guide to Facilitating the Are We There Yet? Follow-up Workshop
Authorship: Brian Parker, PHD
Curtis Wright, BA
Options Sexual Health Association

The Sexual Health DVD

The Are We There Yet? Follow-up Workshop
Authorship: Brian Parker, PHD
Options Sexual Health Association

These can be obtained by contacting Options Sexual Health Association, Edmonton, AB, Canada by email at options@optionssexualhealth.ca or visiting their website at http://www.optionssexualhealth.ca/.

2. The Teen Workshop

Outline for the Are We There Yet? Follow-up Workshop

Designed and conducted by Planned Parenthood Association of Edmonton (now Options), March 2006.

This workshop is intended to reinforce messages introduced in the play. These include awareness of the following:

- Factors that influence sexual boundaries
- A broad range of possibilities for sexual expression
- One's own sexual boundaries
- Strategies for communicating sexual boundaries, for getting protection against STI's and unwanted pregnancies

The workshop is forty-five minutes long but can be extended to one hour by adding discussion. In order to cover all the main concepts, in-depth discussion will probably not be possible. Try to focus the discussion on the points in the outline and fill in information that participants do not bring up.

Session Outline

Debriefing the Play (three to five minutes)

- Ask participants what they liked or disliked about the play. After several participants have shared their ideas, explain that this session will continue the topic of sexual decision making except now it will be applied to them instead of to the actors.

Anonymous Questions Part A (three to five minutes)

- Ask participants to write down a question they might have regarding sexual decision making on a piece of paper that you have handed out. Give them permission to ask anything they want. Give them direction of questions that you will not answer:

–Personal information about the facilitator
–Questions targeted toward another person in the room
–Anything dealing with pornography

- Give them time during the next part of the presentation to think about and write their question.

What Influences Sexual Decisions (five to seven minutes)

- Ask participants to tell you what kinds of things influence how we make decisions. Write participants' ideas on the board as they say them. You may need to give examples to generate ideas. Try the following example: "If you are Catholic or Muslim and you are trying to live by those religious guidelines, how could that effect what decisions you make about sex?"
- List all participants' responses on the board. Ensure that the following ideas are present:
–Religious beliefs and values
–Culture
–Gender (if you are a boy or a girl)
–Parents' expectations
–Opinions of friends and peers
–Personal desires
–Past experiences
–Fears
–Knowledge
–Use of alcohol or drugs
–The nature and quality of the relationship
- Ask participants to describe how the items in the list could influence sexual decisions.
- Ask participants to look over the list and decide which are important to them.

Drawing the Line (ten to fifteen minutes)

- Draw a line across the board approximately four to five feet long. Write the following phrases on the line:
–On one end of the line write "abstinence–no touching"

–On the opposite end of the line write "sexual intercourse–several partners"
–At mid-point write "touching partner's genitals with clothing on"

- Explain that the line represents the range of activities a person might choose to express their sexuality depending on their sexual boundaries.
- Ask participants to come to the board and write in activities that fit on the line between "abstinence—no touching" and "sexual intercourse—several partners." Explain that the activities are not necessarily what they have done, but should include what they have heard about. Ensure there is a range of activities on the line. These could include the following:
–Kissing
–French kissing
–Holding hands
–Massage
–Hugging
–Getting naked
–Touching partner's genitals till orgasm
–Oral sex
–Sexual intercourse only with a condom
–Sexual intercourse with condom and another birth control method
–Sexual intercourse without any protection

Alternate Process

Instead of asking participants to write on the board, ask them to call out activities that fit on the line, and write them on the board yourself.

- Once the line has a broad range of activities listed, ask participants if they remember the red marker activity from the play where the instructor asked the couple to make a red line, in their minds, where their sexual boundary lays. Tell the participants to mark their own boundaries, in their minds, as you read out the activities on the line. Explain that this is a private activity and ask that nobody say anything out loud.
- Ask participants to describe strategies for discussing sexual boundaries with a partner (refer to discussion on sunscreen from the play). After you have several responses, suggest alternate strategies. Other questions that could encourage discussion are:

–Do people who are attracted to someone of the same sex have to consider sexual boundaries?
–What can happen if you don't communicate your sexual boundaries?
–What could you say if your partner wants to go further than you?
–How did characters in the play communicate boundaries? Did it work?
–How could you talk about sexual boundaries if you are shy and cannot be direct?
–Where can you get support and information about sexual boundaries? (Ask participants if they could get support from their families, peer group, religious or cultural groups, or in the general community.)

Things to Consider (ten to fifteen minutes)

- Draw a line before sexual intercourse and ask participants what things a couple should consider if they decide to have sexual intercourse. Ensure that protection against STIs and pregnancy and communicating your boundaries are brought up.
- Demonstrate condoms and ask participants where they can get condoms. Ensure that the following sources are mentioned:
  –Planned Parenthood
  –Birth Control Centre
  –Abbotsfield Teen Clinic
  –Your doctor
  –Drugstore
  –Grocery stores
  –At the pharmacy counter instead of the checkout
  –Others
- You will not have time to have in-depth discussion on birth control. Try to focus on the Pill, Depo-Provera, contraceptive foam, pulling out, and chance and bring out the following points:
  –Where you can get it
  –Effectiveness
  –How it is used
  –How does if fail
  –Where to get more information

Anonymous Questions Part B (ten to fifteen minutes)

- Ask a participant to help collect the questions.
- Pick a question and read it aloud to the group.
- You could ask for help answering the question from the group, but it may be faster to answer yourself.
- Caution: read the question to yourself first and determine suitability for answering. If it is not acceptable, just move on to the next question.

Closure and Evaluation (three to five minutes)

- Thank participants for their involvement in the workshop.
- Ask participants to respond to the following questions, or ask individuals to respond:
  –What did you like about the play and this workshop?
  –What was the most useful things you learned from the play and/or the workshop?
  –Describe two reasons why it is a good idea to think about sexual boundaries and what can happen if you don't have any boundaries.
  –Where could you go to get more information or support?
- Leave prepared evaluation package with the teacher for return to Planned Parenthood.

3. Teens' Anonymous Questions

At the beginning of the Teen Workshop, teens are asked to write a question about sex (anonymously). These are a few examples of their responses. The spelling and phrasing is theirs.

- Can guys get a dick surgery to enlarge their dick?
- My friend has obscene amounts of pubic hair, what does that mean?
- Why are men usually more sexually active?
- What is a G-spot? What is a yeast infection?
- When you take birth control it makes your boobs bigger? Right?
- Where's the male G-spot?
- Is there a way to fix a cracked penis?
- How long can sperm survive on hands, fingers, etc.?

- Can you get any diseases through anal sex?
- Is it true that for girls first time it can hurt a lot or bleed?
- What is the cost of abortion?
- Do you need to take a Pap test for birth control?
- How many time should u have sex? Everyday?
- Would you recommend the HPV shot?
- Does morning after make you extremely sick for a while after?
- What if I had sex when I was drunk, had sex, wasn't wearing protection yet had my period and a couple days after had morning sickness...could I be pregnant?
- When you're pregnant, do you stop having your period?
- Is it unhealthy to masturbate?
- What happens to the piece of skin in the vagina when a girl is having her first intercourse? Does it hurt?
- Will it hurt the woman or the man for there first sex?
- What is "tity fucking"?
- Where can you buy a wooden cock?
- What happens if you go limp during bang time?
- If you go down on a girl, can you get a mouth disease?
- Why does it hurt every time he putts in?
- Is it possible to kill a vagina during sex? What if the girl bleeds every time...a lot
- Is it OK to have a harry penis or nipples?
- What's the point of oral sex, when you can just have sex?
- What do you do if a girl bites your dick off?
- What kind of improvised birth control could you use?
- Do women have sperm?
- How to tell your man you want him to fondle your clit?
- What happens if you pee in a girl's vagrn when sex is happening?
- What if you have pimbles around your dick?
- Say if you partner is completely faithful doesn't cheat and if have unprotected sex, and they have only been with each other what STDs can you get beside herpes?
- What's the easiest way to get a girl to have sex with you?

- I heard that if you orgasm you're more likely to become pregnant (meaning the body is more likely to let the semen in to the ovaries, etc...is this true?
- Will doctors give you birth control without parent consent?
- How do you increase girth?
- What's the earliest age a guy can become erect?
- Where would I go to get "checked up" for free and anonymously?
- Is it true that it is sae for a woman to have see before and /or after her period?
- Do guys actually like boobs or is it more of a media type thing? Is there more than one type of orgasm? Is there a amount of time that you are pregnant for so after that you can't have an abortion?
- What does it mean if your boobs aren't the same size?
- What would I have to expect at a physical the doctor?
- Why do girls have two holes, one for menstrual cycle, and one for urination instead of just one?
- Is it bad if the skin covered the penis when not erected?
- Why do I have wet dreams?
- If you have an STD how can you have a child without transferring a STD or STI?
- Is it true that people can actually get stuck while having sex?
- Does taking birth control reduce the chance of a person being able to get pregnant in the future?
- Is it bad not to get your period all together?
- Do you need parental consent for an abortion?
- Can a girl be pregnant and still get her period every month?
- Can a girl get pregnant from wearing a guys boxers?
- Why does it hurt when someone kicks your testicals?
- Could I run out of sperm?
- First, great presentation! Second how often do guys get boners?Is it normal to get a random boner all of a sudden during the day?
- How many oranges can a woman fit in her vagina?
- Hów does sex feel like?
- If you have had sex with over 20 people is that bad? What are the chances of an STI?

- Do most guys ejaculate within seconds of having sex on their first time??? How is Lesbos be doin the nasty without any love toys or naturals? What if the guy is too wide and it hurts for the girls still, after a long time?
- Does a girl condom hurt?
- Can you use aluminium foil as a condom?
- What happens if you get fingered, what happens?
- What are the signs of a vaginal infection?
- How do lesbians have sex?
- If a girl masturbates can she break her own cherry?
- How can you make your penis bigger?
- If you have sex unprotected, and you think your pregnant already can you on the pill and hope it goes away?
- What happens if you can't feel your hands during sex?
- Does it hurt every single time the girl first has sex?
- What is the easiest way to make girls organism with fingers?
- What makes a vag tight? Can you stretch it by regular sex?
- What happens when you "pop the cherry"? What do you do? Continue sex? Stop? Blood?
- The more you masturbate, the less time you can last in sex?
- What are the effects of using penis enlargement products?
- Is it true that the best way to deal with crabs is to lie in the sun with magnifying glass?
- Can you get blind from masturbating?
- What is a tubal ligation?
- Is it OK to have a boner every 20 minuets?
- Is it true if you don't use it you lose it?
- If you shoved a copper wire up our penis could it conduct electricity? Would it feel good?

APPENDIX 3

Community Meeting

1. The AWTY Community Meeting: Sample Outline

In some communities, people felt it was important to include the full community in the program. The original program consists of the participatory play for teens and a follow-up sexuality education workshop. The teens gain from having spaces where they can work as peers on this sensitive topic, so we wanted to find a way to involve adults, particularly parents, in the program, without losing the peer-to-peer core of the participatory performance. This community meeting and variations were designed for SNTC and the Aboriginal adaptations.

The Facilitator

The community meeting can be led by an individual or a partnership of individuals. For example, it has been led by various combinations: an elder who assisted with the development of the program; a sexual health educator who also participated in rehearsals, actor orientation, and the play and conducted the follow-up workshop; and a community-based health educator.

Outline for Facilitator

This is a short script meant to show the kind of setup and introductions the actors will need before they present their scenes. It is intended as a road map only and does not need to be offered exactly as written.

Please note that this is only for the theatre portion of the meeting, and there may be more to the meeting before and after the scenes. In most cases, other components included introductions, an outline of sex education provided by schools or health providers, and a discussion on various related issues.

Theatre Portion of the Meeting

FACILITATOR *gives brief background info on the play and program, the goals, etc. Then:*

Facilitator: Here is a short scene from the play that the youth are going to see tomorrow. The play is called *Are We There Yet?* and it asks the question: "What if we put the same care and attention into teaching young people about sex as we put into teaching them to drive?"

Here are the actors (*introduce by name if not already done at beginning of meeting*):

ACTORS *do short* SCENES *from* Are We There Yet?
1. *Lesson One: Know Your Vehicle (body parts)*
2. *"Puberty and You"*
3. *Boy/Girl Ask Questions: "What is oral sex exactly?" to "Am I normal?"*

Facilitator: This was a short section from *Are We There Yet?*

FACILITATOR *talks about the issues and teaching that are in the play.*

FACILITATOR *talks about how much of the play is participatory;* CHARACTERS *ask the* AUDIENCE *for advice and help negotiating through a relationship.* AUDIENCE *gets to try out their ideas using communication skills learned throughout the play, and then they can apply these skills in their own lives. Then:*

Facilitator: Talking about sex can be hard for everyone, not just for young people. We're going to bring the actors back, and they're going to be doing a couple of scenes where characters are going to need your advice.

In this first scene, (actor name) will be playing Twilla, aged twelve; (actor name) will be playing Rose, her thirteen-year-old sister; (actor name) will be playing their dad.

ACTORS *do Parent Scene One and Participation. In this scene, the two sisters are looking at a pornographic magazine and discussing the images. A parent comes in from shopping and now needs help from the* AUDIENCE *to decide what to say to his daughters.*

Although AUDIENCE *has participated in the scene itself, a* FACILITATOR *may choose to debrief issues in the scene further. Then, if a second adult participation scene is warranted:*

Facilitator: In this next scene (actor name) and (actor name) are two young kids, Arron is their seventeen-year-old brother and Mitchell will be playing their dad.

ACTORS *do Parent Scene Two (What if I have an* STI?*) and Participation.*

FACILITATOR *thanks* ACTORS, *debriefs issues in the scene as needed.*

Continue with meeting.

2. Sample Participatory Scene for Adults

Note: Other sample scenes are available from the playwright.

What if I Have an STI?

AWTY Community Workshop Scene (Participatory Scene for Adults)
by Jane Heather

PART 1

ADULT *is watching* TV *on couch. Two younger kids are running around.*

KID 1 *climbs on couch jumps off yells,* KID 2 *tries to do same but falls, takes after* KID 1.

Kid 2: You made me fall!

Kid 1: Did not! You fell yourself you big baby.

KID 2 chases KID 1 around the couch, both yelling.

Adult: Hey! I'm trying to watch this! Go outside and run around.

KID 1 and 2 go outside, shoving each other.

Enter RILEY, 17 years old. He stands there.

Adult: What?

Riley: Nothing.

Adult: You home now?

Riley: Yeah.

Adult: Okay, watch the kids, I'm going out after this.

(He is watching TV and makes some comment about a current plot twist, such as) That fat guy looks like Uncle Chubs, eh?)

Riley: Yeah.

Adult: Sit down! Don't hang over me like that.

He keeps standing.

Adult: What are you all mopey about?

Riley: I need to talk to you.

Adult: So talk.

KID 2 runs into the house with KID 1 close behind, both are yelling: "Gimme that!" "It's mine," "Go suck a rock!" etc.)

Adult: You kids shut up! Quit running around!

KIDS retreat to upstage, play quietly

Adult: Okay, what?

Riley: I got...there's stuff coming out of my penis.

Adult: What? What stuff?

Riley: I don't know.

Adult: Has this happened before?

Riley: No.

ADULT goes to AUDIENCE for advice.

Participation

Intention 1: *To explore how to get the crucial information from the teen.*

The teen is very afraid, suicidal, and so almost non-verbal. The adult may assume this is about a wet dream; he then needs to ask more questions to determine whether this may be a STI. *Adult needs to know* (COACHED *by* AUDIENCE) *if the teen has had sex and if it was protected sex. Then adult moves onto symptoms, ("Does it hurt when you pee?" etc.)*

Intention 2: *To get information/advice from the adults in the audience.*

Techniques: *What should I do? What should we do? (The audience will likely recommend testing and maybe treatment if the symptoms are consistent with a* STI. *Also contacting the girl and other partners.)*

PART 2

RILEY *thinks he has* HIV/AIDS.

Adult: Okay, okay, we'll go to the doctor tomorrow and get some tests.
Riley: I don't know.
Adult: I do.
Riley: I don't think I'll be around here tomorrow.
(ADULT *to* AUDIENCE.) What now?

Intention: *This participation is about support. The adult will need to uncover Riley's fears about hiv and convince him to get tested. Also must acknowledge and address that Riley is at risk for suicide. Work with audience to learn this and come up with plan to support Riley.*

APPENDIX 4

Promoting the AWTY Program

1. Copy for Promoting the AWTY Program

Are We There Yet? partners found that the following copy is useful in promoting the program with schools, public health organizations, community groups and potential funders. Along with the script, this copy is available as a PDF from the University of Alberta Press.

A Workshop and Play for Teens

What would happen if we put the same care and attention into teaching young people about sex as we put into teaching them to drive?

Are We There Yet? is a compelling participatory play and workshop about sexuality health education for fourteen- to sixteen-year-olds. Using the metaphor of learning to drive to frame realistic scenes of relationship dilemmas, the play creates instant ease amongst teenagers, and between teenagers and adults. Humour is used to release tension and creates an atmosphere in which young people feel safe and free to talk about the topical dilemmas presented on stage, and by proxy, in their lives.

Are We There Yet? was developed jointly by Concrete Theatre, Planned Parenthood Association of Edmonton, and playwright Jane Heather. Since 1998, the play and workshop has toured Edmonton area junior high schools (suburban, inner city, youth detention centres, hearing impaired, etc.), meeting the sexuality curriculum requirements for grade nine in Alberta, and will soon tour *[insert tour information here]*.

How can Are We There Yet? *help teach sexuality and sexual health? The play and workshop:*

- Identify, develop, and model communication strategies necessary for the healthy sexual choices. These include: naming and negotiating personal boundaries with a partner; naming and negotiating condom use with a partner; negotiating changes in personal boundaries.
- Encourage youth to reflect upon the consequences of uninformed, poor decision making in sexual relationships.
- Provide information about the agencies and organizations that supply services to adolescents, and encourage them to use these services.

How will students benefit from seeing Are We There Yet?

- They will be able to safely ask questions about issues of sexuality, explore how to communicate their sexual feelings, develop strategies for safe and respectful behaviour, and learn about community resources and supports for teens.
- The follow-up workshop, conducted by a youth counsellor/educator, will allow students to deal with questions and issues revealed in the play, provide information, reinforce positive behaviours, and address barriers to healthy relationships.
- They will learn how to make better sexual choices, to reduce the chances of contracting STIs, and to avoid unplanned pregnancies.

What are teens saying about Are We There Yet?

- "I really enjoyed the play. I thought it was an interesting way to learn about sexuality."
- "I liked the comparison of driving and sex. It was a good way of relating to a topic that my age group is comfortable with."

- "The play made me more aware of diseases and consequences of sex."
- "It helped me realize that people have to respect my body and boundaries."

2. Adapting Promotional Materials

As with the play and workshop, some adaptation of materials is useful to best suit your community and audiences. For example, this is how these materials were redeveloped for Aboriginal communities.

An Interactive Play and Workshop for Teens

What if learning about sex was like learning to drive?

Everybody talks about driving: how to drive, when to drive, what driving is like, drinking and driving, accidents, good drivers, stupid drivers...but sex? Well, that's a different story...

Are We There Yet? by Jane Heather is a funny, participatory play and workshop about sexuality health education for fourteen- to sixteen-year-olds. In 2006, Jane Heather and Kenneth Williams created a new version of this award-winning play for Aboriginal teens. The play draws a parallel between mastering driving skills and negotiating relationships, and humorously opens a dialogue about sexuality. As teens are invited to advise characters on stage, they feel safe and free to talk about sexuality and relationship issues. Road testing their knowledge in the environs of theatre, they become better and safer drivers of their own sexual growth.

How can Are We There Yet? *help teach sexuality and sexual health to Aboriginal teens?*

- The program includes the play, produced by Saskatchewan Native Theatre Company, a follow-up sexual health education workshop facilitated by a local or regional health educator, and a community meeting. The community meeting, led by an elder and health educator, provides an opportunity for parents and community to learn about and reinforce the program.

- It identifies, develops, and models communication strategies necessary for healthy sexual choices. These include naming and negotiating personal boundaries with a partner; naming and negotiating condom use with a partner; and negotiating changes in personal boundaries.
- It encourages youth to reflect upon the consequences of uninformed, poor decision making in sexual relationships.
- It provides information about agencies and organizations that supply services to adolescents, and encourages them to use these services.

How will teens benefit from seeing Are We There Yet?

- They can safely ask questions about sexuality, explore how to communicate their sexual feelings, develop strategies for safe and respectful behaviour with partners, and learn about community resources and supports.
- They learn how to make good sexual choices, reduce their chances of contracting STIS/STDS, and avoid unplanned pregnancies.
- The follow-up workshop allows students to deal with questions and issues raised by the play, and provides information, reinforces positive behaviours, and addresses barriers to healthy relationships.

What are Aboriginal teens saying about Are We There Yet?

- "I just thought that it was really enjoyable and that I actually learned something from it."
- "It gets kids interested into it and so they want to learn it more—instead of just forgetting it they'll remember the play so they'll remember things about sexual education."
- "I learned to talk before you...act."

APPENDIX 5

The Are We There Yet? Community-University Research Alliance Partners

Theatre Company Partners

Concrete Theatre, Edmonton, AB (founding partner)
Mulgrave Road Theatre, Guysborough, NS
Neworld Theatre, Vancouver, BC
Saskatchewan Native Theatre Company, Saskatoon, SK

Playwrights

Jane Heather, Edmonton, AB (founding partner)
Kenneth T. Williams, Saskatoon, SK

Health Organization Partners

Options Sexual Health Association of Edmonton (formerly Planned Parenthood of Edmonton) (founding partner)
Lac La Ronge Indian Health Band Services, Lac La Ronge, SK
Mamawetan Churchill River Health Region, Lac La Ronge, SK
Native Counselling Services of Alberta, Edmonton, AB
Northern Inter-Tribal Health Association, Prince Albert, SK

Public Health Services, Guysborough Youth Health and Services Centre, Guysborough, NS
Saskatoon Health Region, Saskatoon, SK
Vancouver Coastal Health, Vancouver, BC

University Partners

University of Alberta

Jan Selman, Principal Investigator, Department of Drama (founding partner)
Brenda Munro, Department of Human Ecology
Shaniff Esmail, Department of Occupational Therapy
Kate Nunn, Project Administrator (founding administrator)
Anne Bailey, Project Administrator
Liz Ludwig, Project Administrator

University of British Columbia

Jim Ponzetti, School of Social Work and Family Studies

University of Guelph

Gerald Adams, Department of Family Relations and Applied Nutrition, College of Social and Applied Human Sciences

BIBLIOGRAPHY

AADAC (Alberta Alcohol and Drug Abuse Commission). 2011. Alberta Health Services. Accessed July 27. http://www.albertahealthservices.ca/?from=aadac.

Aboriginal Nurses Association of Canada. 1999. *Aboriginal Round Table on Sexual and Reproductive Health*. Ottawa: Aboriginal Nurses Association of Canada.

Adams, Gerald. 2005. "Adolescent Development." In *Handbook of Adolescent Behavior Problems: Evidence-based Approaches to Assessment and Treatment*, edited by Thomas P. Gullotta, and Gerald Adams, 3–16. New York: Kluwer Academic.

Agrell, Siri. 2008. "The Death of Sex Education." *Globe and Mail*, March 13. http://www.theglobeandmail.com/life/the-death-of-sex-education/article668962/.

Alberta Learning. 2009. "Health and Life Skills, Kindergarten to Grade 9." http://www.education.alberta.ca/teachers/program/health/programs.aspx.

AREPP: Theatre for Life. 2010. Accessed June 15. http://www.arepp.org.za.

Are We There Yet? Community-University Research Alliance. 2011. "About Us." Accessed June 15. http://www.ualberta.ca/AWTY/about.html.

Asher, Herbert B. 1983. *Causal Modeling*. 2nd ed. Newbury Park, CA: Sage.

Assembly of First Nations. 2009. "A History of Residential Schools." Accessed August 9. http://www.afn.ca/residentialschools/history.html.

Atwood, Margaret. 1982. "Writing the Male Character." In *Second Words: Selected Critical Prose*, 412–30. Toronto: House of Anansi Press.

Auger, Josie, and Jane Heather. 2009. "My People's Blood: Mobilizing Rural Aboriginal Populations in Canada around Issues of HIV." In *The Applied Theatre Reader*, edited by Tim Prenki and Sheila Preston, 283–90. London: Routledge.

Babbage, Frances. 2004. *Augusto Boal*. New York: Routledge.

Baim, Clark, Sally Brookes, and Alun Mountford. 2002. *The Geese Handbook*. London: Waterside Press.

Bain, Ken. 2004. *What the Best College Teachers Do.* Cambridge, MA: Harvard University Press.

Bakhtin, Mikhail. 1981. "Epic and the Novel: Towards a Methodology for the Study in the Novel." In *The Dialogic Imagination,* translated by Michael Holquist and Caryl Emerson, 3–40. Austin: University of Texas Press.

———. 1984. *Rabelais and His World,* translated by Hélène Iswolsky. Bloomington: Indiana University Press.

Balfour, Michael, and John Somers. 2006. *Drama as Social Intervention.* Concord, ON: Captus University Publications.

Bandura, Albert. 1999. "Social Cognitive Theory of Personality." In *Handbook of Personality: Theory and Guide to Research.* 2nd ed., edited by Lawrence A. Pervin and Oliver P. John, 154–96. New York: Guilford Press.

Bennett, Susan. 1990. *Theatre Audiences: A Theory of Production and Reception.* London: Routledge.

Berzonsky, Michael D. 1989. "Identity Style: Conceptualization and Measurement." *Journal of Adolescent Research* 4:267–81.

———. 1990. "Self-construction Over the Life-span: A Process Perspective on Identity Formation." *Advances in Personal Construct Psychology* 1:55–86.

Berzonsky, Michael D., and Colleen Sullivan. 1992. "Social-Cognitive Aspects of Identity Style: Need for Cognition, Experiential Openness, and Introspection." *Journal of Adolescent Research* 7:140–55.

Blalock, Hubert M. Jr. 1985. *Causal Models in the Social Sciences.* 2nd ed. Chicago: Aldine.

Bloom, Benjamin S., ed. 1956. *Taxonomy of Educational Objectives: The Classification of Educational Goals.* Boston: Allyn and Bacon:

Boal, Augusto. 1979. *Theatre of the Oppressed.* New York: Theatre Communications Group.

———. 1992. *Games for Actors and Non-Actors.* New York: Routledge.

———. 2002. *Games for Actors and Non-Actors.* 2nd ed. New York: Routledge.

Boal, Augusto, and Adrian Jackson. 2006. *The Aesthetics of the Oppressed.* London: Routledge.

Booth, David W., and Kathleen Gallagher. 2003. *How Theatre Educates: Convergences and Counterpoints with Artists, Scholars and Advocates.* Toronto: University of Toronto Press.

Boyce, William, Maryanne Doherty, Christian Fortin, and David Mackinnon. 2003. *Canadian Youth, Sexual Health and HIV/AIDS Study: Factors Influencing Knowledge, Attitudes and Behaviours.* Toronto: Council of Ministers of Education.

Boyd, J.R., and M. Hunsberger. 1998. "Chronically Ill Children Coping with Repeated Hospitalizations: Their Perceptions and Suggested Interventions." *Journal of Pediatric Nursing* 13:330–41.

Brecht, Bertolt. [1951] 1972. *Collected Plays,* edited and translated by Ralph Manheim and John Willett. Vol. 9. Pantheon Books: New York.

———. 1964a. "A Short Organum for the Theatre." In *Brecht on Theatre,* translated by John Willett, 179–208. New York: Hill and Wang.

———. 1964b. "Theatre for Pleasure or Theatre for Instruction." In *Brecht on Theatre,* translated by John Willett, 69–76. New York: Hill and Wang.

Bristol, Michael D. 1989. *Carnival and Theatre*. London: Routledge.

Budhan Theatre. 2013. Accessed October 5. www.budhantheatre.org.

Burnard, Phillip. 1991. "A Method of Analyzing Interview Transcripts in Qualitative Research." *Nurse Education Today* 11(6):461–66.

Burnham, Linda Frye, and Steven Durland, eds. 1998. *The Citizen Artist: 20 Years of Art in the Public Arena An Anthology from High Performance Magazine 1978–1998*. New York: Critical Press.

Butterwick, Shauna, and Jan Selman. 2003. "Intentions and Context: Popular Theatre in a North American Context." *Convergence* 36(2):51–66.

Cairns, K., S. Collins, and B. Hiebert. 1994. "Gender Differences in Adolescent Self-perceived Needs for Sexuality Education." *Canadian Journal of Human Sexuality* 3:245–51.

Canadian Association for Adolescent Health. 2006. "Many Canadian Teens Are Engaging in Sexual Behaviours That Pose a Threat to Their Health." *Prcteen* 15(1–2):4–9.

Cannon, Martin. 2004. "The Regulation of First Nations Sexuality." In *I Could Not Speak My Heart: Education and Social Justice for Gay and Lesbian Youth*, edited by James McNinch and Mary Cronin, 95–108. Regina, SK: University of Regina Press.

Cardboard Citizens. 2009. Accessed June 15. http://www.cardboardcitizens.org.uk.

Carlson, Marvin. 1993. *Theories of the Theatre*. Ithaca, NY: Cornell University Press.

Catalyst Theatre. 2010. Accessed June 15. http://www.catalysttheatre.ca.

CBC News. 2009. "Alberta Passes Law Allowing Parents to Pull Kids out of Class." *cbc.ca*. June 2. http://www.cbc.ca/news/canada/alberta-passes-law-allowing-parents-to-pull-kids-out-of-class-1.777604.

Cernerud, Lars, and Henny Olsson. 2004. "Humour Seen From a Public Health Perspective." *Scandinavian Journal of Public Health* 32:396–98.

Certain Curtain Theatre Company. 2010. Accessed June 15. http://www.cctheatre.co.uk.

Chapman, Antony J., and Hugh C. Foot, eds. 1976. Preface to *Humor and Laughter: Theory, Research and Applications*, xxvii–xxix. Edison, NJ: Transaction.

Christopher, Scott, and Rodney. M. Cate. 1984. "Factors Involved in Premarital Sexual Decision-Making." *Journal of Sex Research* 20:363–76.

Clurman, Harold. 1972. *On Directing*. New York: Collier Books.

Cobain, Ian, and Peter Walker. 2011. "Secret Memo Gave Guidelines on Abuse of Mau Mau in 1950s." *Guardian* (UK), April 11, 8. http://www.guardian.co.uk/world/2011/apr/11/mau-mau-high-court-foreign-office-documents?INTCMP=SRCH#history-link-box.

Cohen, Jonathan. 2006. *A Tale of Two Presidential Initiatives: Changes in an HIV Prevention Program in Uganda*. http://www.hrw.org/english/docs/2006/02/01/uganda12591.htm.

Cohen-Cruz, Jan. 2005. *Local Acts: Community-Based Performance in the United States*. Piscataway, NJ: Rutgers University Press.

———. 2010. *Engaging Performance: Theatre as Call and Response*. New York: Routledge.

Concrete Theatre. 2010. "Are We There Yet?" Accessed June 15. http://www.concretetheatre.ca/Arewethereyet2011.html.

Conn, Kathleen. 2009. "Parents' Right to Direct Their Children's Education and Student Sex Surveys." *Journal of Law and Education* 38(1):139–50.

Couzin, Jennifer. 2007. "Opening Door to Native Knowledge." *Science* 315:1518–19.

Critchley, Simon. 2002. *On Humor: Thinking in Action*. New York: Routledge.

Crockett, Lisa J., Marcela Raffaelli, and Kristin L. Moilanen. 2003. "Adolescent Sexuality: Behavior and Meaning." In *Blackwell Handbook of Adolescence*, edited by G.R. Adams, and M.D. Berzonsky, 371–92. Malden, MA: Blackwell.

Cruikshank, Julie. 1994. "Oral Tradition and Oral History: Reviewing Some Issues." *Canadian Historical Review* 75(3):403–18.

———. 1998. *The Social Life of Stories: Narrative and Knowledge in the Yukon Territory*. Vancouver: University of British Columbia Press.

Curran, Angela. 2001. "Brecht's Criticisms of Aristotle's Aesthetics of Tragedy." *Journal of Aesthetics and Art Criticism* 59(2):165–84.

Dalrymple, Lynn. 2006. "Has it Made a Difference? Understanding and Measuring the Impact of Applied Theatre With Young People in the South African Context." *Research in Drama Education* 11(2): 201–18.

Dean, Ruth, Anne Kinsman, and David M. Gregory. 2005. "More Than Trivial: Strategies for Using Humor in Palliative Care." *Cancer Nursing* 28(4):292–300.

Deavere Smith, Anna. 2000. *Talk to Me: Listening Between the Lines*. New York: Random House.

Defraeye, Piet. 1999. "The Romans in Britain and the Effect of Male/Male Sexual Iconography at London's National Theatre." *Torquere* 1:60–86.

Diamond, David. 2007. *Theatre for Living: The Art and Science of Community-Based Dialogue*. Victoria, BC: Trafford.

Dolan, Jill. 2001. *Geographies of Learning: Theory and Practice, Activism and Performance*. Middleton, CT: Wesleyan University Press.

———. 2005. *Utopia in Performance: Finding Hope in the Theatre*. Michigan: University of Michigan Press.

Duran, Bonnie M., and K.L. Walters. 2004. "HIV/AIDS Prevention in 'Indian Country': Current Practice, Indigenist Etiology Models, and Postcolonial Approaches to Change." *International Society for AIDS Education* 16(3):187–201.

Each One Reach One. 2013. Accessed October 5. http://www.eoro.org.

Eisen, Marvin, Gail L. Zellman, and Alfred L. McAlister. 1990. "Evaluating the Impact of a Theory-Based Sexuality and Contraceptive Education Program." *Family Planning Perspectives* 22:261–71.

Etherton, Michael, and Tim Prentki. 2006. "Drama for Change? Prove it! Impact Assessment in Applied Theatre." *Research in Drama Education* 11(2):139–55.

Finklea, Lorraine, Gail Gruendemann, and Debra C. Harris. 2004. "Abstaining from Abstinence." *American Journal of Health Education* 35(2):100–2.

Fisher, Jeffrey D., and William A. Fisher. 2000. "Theoretical Approaches to Individual-Level Change in HIV Risk Behavior." In *HIV Prevention Handbook*, edited by John L. Peterson, and Ralph DiClements, 3–55. New York: Kluwer Academic.

Fisher, William A., and Jeffrey D. Fisher. 1992. "Understanding and Promoting AIDS Preventive Behaviour: A Conceptual Model and Educational Tool." *Canadian Journal of Human Sexuality* 1:99–106.

———. 1998. "Understanding and Promoting Sexual and Reproductive Health Behavior: Theory and Method." *Annual Review of Sex Research* 9:39–76.

Flicker, Sarah, Susan Flynn, June Larkin, Robb Travers, Adrian Guta, Jason Pole, and Crystal Labine. 2009. *Sexpress: The Toronto Teen Survey Report*. Toronto: Planned Parenthood.

Foon, Dennis, Wendy Van Reisen, and Fran Gebhard. 1982. "Feeling Yes, Feeling No." Unpublished manuscript, Green Thumb Theatre.

Fortier, Mark. 1997. *Theory/Theatre: An Introduction*. London: Routledge.

Forum for African Women Educationalists (FAWE). 2009. "Tuseme Youth Empowerment." http://www.fawe.org/activities/interventions/tuseme/index.php.

Fournier, Suzanne, and Ernie Crey. 2006. "Killing the Indian Child Four Centuries of Church-Run Schools." *The Indigenous Experience: Global Perspectives*, edited by Roger Maaka and Chris Anderson, 141–49. Toronto: Canadian Scholars' Press.

Freire, Paolo. 1983. *Pedagogy of the Oppressed*. Translated by Myra Bergman Ramos. New York: Continuum.

Gavin, Loretta E., Richard F. Catalano, Corinne David-Ferdon, Kari M. Gloppen, and Christine M. Markham. 2010. "A Review of Positive Youth Development Programs that Promote Adolescent Sexual and Reproductive Health." *Journal of Adolescent Health* 46:S75–91.

Geese Theatre Company. 2010. Accessed June 15. http://www.geese.co.uk/HTML/index.html.

Gilley, Brian Joseph. 2006. "Snag Bags: Adapting Condoms to Community Values in Native American Communities." *Culture, Health and Sexuality* 8(6):559–70.

Government of Mexico. 2008. "1st Meeting of Ministers of Health and Education to Stop HIV and STIs in Latin America and the Caribbean." Unpublished ministerial declaration. http://data.unaids.org/pub/BaseDocument/2008/20080801_minsterdeclaration_en.pdf.

Gramsci, Antonio. 1994. *Letters from Prison*. Vol. 1, edited by Frank Rosengarten and translated by Raymond Rosenthal. New York: Columbia University Press.

Great Canadian Theatre Company. 2010. Accessed June 15. http://www.gctc.ca.

Green Thumb Theatre for Young People. 2010. "Feeling Yes, Feeling No." Accessed June 15. http://www.greenthumb.bc.ca/play_detail.asp?playid=69.

Greene, Maxine. 1995. *Releasing the Imagination: Essays on Education, the Arts, and Social Change*. San Francisco: Jossey-Bass.

Greydanus, Donald, Helen Pratt, and Linda Dannison. 1995. "Sexuality Education Programs for Youth: Current State of Affairs and Strategies for the Future." *Journal of Sex Education and Therapy* 4:238–54.

Ground Zero Productions. 2010. "OCHU." June 15. http://www.gzpedmonton.org/projects/view/ochu.

Gullotta, Thomas P., and Gerald R. Adams, eds. 2003. *Encyclopedia of Adolescence*. Norwell, MA: Kluwer Academic.

Gullotta, Thomas P., Gerald R. Adams, and Carol A. Markstrom. 2000. *The Adolescent Experience*. 4th ed. San Diego, CA: Academic Press.

Gullotta, Thomas P., Robert L. Hampton, Gerald R. Adams, Bruce A. Ryan, and Roger P. Weissberg, eds. 1999. *Children's Health Care: Issues for the Year 2000 and Beyond (Issues in Children's and Families' Lives)*. Thousand Oaks, CA: Sage.

Guttmacher Institute. 2006. "In Brief: Facts on Sex Education in the United States." http://www.guttmacher.org/pubs/fb_sexEd2006.html.

Haedicke, Susan C., and Tobin Nellhaus. 2001. *Performing Democracy: International*. Ann Arbor: University of Michigan Press.

Haydon Taylor, Drew, ed. 2008. *Me Sexy: An Exploration of Native Sex and Sexuality*. Toronto: Douglas and McIntyre.

Headlines Theatre. 2011. Accessed June 15. http://www.headlinestheatre.com/intro.htm.

Health Canada. 1994. *Canadian Guidelines for Sexual Health Education*. 1st ed. Ottawa: Population and Public Health Branch, Health Canada.

———. 2003. *Revised Edition of the 2003 Canadian Guidelines for Sexual Health Education*. Ottawa: Population and Public Health Branch, Health Canada.

Heathcote, Dorothy, and Gavin Bolton. 1995. *Drama for Learning: Dorothy Heathcote's Mantle of the Expert Approach to Education*. Portmouth, NH: Heinemann.

Heather, Jane. 1998. "Are We There Yet?" Unpublished play script. www.ualberta.ca/AWTY.

Heather, Jane, and Kenneth T. Williams. 2006. "Are We There Yet?" Unpublished play script. www.ualberta.ca/AWTY.

Hoffman-Goetz, Laurie, Daniela B. Friedman, and Juanne N. Clarke. 2005. "HIV/AIDS Risk Factors as Portrayed in Mass Media Targeting First Nations Metis and Inuit Peoples of Canada." *Journal of Health Communication* 10(2):145–62.

hooks, bell. 1994. *Teaching to Transgress: Education as the Practice of Freedom*. New York: Routledge.

Hope, Anne, and Sally Timmel. 1999. *Training for Transformation: A Handbook for Community Workers*. Zimbabwe: Mambo Press.

Hubbard, Betty M., Mark L. Giese, and Jacquie Rainey. 1998. "A Replication of Reducing the Risk, a Theory-Based Sexuality Curriculum for Adolescents." *Journal of School Health* 68:243–47.

Hyde, Janet S., John D. DeLamater, and Sandra Byers. 2009. *Understanding Human Sexuality*. 4th ed. Toronto: McGraw-Hill.

"India Street Theatre." 2012. *IndiaNetzone*. December 13. http://www.indianetzone.com/5/indian_street_theatre.htm.

Jackson, Anthony. 2007. *Theatre, Education and the Making of Meanings: Art or Instrument?* Manchester: Manchester University Press.

Johansson, Ola. 2010. "The Limits of Community-Based Theatre: Performance and HIV Prevention in Tanzania." *Drama Review* 54(1):59–75.

Johnson, Paige. 2002. "The Use of Humour and its Influence on Spirituality and Coping in Breast Cancer Survivors." *Oncology Nursing Forum* 29:691–95.

Kahn, Si. 1970. *How People Get Power: Organizing Oppressed Communities for Action.* New York: McGraw-Hill.

Kattwinkel, Susan. 2003. *Audience Participation: Essays on Inclusion in Performance.* Santa Barbara, CA: Praeger.

Kershaw, Baz. 1992. *The Politics of Performance: Radical Theatre as Cultural Intervention.* London: Routledge.

———. 1999. *The Radical in Performance: Between Brecht and Baudillard.* London: Routledge.

Kidd, Ross. 1979. "Liberation of Domestication: Popular Theatre and Non-formal Education in Africa." *Educational Broadcasting International* 12(1):3–9.

———. 1983a. "Popular Theatre and Popular Struggle in Kenya: The Story of Kamiriithu." *Race and Class* 24(3):287–304.

———. 1983b. "A Testimony From Nicaragua: An Interview with Nidia Bustos, the Coordinator of Mecate, the Nicaraguan Farm Workers' Theatre Movement." *Studies in Latin American Popular Culture* 2:190–201.

———. 1985. "Popular Theatre, Conscientization and Popular Organization". In *Reaching and Helping Unorganized and Disadvantaged People. Courier* 33, 18–29. Asian South Pacific Bureau of Adult Education Publication.

———. 1987. "Theatre on Its Own." *Participatory Research Newsletter, Special Issue* 4(2):4.

Kidd, Ross, and Martin Byram. 1982. "Demystifying Pseudo Freirian Non-formal Education: A Case Description and Analysis of Laedza Batanani." *Canadian Journal of Development Studies* 3(2): 271–89.

Kirby, Douglas. 1984. *Sexuality Education: An Evaluation of Programs and Their Effects.* Santa Cruz, CA: Network.

———. 1992. "School-Based Programs to Reduce Sexual Risk-Taking Behavior." *Journal of School Health* 62:280–87.

———. 1998. "Math Tech Questionnaires: Sexuality Questionnaires for Adolescents." In *Handbook of Sexuality-Related Measures.* 2nd ed., edited by C.D. Davis, W.L. Yarber, R. Bauserman, G. Schreer, and S.L. Davis, 35–47. Thousand Oaks, CA: Sage.

———. 2001. "Understanding What Works and What Doesn't in Reducing Adolescent Sexual Risk Taking." *Family Planning Perspectives* 33(6):276–81.

———. 2007. *Emerging Answers 2007: Research Findings on Programs to Reduce Teen Pregnancy and Sexually Transmitted Diseases.* The National Campaign to Prevent Teen and Unplanned Pregnancy. http://www.thenationalcampaign.org/resources/pdf/pubs/EA2007_FINAL.pdf.

Kirby, Douglas, B.A. Laris, and Lori Rolleri. 2005. *Impact of Sex and HIV Education Programs on Sexual Behaviors of Youth in Developing and Developed Countries.* Research Triangle Park, NC: Family Health International.

———. 2007. "Sex and HIV Education Programs: Their Impact on Sexual Behaviors of Young People Throughout the World." *Journal of Adolescent Health* 40:206–17.

Klein, Jeanne. 2005. "From Children's Perspectives: A Model of Aesthetic Processing in Theatre." *Journal of Aesthetic Education* 39(4):40–57.

Korza, Pam, Barbara Shaffer-Bacon, and Andrea Assaf. 2005. *Civic Dialogue, Arts and Culture: Findings from Animating Democracy*. Washington, DC: Americans for the Arts.

Krasner, David. 2006. "Empathy and Theater." In *Staging Philosophy: Intersections of Theater, Performance, and Philosophy*, edited by David Krasner, and David Z. Saltz, 255–77. Ann Arbor: University of Michigan Press.

Krasner, David, and David Z. Saltz. 2006. *Staging Philosophy: Intersections of Theater, Performance, and Philosophy*. Ann Arbor: University of Michigan Press.

Kuftinec, Sonja. 2003. *Staging America: Cornerstone and Community-Based Theater*. Illinois: Southern Illinois University Press.

Kuortti, Marjo, and Elise Kosunen. 2009. "Risk-taking Behaviour Is More Frequent in Teenage Girls with Multiple Sexual Partners." *Scandinavian Journal of Primary Health Care* 27(1):47–52.

Kuppers, Petra, and Gwen Robertson. 2007. *The Community Performance Reader*. London: Routledge.

Kvale, Steinar. 1996. *Interviews: An Introduction to Qualitative Research Interviewing*. Thousand Oaks, CA: Sage.

Kvalem, Ingela L., Jon M. Sundet, Kate I. Rivo, Dag E. Eilertsen, and Leiv S. Bakketeig. 1996. "The Effect of Sex Education on Adolescents' Use of Condoms: Applying the Solomon Four-Group Design." *Health Education Quarterly* 23(1):34–47.

Lancaster, Kurt. 1997. "When Spectators Become Performers: Contemporary Performance-Entertainments Meet the Needs of an 'Unsettled' Audience." *Journal of Popular Culture* 30(4): 75–88.

Langer, Susanne K. 1953. *Feeling and Form*. New York: Charles Scribners.

Langille, Donald B., Gail T. Murphy, Jean Hughes, and Janet A. Rigby. 2001. "Nova Scotia High School Students' Interactions with Physicians for Sexual Health Information and Services." *Canadian Journal of Public Health* 92(3):219–22.

Law Society of Alberta. 2010. http://www.lawsociety.ab.ca.

The Lawnmowers Theatre. 2010. "What We Do." Accessed June 15. http://www.thelawnmowers.co.uk/actors/whatwedo.php.

Levy, Jonathan. 2005. "Reflections on How The Theatre Teaches." *Journal of Aesthetic Education* 39(4):20–30.

Lightning, Walter. 1992. "Compassionate Mind: Implications of a Text Written by Elder Louis Sunchild." *Canadian Journal of Native Education* 19:215–35.

Lindsay, William G. 2007. "Gathering Dust Not Saving Lives: The Call for Texts Which Honestly and Straightforwardly Teach Aboriginal Children About HIV/AIDS and Other Important Issues." *Canadian Journal of Native Studies* 27(2):503–8.

Lorde, Audre. 1984. "The Master's Tools Will Never Dismantle the Master's House." In *Sister Outsider: Essays and Speeches*. New York: Crossing Press.

Los Angeles Poverty Department. 2010. Accessed June 15. http://lapovertydept.org.

Lowes, Lesley, and Morag A. Prowse. 2001. "Standing Outside the Interview Process? The Illusion of Objectivity in Phenomenological Data Generation." *International Journal of Nursing Studies* 38:471–80.

Mabray, Debbie, and Bill Labauve. 2002. "A Multidimensional Approach to Sexual Education." *Sex Education* 2(1): 31–44.

Malibo, Rethabile Khantse. 2008. "Using Popular Participatory Theatre Research Method to Expose the Relationship Between HIV/AIDS and Silence in Malealea Valley, Lesotho." MA thesis, University of KwaZulu, Durban. http://researchspace.ukzn.ac.za/xmlui/handle/10413/926.

Manossa, Geraldine. 2001. "The Beginning of Cree Performance Culture." In *(Ad)dressing Our Words: Aboriginal Perspectives on Aboriginal Literatures*, edited by Armand Garnet Ruffo, 169–80. Penticton, BC: Theytus Books.

Marion, Frank. 1995. *AIDS Education Through Theatre*. Beyreuth, Germany: Beyreuth African Studies.

Marshall, Gordon. 1998. "Causal Modelling." *A Dictionary of Sociology. Encyclopedia. com*. Accessed August 4, 2010. http://www.encyclopedia.com/doc/1088-causalmodelling.html.

Matarasso, Francois. 1997. *Use or Ornament? The Social Impact of Participation in the Arts*. London: Comedia.

Maticka-Tyndale, Eleanor. 1997. "Reducing the Incidence of Sexually Transmitted Disease Through Behavioural and Social Change." *Canadian Journal of Human Sexuality* 6(2):89–104.

Maticka-Tyndale, Eleanor, M. Barrett, and Alexander McKay. 2000. "Adolescent Sexual and Reproductive Health in Canada: A Review of National Data Sources and Their Limitations." *Canadian Journal of Human Sexuality* 9(1):42–65.

"Mau Mau Torture Files Were 'Guilty Secret.'" 2011. *BBC News UK*. May 9. http://www.bbc.co.uk/news/uk-13336343.

Mayan, Maria. 2001. "An Introduction to Qualitative Methods: A Training Module for Students and Professors." Unpublished manuscript. Edmonton, AB: International Institute for Qualitative Methodology.

Maykut, Pamela, and Richard Morehouse. 2001. *Beginning Qualitative Research: A Philosophical and Practical Guide*. Washington, DC: Falmer.

McCabe, Marita P., and Eoin J. Killackey. 2004. "Sexual Decision Making in Young Women." *Sexual and Relationship Therapy* 19(1):15–27.

McCosker, Heather, Alan Barnard, and Rod Gerber. 2001. "Undertaking Sensitive Research: Issues and Strategies for Meeting the Safety Needs of all Participants." *Forum: Qualitative Social Research* 2(1), Article 22. http://www.qualitative-research.net/index.php/fqs/article/viewArticle/983/2142.

McGrath, John. 1981. *A Good Night Out: Popular Theatre, Audience, Class and Form*. London: Methuen.

———. 1990. *The Bone Won't Break: On Theatre and Hope in Hard Times*. London: Methuen.

McKay, Alexander. 1993. "Research Supports Broadly-Based Sex Education." *Canadian Journal of Human Sexuality* 2(2):89–98.

———. 2000. "Prevention of Sexually Transmitted Infections in Different Populations: A Review of Behaviourally Effective and Cost-Effective Interventions." *Canadian Journal of Human Sexuality* 9:95–120.

McKay, Alexander, Mary-Anne Pietrusiak, and Phillippa Holowaty. 1998. "Parents' Opinions and Attitudes Towards Sexuality Education in the Schools." *Canadian Journal of Human Sexuality* 7:139–45.

McLeod, Neal. 2007. *Cree Narrative Memory: From Treaties to Contemporary Times.* Saskatoon, SK: Purich.

McRanor, Shauna. 1997. "Maintaining the Reliability of Aboriginal Records and Their Material Implications: Implications for Archival Practice." *Archivaria* 43. http://journals.sfu.ca/archivar/index.php/archivaria/article/view/12176.

Mill, Judy E., Randy Jackson, Catherine Worthington, Chris Archibald, Tom Wong, Ted Myers, Tracey Prentice, and Susan Sommerfeldt. 2008a, January. *The Diagnosis and Care of* HIV *Infections in Canadian Aboriginal Youth, Final Report.* Canadian Aboriginal AIDS Network, Toronto. http://www.caan.ca/wp-content/uploads/2012/05/The-Diagnosis-and-Care-of-HIV-Infection-of-Canadian-Aborignal-Youth.pdf.

———. 2008b. "HIV Testing and Care in Canadian Aboriginal Youth: A Community Based Mixed Methods Study." BMC *Infectious Diseases* 8(132). doi:10.1186/1471-2334-8-132.

Miller, Brent C., Bruce K. Bayley, Mathew Christensen, Spencer C. Leavitt, and Diana D. Coyl. 2003. "Adolescent Pregnancy and Childbearing." In *Blackwell Handbook of Adolescence*, edited by Gerald R. Adams, and Michael D. Berzonsky, 415–49. Oxford, UK: Blackwell.

Mishel, Merle H. 1989. "Methodological Studies: Instruments Development." In *Advanced Design in Nursing Research.* 2nd ed., edited by P. Brink and M.J. Wood, 235–82. Newbury Park, CA: Sage.

Mooney, Nancy. 2000. "The Therapeutic Use of Humour." *Orthopaedic Nurse* 19:88–92.

Moore, Kristin A., Jennifer Manlove, and Dana Glei. 1998. "Nonmarital School-Age Motherhood: Family, Individual, and School Characteristics." *Journal of Adolescent Research* 13(4):433–57.

Mulgrave Road Theatre. 2011. "Home." Accessed June 15. http://www.mulgraveroad.ca.

Munier, Asif, and Michael Etherton. 2006. "Child Rights Theatre for Development in Rural Bangladesh: A Case Study." *Research in Drama Education: Journal of Applied Theatre and Performance* 11(2):175–83.

Munro, Brenda, Jan Selman, Shaniff Esmail, and Jane Heather. 2009. "Identity: Is Theatre an Asset in Dealing with Hard-to-Reach Youth?" *International Journal of Learning* 16(6):101–15.

Munro, Brenda, Jan Selman, Shaniff Esmail, and James Ponzetti. 2007. "Are We There Yet? Using Theatre in Sexual Education: A Combination of Academic and Theatre Groups." *International Journal of Diversity in Organizations, Communities and Nations* 7(3):131–38.

Myers, Ted, Sandra L. Bullock, Liviana M. Calzavara, Rhoda Cokerill, Victor W. Marshall, and Cathryn George-Mandoka. 1999. "Culture and Sexual Practices in Response to HIV Among Aboriginal People Living On-Reserve in Ontario." *Culture, Health and Sexuality* 1(1):19–37.

Nelhaus, Tobin, and Susan Haedicke, eds. 2001. *Performing Democracy: International Perspectives on Urban Community-Based Performance.* Ann Arbor: University of Michigan Press.

Neworld Theatre. 2010. Accessed June 15. http://www.neworldtheatre.com/index.html.

Nicholson, Helen. 2005. *Applied Drama: The Gift of Theatre.* Basingstoke, UK: Palgrave Macmillan.

———. 2009. *Theatre and Education.* Basingstoke, UK: Palgrave Macmillan.

Norris, Anne E., and Barbara H. Munro, eds. 1997. *Path Analysis: Statistical Methods for Health Care Research,* 3rd ed. Philadelphia: Lippincott.

O'Neill, Geraldine, and Tim McMahon. 2005. "Student-Centred Learning: What Does It Mean for Students and Lecturers?" In *Emerging Issues in the Practice of University Learning and Teaching,* edited by Geraldine O'Neill, Sarah Moore, and Barry McMullin. Dublin: All Ireland Society for Higher Education. http://www.aishe.org/readings/2005-1/oneill-mcmahon-Tues_19th_Oct_SCL.html.

Ong, Walter. 2002. *Orality and Literacy: The Technologizing of the Word.* 2nd ed. New York: Routledge.

Options Sexual Health Association. 2011. Accessed February 10. http://www.optionssexualhealth.ca.

Ottawa Planned Parenthood. 2009. "Programs—Insight Theatre." http://www.ppottawa.ca/programs.aspx.

Pamoja Youth Foundation. 2013. "Home." http://www.pamoja.help-kenya.org/pamoja/.

PHAC (Public Health Agency of Canada). 2007. *HIV and AIDS in Canada: Surveillance Report to December 31, 2006.* Surveillance and Risk Assessment Division, Centre for Infectious Disease Prevention and Control, Public Health Agency of Canada. www.phac-aspc.gc.ca/aids-sida/populations-eng.php#ab.

Postman, Neil, and Charles Weingartner. 1969. *Teaching as a Subversive Activity.* New York: Dell Publishing.

Powell, J. P., and L.W. Anderson. 1985. "Humour and Teaching in Higher Education." *Studies in Higher Education* 10(1):79–90.

Prendergast, Monica, and Juliana Saxton. 2009. *Applied Theatre: International Case Studies and Challenges for Practice.* Bristol: Intellect.

Prentki, Tim. 2009. "Introduction to Poetics of Representation." In *The Applied Theatre Reader,* edited by Tim Prentki and Sheila Preston, 19–21. New York: Routledge.

Prentki, Tim, and Sheila Preston, eds. 2009. *The Applied Theatre Reader.* London: Routledge.

Prentki, Tim, and Jan Selman. 2000. *Popular Theatre in Political Culture: Britain and Canada in Focus.* Bristol: Intellect.

Pritchard, Alan. 2007. *Effective Teaching with Internet Technologies: Pedagogy and Practice.* London: Paul Chapman.

———. 2009. *Ways of Learning: Learning Theories and Learning Styles in the Classroom.* 2nd ed. New York: Routledge.

Pritchard, Alan, and John Woollard. 2010. *Psychology for the Classroom: Constructivism and Social Learning.* London: Routledge.

Project Humanity. 2011, June 6. http://www.projecthumanity.ca/index.html.

Queen, Carol, and Lynn Comella. 2008. "The Necessary Revolution: Sex-Positive Feminism in the Post-Barnard Era." *Communication Review* 11(3):274–91.

Roadside Theater. 2013. Accessed October 5. www.roadside.org.

Rohd, Michael. 1998. *Theatre for Community, Conflict and Dialogue: The Hope is Vital Training Manual.* Portsmouth, NH: Heinemann.

Royal Commission on Aboriginal Peoples. 1996. *Report of the Royal Commission on Aboriginal Peoples.* Ottawa: Indian and Northern Affairs Canada. http://www.ainc-inac.gc.ca/eng/1100100014597/1100100014637.

Salverson, Julie. 1996. "Performing Emergency: Witnessing, Popular Theatre, and the Lie of the Literal." *Theatre Topics* 6(2):181–91.

Saskatchewan Education. 2009. "Health Education 9." http://www.progetudes.gov.sk.ca/index.jsp?lang=en&subj=health_education&level=9.

Saskatchewan Native Theatre Company. 2010. Accessed June 15. http://www.sntc.ca/net/desktopdefault.aspx.

Schechner, Richard. 1989. "Race Free, Gender Free, Body-Type Free, Age Free Casting." Drama Review 33(1):4–12.

———. 2002. *Performance Studies: An Introduction.* London: Routledge.

Schutzman, Mady, and Jan Cohen-Cruz. 1994. *Playing Boal.* New York: Routledge.

Selman, Jan. Unpublished journal: Community Arts, Kenya. January 2011–May 2013.

Serafini, Toni, and Gerald R. Adams. 2002. "Functions of Identity: Scale Construction and Validation." *Identity: An International Journal of Theory and Research* 2:361–89.

Shercliffe, Regan J., Mary Hampton, Kim McKay-McNabb, Bonnie Jeffery, Pamela Beattie, and Barb McWatters. 2007. "Cognitive and Demographic Factors that Predict Self-Efficacy to Use Condoms in Vulnerable and Marginalized Aboriginal Youth." *Canadian Journal of Human Sexuality* 16:1–2.

Sistren Theatre Collective. 2013. Accessed October 5. http://sistrentheatrecollective.org/.

SPARC (Social Planning and Research Council), BC. 2010. Accessed December 1. http://www.sparc.bc.ca.

Spratt, Mary, and Benji Leung. 2000. "Peer Teaching and Peer Learning Revisited." *ELT Journal* 54(3):218–26.

Starr, Floyd Favel. 1997. "The Artificial Tree: Native Performance Culture Research 1991–1996." *Canadian Theatre Review* 90 (Spring):83–85.

Tavakol, Mohsen, and Reg Dennick. 2011. "Making Sense of Cronbach's Alpha." *International Journal of Medical Education* 2:53–55.

Taylor, Philip. 2003. *Applied Theatre: Creating Transformative Encounters in the Community.* Portsmouth, NH: Heinemann.

Theatre for Life. 2010. Accessed June 10. http://www.arepp.org.za/index.html.

Thomas, Robina Anne. "Honouring the Oral Traditions of My Ancestors through Storytelling." In *Research as Resistance: Critical, Indigenous and Anti-Oppressive Approaches,* edited by Lesley Brown and Susan Strega, 237–54. Toronto: Canadian Scholars' Press.

Thompson, James. 2006. *Applied Theatre: Bewilderment and Beyond.* Bern: Peter Lang.

Truth and Reconciliation Commission of Canada. 2014a. Introduction to "Schedule N of the Indian Residential Schools Settlement Agreement." Accessed January 6. http://www.trc.ca/websites/trcinstitution/index.php?p=7#Principles.

———. 2014b. "Mandate." Accessed January 6. http://www.trc.ca/websites/trcinstitution/index.php?p=7.

Turner, Victor. 1967. "Betwixt and Between: The Liminal Period in *Rites de Passage*." *The Forest of Symbols: Aspects of Ndembu Ritual*. Ithaca, NY: Cornell University Press.

———. 1974. *Dramas, Fields, and Metaphors: Symbolic Action in Human Society*. Ithaca, NY: Cornell University Press.

Ubersfeld, Anne. 1982. "The Pleasure of the Spectator." *Modern Drama* 25(1):27–39.

Ubersfeld, Anne, and Frank Collins, trans. 1999. *Reading Theatre*, edited by Paul Perron and Patrick Debbèche. Toronto: University of Toronto Press.

UNFPA (United Nations Population Fund). 2002. "State of World Population." http://www.unfpa.org/public/cache/offonce/publications/pid/3206.

Van Erven, Eugene. 2001. *Community Theatre: Global Perspectives*. London: Routledge.

Walker, Damian. 2003. "Cost and Cost-effectiveness of HIV/AIDS Prevention Strategies in Developing Countries: Is There an Evidence Base?" *Health Policy and Planning* 1:4–17.

Wallace, David Foster. 2008. "David Foster Wallace on Life and Work/This is Water: Some Thoughts, Delivered on a Significant Occasion, About Living a Compassionate Life." *Wall Street Journal*, September 19, book edition, W14.

WarGames. 1983. Dir. John Badham. USA: MGM.

Wareham, Evelyn. 2001. "Our Own Identity, Our Own Taonga, Our Own Self Coming Back: Indigenous Voice in New Zealand Record-Keeping." *Archivaria* 52:26–46.

Washburn, Frances. 2006. *American Indian Culture and Research Journal* 30(4):109–19.

Weigler, Will. 2001. *Strategies for Play Building: Helping Groups Translate Issues into Theatre*. Portsmouth, NH: Heinemann.

Weiten, Wayne. 2001. *Psychology Themes and Variations*, 5th ed. Belmont, CA: Wadsworth Thompson Learning.

Wellings, Kaye, Julia Field, Anne M. Johnson, and Jane Wadsworth. 1994. *Sexual Behavior in Britain*. London: Penguin.

Wellings, Kaye, Kirsti Mitchell, Anne M. Johnson, and Jane Wadsworth. 1998. "Risks Associated With Early Sexual Activity and Fertility." *Teenage Sexuality: Health Risks and Education*, edited by John Coleman, and Debi Roker, 81–100. London: Routledge.

West, Malcolm, M.S. Rose, Sheila Spreng, A. Sheldon-Keller, and Kenneth Adam. 1998. "Adolescent Attachment Questionnaire: A Brief Assessment of Attachment in Adolescence." *Journal of Youth and Adolescence* 27:661–73.

WHO (World Health Organization). 2000. *Reproductive Health During Conflict and Displacement: A Guide for Programme Managers*. Geneva.

———. 2006. *Youth Sex Education in a Multicultural Europe*. Retrieved from Mexico, Minister Declaration, 2008. http://data.unaids.org/pub/BaseDocument/2008/20080801_minsterdeclaration_en.pdf.

Willett, John. 1959. *The Theatre of Bertolt Brecht: A Study from Eight Aspects*. London: Methuen.

Willett, John, ed. and trans. 1964. *Brecht on Theatre: The Development of an Aesthetic*. London: Eyre Methuen.

Willett, Rebekah. 2007. "Technology, Pedagogy and Digital Production: A Case Study of Children Learning New Media Skills." *Learning, Media and Technology* 32(2):167–81.

Women's Circus. 2013. Accessed October 5. http://womenscircus.org.au.

Workman Arts. 2007. "About Us." http://www.workmanarts.com/About.

Zabin, Laurie, Marilyn Hirsch, Edward Smith, and Janet Hardy. 1984. "Adolescent Sexual Attitudes and Behavior: Are They Consistent?" *Family Planning Perspectives* 16(4):181–85.

Interviews and Personal Communication[1]

Alcorn, Emmy (artistic director, Mulgrave Road Theatre, Guysborough, NS). Interview by Jane Heather, April 1, 2008.

Alexander, Ryland (AWTY actor, Concrete Theatre, Edmonton, AB). Interview by Mieko Ouchi, August 29, 2010.

———. Interview by James McKinnon, February 3, 2011.

Bear, Tracy L. (graduate researcher). Personal communication by email with Jan Selman, September 27, 2010.

Bishop, Jennifer (actor, Saskatchewan Native Theatre Company, Saskatoon, SK). Interview by Tracy L. Bear, July 27, 2008.

Brockman, Larry (executive director, Options Sexual Health Association, Edmonton, AB). Interview by Jane Heather, December 1, 2009.

Brooks, Leslie (communicable disease control nurse, Northern Inter-Tribal Health Authority, Prince Albert, SK). Interview by Tracy L. Bear, May 16, 2007, Saskatoon, SK.

———. Interview by Tracy L. Bear, July 13, 2008.

Chamale, Pedro (AWTY actor, Neworld Theatre, Vancouver, BC). Interview by Jan Selman, November 8, 2010.

Chu, Evelyn (AWTY actor, Neworld Theatre, Vancouver, BC), Interview by Jan Selman, November 8, 2010.

Chu, Nadien (AWTY actor, Concrete Theatre, Edmonton, AB). Interview by Jan Selman, August 28, 2010.

Cuckow, Nathan (AWTY actor, Concrete Theatre, Edmonton, AB). Interview by Mieko Ouchi, August 28, 2010.

Dow, Brett (public health nurse, Sexual Health Program, Saskatoon Health Region). Interview by Tracy L. Bear, May 15, 2007, Saskatoon, SK.

Elter, Sheldon (AWTY actor, Concrete Theatre, Edmonton, AB). Interview by Jan Selman, August 28, 2010.

Hansen, Kristi (AWTY actor, Concrete Theatre, Edmonton, AB.) Interview by Jan Selman, August 25, 2010.

———. Interview by Mieko Ouchi, August 27, 2010.

Howarth, Caroline (artistic co-director, Concrete Theatre; director, AWTY Concrete Theatre, Edmonton, AB). Interview by Mieko Ouchi, January 5, 2011.

Lee, Richard (AWTY actor, Concrete Theatre, Edmonton, AB). Interview by Jan Selman, August 28, 2010.

Maeda, Kenji (sexual health educator for AWTY Neworld Theatre, Vancouver, BC). Interview by Jan Selman, November 8, 2010.

Matsunaga-Turnbull, Jared (AWTY actor and director, Concrete Theatre, Edmonton, AB). Interview by Mieko Ouchi, January 5, 2011.

McPhail, Wendy (sexual wellness co-ordinator, Mamawetan Churchill River Health Region, SK). Interview by Tracy L. Bear, May 17, 2007, La Ronge, SK.

Naytowhow, Arron (AWTY actor, Saskatchewan Native Theatre Company, Saskatoon, SK). Interview by Tracy L. Bear. July 27, 2008.

Omondi, Raphael (director, Pamoja Youth Foundation, Nairobi, Kenya). Interview by Jan Selman, March 5, 2011.

———. Interview by Jan Selman, July 23, 2011.

Ouchi, Mieko (artistic co-director, Concrete Theatre; director, AWTY). Interview by Jan Selman, January 5, 2011, Edmonton, AB.

Parker, Brian (sexual health educator, Options Sexual Health Association, Edmonton, AB). Interview by Jane Heather, February 15, 2010.

Pederson, Krystle (AWTY actor, Saskatchewan Native Theatre Company, Saskatoon, SK). Interview by Tracy L. Bear, July 27, 2008.

Puntil, Gina (stage manager, AWTY Concrete Theatre, Edmonton, AB). Interview by Mieko Ouchi, August 25, 2010.

Purcell, Leona (public health nurse and co-ordinator, Guysborough Youth Health and Services Centre, Guysborough, NS). Interview by Jane Heather, April 21, 2008.

Williams, Kenneth T. (co-playwright). Interview by Tracy L. Bear, November 16, 2010, Edmonton, AB.

Wong, Adrienne (artistic associate, Neworld Theatre; director, AWTY 2010 production). Interview by Jan Selman, November 7, 2010, Vancouver, BC.

NOTE

1. Interviewees' titles are given with reference to their position at the time of interview or role in the AWTY project.

CONTRIBUTORS

The Authors

Jan Selman is a professor of acting, directing, and community-based theatre in the Department of Drama at University of Alberta in Edmonton, Canada. A theatre director who specializes in new and contemporary work, she also has facilitated and directed many community-based theatre projects and participatory theatre events. Much of her early popular theatre and community work was with Catalyst Theatre where she was artistic director for its first eight years. Based in this work, she co-wrote and edited the book, *Popular Theatre in Political Culture: Britain and Canada in Focus*, and a variety of other articles in venues such as *Canadian Theatre Review*, Routledge's *Applied Theatre Reader*, *Adult Education Quarterly*, and the *New Zealand Journal of Adult Learning*. Jan led the Are We There Yet? Community-University Research Alliance, which informs this book and was executive producer of the accompanying DVD.

Jane Heather is an associate professor in the Department of Drama at the University of Alberta, in Edmonton, Canada. She teaches acting, directing, playwriting, and performer-created and community-based theatre. Jane has created and/or written community-based theatre projects with prison inmates, Aboriginal youth, unions, teachers, seniors, counsellors, women's groups, new immigrants, adults with disabilities, and many social agencies and organizations. Two of her plays are performed each year in Canadian schools, *Are We There Yet?* and *Work Plays*, which is for fifteen- to eighteen-year-olds about workers' rights. Recent popular theatre work includes *A Musta Be* (with Old Earth Productions), a play about Aboriginal women and incarceration, and *Seasons*, a play about poor youth and elders in the inner city. She has written or co-written articles about her work, published in *Canadian Theatre Review*, Routledge's *Applied Theatre Reader*, and University of Michigan's *Performing Democracy*. She is interested in how playwriting and playwrights can animate communities and foster social change.

Co-Researchers and Contributors

Shaniff Esmail, PHD, MSC OT (C), is associate chair and associate professor in the Department of Occupational Therapy, University of Alberta. Dr. Esmail is an occupational therapist with clinical and research interests focusing primarily on sexuality and disability. Specific research areas include sexuality counselling and intervention for couples impacted by disability or illness and sexuality training and education for children with disabilities and their parents. Dr. Esmail teaches an array of physical assessment courses in the Department of Occupational Therapy as well as human sexuality courses for the faculties of Rehabilitation Medicine, Medicine, and Human Ecology.

Brenda Munro, professor emeritus, Department of Human Ecology, University of Alberta, has worked in the area of youth at risk for some years. This focus has included areas such as health and risk behaviours participated in by junior and senior high students. Brenda's focus with the Are We There Yet? Community-University Research Alliance is on the assessment of dimensions such as decision making, boundary setting, self-efficacy, emotional response, motivation, and the evaluation of what is a safe environment. Brenda is also involved in a research project that links university students with homeless youth. Rather than a mentorship program, it is a cultural exchange program that allows university students to learn about the realities of homelessness and the homeless youth to understand university students.

Tracy L. Bear is a member of the Montreal Lake Cree Nation. She currently works as a senior advisor to the provost/vice president (academic) on Aboriginal initiatives at the University of Alberta while she completes her PHD in English and Native Studies.

Tracy holds two degrees: a Bachelor of Education and a Bachelor of Arts in Native Studies (both with distinction). She is the recipient of numerous awards including the first Chancellor's Citation in the Faculty of Native Studies. She co-wrote two successful SSHRC grants as an undergraduate student. Her research interests include teaching healthy sex and sexuality through participatory theatre and storytelling and exploring how literature and art forms of Indigenous erotica function in contemporary contexts.

James McKinnon is a lecturer at Victoria University of Wellington (VUW), New Zealand. James has a PHD in drama from the University of Toronto, an MA in drama from the University of Alberta, and a BA in English from McGill University. His writing has appeared in *alt.theatre*, *Canadian Theatre Review*, and other publications, and his research interests include adaptation, theatre pedagogy, Canadian appropriations of Shakespeare and Chekhov, and dramaturgy. Prior to his scholarly pursuits, James enjoyed a career in theatre that took him across Canada and back several times, working as a dramaturge, designer, director, and production manager, among other things. He currently teaches theatre in the School of English, Film, Theatre, and Media Studies at VUW.

The DVD

Mieko Ouchi, director of the accompanying DVD, is an Edmonton-based actor, writer, and director who works in both theatre and film/TV. As a director, she has been nominated five times at the Sterling Awards for her work in Edmonton. As co-founder and artistic co-director of Concrete Theatre, she has directed productions that have toured to the National Arts Centre, Persephone Theatre, Young People's Theatre, and the Grand Theatre in London as well as throughout Alberta. She wrote and directed the award-winning documentaries *Minor Keys* (NFB/CBC's *The Nature of Things*), *Shepherd's Pie and Sushi* (NFB), as well as shorts *Assembly*, *Paper Cut*, *By This Parting*, and *Samurai Swing*, which have screened at over thirty festivals across North America and Europe.

Research Assistants

Many student assistants contributed to the AWTY CURA research program, and fruits of their work have certainly informed parts of this book. While a more complete list of students can be found on the project website, the authors particularly acknowledge the following people for their contributions to the development of this publication:

Anamaria Antonescu, Roger S. Smith student researcher

Darlene Auger, independent research assistant

and graduate students:

John Battye, University of Alberta, Drama

Tracy L. Bear, University of Alberta, English and Native Studies

Sherri C. Brown, University of Alberta, Rehabilitation Medicine

Evelyn Derus, University of Alberta, Human Ecology

Matthew Gusal, University of Alberta, Drama

Heidi Knupp, University of Alberta, Rehabilitation Medicine

Courtney Lohnes, University of Alberta, Drama

Jessica Peverett, University of Alberta, Drama

Janine Plummer, University of Alberta, Drama

INDEX

Page numbers in italics refer to photographs. Page numbers with **t** refer to tables; page numbers with **f** refer to figures.

AWTY (in italics) refers to the play. AWTY (in normal text) refers to the program: the play, the research, and the workshops.